Outpatient Nutrition Care and Home Nutrition Support

Practical Guidelines for Assessment and Management

Outpatient Nutrition Care and Home Nutrition Support

Practical Guidelines for Assessment and Management

edited by

Carol Ireton-Jones, PhD, RDN

CRC Press
Taylor & Francis Group
Boca Raton London New York

CRC Press is an imprint of the
Taylor & Francis Group, an **informa** business

CRC Press
Taylor & Francis Group
6000 Broken Sound Parkway NW, Suite 300
Boca Raton, FL 33487-2742

Printed on acid-free paper
Version Date: 20160603

International Standard Book Number-13: 978-1-4987-1102-9 (Paperback)

Library of Congress Cataloging-in-Publication Data

Names: Ireton-Jones, Carol S., editor.
Title: Outpatient nutrition care and home nutrition support : practical
guidelines for assessment and management / edited by Carol Ireton-Jones.
Description: Boca Raton : CRC Press, 2017. | Includes bibliographical
references and index.
Identifiers: LCCN 2016004059 | ISBN 9781498711029 (alk. paper)
Subjects: | MESH: Nutrition Therapy--methods | Nutrition Assessment | Home
Care Services | Ambulatory Care | Outpatients
Classification: LCC RM217 | NLM WB 400 | DDC 615.8/54--dc23
LC record available at http://lccn.loc.gov/2016004059

Visit the Taylor & Francis Web site at
http://www.taylorandfrancis.com

and the CRC Press Web site at
http://www.crcpress.com

Printed and bound in the United States of America by Publishers Graphics,
LLC on sustainably sourced paper.

First and foremost to Mom, your support, love, and inspiration are why I am successful today;

and to

Jim, your support and love make everything possible;

Lauren and Krissy, such amazing daughters, and son-in-law Cody, love you tons;

Finally, to the nutrition profession that continues to provide the greatest colleagues ever.

Contents

SECTION II Home Nutrition Support

SECTION III Summary

Introduction

Nutrition has always been important to me—it became my career. It is a vital part of life—in fact, without nutrition, there is no life. Food can be satisfying and it can also be healing. There are a wide range of ways that nutrition can be healing from a simple broth that provides fluids and electrolytes to therapeutic nutrition for diabetes, irritable bowel syndrome, or osteoporosis. Registered Dietitian Nutritionists (RDNs) have expertise in disease management and translation of nutrition requirements to foods to consume. However, nutrition care often does not receive the attention in the outpatient setting that is needed to achieve nutrition goals.

For example, a patient may receive a diet instruction in the hospital, often right before discharge. This does not give the patient or family time to synthesize the information. An individual seen in the general practitioner or specialist's office may be given information on "diet" but this is not fully explained or is provided as a handout to take home. Even with complex diagnoses and therapies such as oncology and inflammatory bowel disease or home parenteral or enteral nutrition, nutrition knowledge provided to the patient is often lacking.

The purpose of this book is to provide pertinent and concise nutrition care information for dietitians and other professionals working with individuals outside the hospital. The authors were chosen because of their expertise in the topics covered. It is assumed that the reader is at a level to understand the basics of nutrition and will be able to implement nutrition care at a higher level. Starting with nutrition care in the outpatient setting to home nutrition support, in each chapter, the reader will learn more about the disease process as well as the management of the disease or therapy.

The subject matter in this book covers complex health issues. The chapter on oncology encompasses many specific areas of the disease process. The chapters on osteoporosis and inflammatory bowel disease are comprehensive in scope. Home enteral nutrition considers adults and pediatric patients. Parenteral nutrition access is not only explained but depicted in a graphic for ease of understanding. Nutrition services in the outpatient setting discuss the RDN in private practice as well as how to find an RDN.

Nutrition care outside the hospital is important. Reimbursement for outpatient nutrition services may be a challenge and is being addressed at many levels; however, the valuable services provided are evidence and science based and make a difference. The experts agree:

> Let food be thy medicine and medicine be thy food.

Hippocrates

> The doctor of the future will no longer treat the human frame with drugs, but rather will cure and prevent disease with nutrition.

Thomas Edison

> It is time for Good Nutrition for Good Living©.

Carol Ireton-Jones
PhD, RDN, LD, CNSC, FAND, FASPEN

Editor

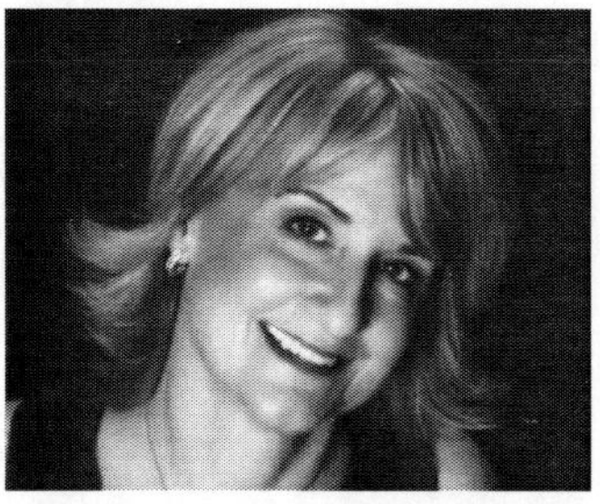

Carol Ireton-Jones, PhD, RDN, LD, CNSC, FAND, FASPEN, earned her PhD and master's in nutrition from Texas Woman's University. Her undergraduate degree in nutrition and dietetics came from Texas Tech University where she also received her clinical training. She developed the Ireton-Jones equations for estimating the energy requirements in hospitalized patients that are widely used nationally and internationally.

Dr. Ireton-Jones is a consultant/speaker and in private practice currently managing patients with gastrointestinal (GI) disorders including irritable bowel syndrome (IBS), gastroparesis, and inflammatory bowel disease (IBD), as well as home parenteral and enteral nutrition patients. She teaches graduate and undergraduate nutrition courses at Texas Tech University and Rutgers University. Dr. Ireton-Jones is also a cofounder and chief nutrition officer for Utopia Food and Fitness headquartered in Plano, Texas.

She has extensively lectured nationally and internationally on a variety of nutrition topics and authored three previous books and numerous book chapters and peer-reviewed papers. Dr. Ireton-Jones is an active member of several local and national nutrition-related organizations. She has received many honors and awards including the prestigious Medallion Award from the Academy of Nutrition and Dietetics, the Texas Distinguished Scientist Award and the Texas Distinguished Dietitian Award from the Texas Academy of Nutrition and Dietetics, and the Lifetime Achievement Award from the Dallas Academy of Nutrition and Dietetics.

Balancing evidence-based nutrition with sensible and *practical* applications is her strong point!

Contributors

Elizabeth Bobo, MS, RDN, LDN, CNSC
Nemours Children's Specialty Care
Jacksonville, Florida

Kalli Castille, MS, RDN, LD, FAND
Cancer Treatment Centers of America at
Southwestern Regional Medical Center
Tulsa, Oklahoma

Marianne Duda, MS, RDN, LDN, CNSC
Thrive RX
Cincinnati, Ohio

Jessica Engelbrecht, MS, RDN, CSR, LD, CNSC
Cancer Treatment Centers of America at
Southwestern Regional Medical Center
Tulsa, Oklahoma

Julia Fechtner, RDN, CSO, CNSC, LDN
Cancer Treatment Centers of America at
Midwestern Regional Medical Center
Zion, Illinois

Trisha Fuhrman, MS, RDN, LD, FAND, FASPEN
Malnutrition Antagonists
St. Louis, Missouri

Maureen Geboy, RDN, LD
Cancer Treatment Centers of America at
Southeastern Regional Medical Center
Newnan, Georgia

Brenda Gray, PharmD, CNSC, BCNSP, CVAA(c), PRS
Clinical Pharmacy Partners
Tampa, Florida

Eileen Heffernan-Swingle, MS, RDN
Department of Nutritional Sciences
School of Health Related Professions
Rutgers Biomedical and Health Sciences
Rutgers University
Newark, New Jersey

Carol Ireton-Jones, PhD, RDN, LD, CNSC, FAND, FASPEN
Good Nutrition for Good Living
Carrollton, Texas

Maryann King, MPH, RDN, LD, CNSC, CSO
Consultant
Downingtown, Pennsylvania

Crystal Langlois, RDN, CSO, LD
Cancer Treatment Centers of America at
Southeastern Regional Medical Center
Newnan, Georgia

Angela Matthewson, MPH, RDN
Cancer Specialists of North Florida
Jacksonville, Florida

Martha McHenry, RDN, LD, CDE
North Texas Nutritional Care
Dallas, Texas

Brooke McIntyre, RDN, CSO, LD, CNSC
Cancer Treatment Centers of America at
Southwestern Regional Medical Center
Tulsa, Oklahoma

Kevn McNamara, PharmD, RPh, CNSC, PRS, CVAA(c)
Clinical Pharmacy Partners
Tampa, Florida

Marianne Opilla, RN, BSN, CNSC
Nutrishare, Inc.
Elk Grove, California

David Orozco, MS, RDN, LD
td wellness, llc
Decatur, Georgia

Stephanie Paver, RDN, CSO, CNSC
Cancer Treatment Centers of America at
Western Regional Medical Center
Goodyear, Arizona

Deborah Pfister, MS, RDN, CNSC
Thrive Rx
Cincinnati, Ohio

Renee Pieroth, RDN, CSO, LDN
Cancer Treatment Centers of America at
Eastern Regional Medical Center
Philadelphia, Pennsylvania

Matt Rinehart, MS, RDN, CSO, LD
Cancer Treatment Centers of America at
Southwestern Regional Medical Center
Tulsa, Oklahoma

Nancy Robinson, RDN, LD
Food 4 Osteoporosis
Arlington, Texas

Kristen Roberts, PhD, RDN, LD
Thrive Rx
Cincinnati, Ohio

Michelle Romano, RDN, LD/N, CNSC
Fresenius Kabi USA
Glenview, Illinois

Kamorin Samson, RDN, CSO, LDN
Cancer Treatment Centers of America at
Eastern Region Medical Center
Philadelphia, Pennsylvania

Roberta Scheuer, RDN, LD
Cancer Treatment Centers of America at
Southeastern Regional Medical Center
Newnan, Georgia

Nathan Schober, MS, RDN, CNSC
Cancer Treatment Centers of America at
Southeastern Regional Medical Center
Newnan, Georgia

Jessica Smith, MS, RDN, CSO, LD
Cancer Treatment Centers of America at
Southwestern Regional Medical Center
Tulsa, Oklahoma

Jody Strain
Nutrishare, Inc.
Elk Grove, California

Andrea Swartz, RDN, LD
Cancer Treatment Centers of America at
Southeastern Regional Medical Center
Newnan, Georgia

Gabrielle Taylor, MS, RDN, LD
Cancer Treatment Centers of America at
Southwestern Regional Medical Center
Tulsa, Oklahoma

Kristen Trukova, MS, RDN, CSO, CNSC, LDN
Cancer Treatment Centers of America at
Midwestern Regional Medical Center
Zion, Illinois

Pankaj Vashi, MD, CNSC
Cancer Treatment Centers of America at
Midwestern Regional Medical Center
Zion, Illinois

Jasmyn Walker, MS, RDN, LD, CSO, CNSC
Cancer Treatment Centers of America at
Southwestern Regional Medical Center
Tulsa, Oklahoma

Rachel Winston, MS, RDN, CSO
Cancer Treatment Centers of America at
Western Regional Medical Center
Goodyear, Arizona

Section I

Outpatient Nutrition Care

1 Nutrition Screening, Assessment, and Monitoring

Trisha Fuhrman, MS, RDN, LD, FAND, FASPEN

CONTENTS

INTRODUCTION

Patients are referred to home care and outpatient care from hospitals, healthcare facilities, primary care providers, and patient self-referral. No matter what brings the patient to the outpatient or home care setting, the patient's current nutritional status should be evaluated. Sometimes, the clinician receiving the referral is given an extensive amount of information about the patient and sometimes, there is little or no information provided. Regardless of the quantity and quality of the information provided with the referral, the clinician should perform his/her own nutrition screening and assessment.

NUTRITION SCREENING

A nutrition screen should be a simple and quick means of determining which patient will require an in-depth nutrition assessment. It can also be used to collect information on what the patient hopes to accomplish, or goals of therapy, through interactions with the nutrition-focused clinician. For the dietitian working in an outpatient clinic or private practice, the initial form(s) completed by the patient prior to a consult may include nutrition-screening questions.

There are several validated tools available for nutrition screening.[1] However, if the clinician changes the screening tool, it is no longer validated and the clinician should validate the changed tool to determine if it still enables the clinician to identify the patients who require a nutrition intervention versus those who do not. The information generally collected in a nutrition screen includes nonquantified changes in weight and appetite, chewing and/or swallowing problems, and diagnosis or reason for an admission or visit. In the outpatient setting, it is reasonable to have the patient and/or caregiver to complete the nutrition screen. Each facility/practice needs to identify who will perform the screen and how the referral to the registered dietitian nutritionist (RDN) or to the nutrition-trained qualified individual will be done. Identification of a patient who requires a nutrition assessment leads to initiation of the nutrition care process (NCP), a standardized process that includes assessment, nutrition diagnosis, nutrition intervention, and monitoring and evaluation.[2] Standards of practice indicators for RDNs working in nutrition support performing the NCP are delineated by the level of practice (competent, proficient, and expert) and apply to all practice settings.[3] There are also standards of practice for clinicians working in home care and an alternate site.[4]

NUTRITION ASSESSMENT

The nutrition assessment incorporates medical and surgical history, laboratory data, medications, anthropometrics, functional status, nutrient intake, nutrition-focused physical exam, and clinical judgment.[3–5] The goal is not only to determine the individualized nutritional and educational needs of the patient, but also to identify whether or not the patient is malnourished. Although malnutrition is typically associated with patients in either a hospital or long-term care facility, shorter hospital stays and preference for keeping patients at home increases the risk for malnutrition in the outpatient setting, emphasizing the importance of evaluating all patients for malnutrition. In addition, chronic diseases such as an inflammatory bowel disease, diabetes, or renal disease may detrimentally affect the nutritional status.

The nutrition assessment components that are used to diagnose malnutrition include anthropometrics, functional status, nutrient intake, and nutrition-focused physical exam (Table 1.1). If the patient is malnourished, the degree of malnutrition and the planned nutrition intervention must be delineated in the care plan and communicated with the entire healthcare team. The clinician should evaluate the patient/caregivers nutrition-counseling needs and the readiness to make nutrition and lifestyle changes.

MALNUTRITION

The Academy of Nutrition and Dietetics and the American Society of Parenteral and Enteral Nutrition created a Malnutrition Workgroup that published the definitions and the characteristics of adult malnutrition.[6] The definitions of malnutrition are etiology based and are divided into three categories: (1) chronic starvation due to societal and environmental conditions, (2) a chronic disease with mild-to-moderate inflammation, and (3) an acute disease, illness, or injury with severe inflammation. Malnourished patients in the outpatient and home care setting are more likely to suffer from chronic malnutrition without inflammation or chronic disease-related malnutrition with mild-to-moderate inflammation. Six characteristics that are used to determine the degree of malnutrition (severe vs. nonsevere) include the amount/degree of weight loss, insufficient nutrient intake, loss of body fat, loss of subcutaneous fat, fluid accumulation, and diminished functional capacity (Table 1.1). Two characteristics are needed to assign the diagnosis of malnutrition. The assessment of weight loss over time and the percent of intake compared to estimated needs are the skills regularly used by RDNs. It is not surprising that these characteristics were the most-often used to diagnose malnutrition in a recent study.[7] The challenge is to increase the competency in nutrition-focused physical assessment to assess the patient's lean body mass, subcutaneous fat mass, and fluid status. In general, the clinician can examine the upper body to obtain the indicators of lean body mass and subcutaneous fat losses. This is often more feasible in the outpatient setting where patients are wearing their usual clothing versus wearing a hospital gown. It is important for clinicians to be cognizant of the potential for the presence of malnutrition in patients who are obese. For example, an obese patient's temporal muscle may not be visibly sunken, but may depress quickly and feel watery above the bone.

TABLE 1.1
Characteristics Associated with a Chronic Disease and Mild-to-Moderate Inflammation

	Severe Malnutrition		Nonsevere Malnutrition	
Characteristics	**Starvation Related**	**Chronic Disease Related**	**Starvation Related**	**Chronic Disease Related**
Energy needs (compare the estimated energy needs to the patient's past and the current intake to an estimated adequacy of intake over time)	≥1 month consuming <50% energy needs	≥1 month consuming <75% energy needs	>3 months consuming ≤75% energy needs	>1 month consuming ≤75% energy needs
Actual body weight (consider the hydration status when interpreting weight changes from the baseline. Fluid accumulations can mask weight changes and the loss of fat and lean body mass)	>5%, >7.5%, >10%, and >20% weight loss over 1, 3, 6, and 12 months, respectively	>5%, >7.5%, >10%, and >20% weight loss over 1, 3, 6, and 12 months, respectively	5%, 7.5%, 10%, and 20% weight loss over 1, 3, 6, and 12 months, respectively	>5%, >7.5%, >10%, and >20% weight loss over 1, 3, 6, and 12 months, respectively
Muscle mass (examine the temples, clavicles, shoulders, interosseous muscle, scapula, thigh, and calf muscle for visible signs of losses)	Severe loss of lean body mass		Mild loss of lean body mass	
Body fat (examine orbital, triceps [role of the skin between the thumb and forefinger to separate fat from the muscle in the upper arm with the arm bent], and ribs for the loss of subcutaneous fat)	Severe loss of subcutaneous body fat		Mild loss of subcutaneous body fat	
Fluid accumulation (examine for signs of fluid retention in extremities, vulvar/scrotal edema, or ascites. Physician and nursing notes may provide information on the fluid status)	Severe, localized, or generalized fluid accumulation		Mild, localized, or generalized fluid accumulation	
Functional capacity (compare measurement to normative standards as provided by the manufacturer of the measurement device. Occupation therapy evaluation may provide information on the functional status and capacity)	Measurably reduced functional measures, such as hand grip strength		Nonapplicable	

Source: Adapted from White JW et al., *JPEN J Parenter Enteral Nutr.* 2012;36(3):275–283. With permission.

Medical and Surgical History

The patient's medical and surgical history is often obtained from the medical chart or through discussion with the referring physician. However, there may be times when the clinician must obtain data from the patient and the patient's family. The more the clinician knows about the patient's medical and surgical history, the more comprehensive the nutrition care plan for the present and future can be developed. The patient's primary reason for referral as well as existing comorbidities impacts the plan of care. Past gastrointestinal surgical procedures as well as chronic conditions can affect consumption, digestion, absorption, and excretion of nutrients.

Laboratory Data

Laboratory data may have been collected during a hospitalization or the most recent physician office visit and may be useful in the current situation. It can provide a historic perspective of the patient's overall health and trends in improvement or deterioration, such as those that can be seen with sequential lipid panels or HgbA1C levels. Historically, malnutrition was determined by hepatic protein levels. Unfortunately, this quick and easy way to categorize malnutrition is neither specific nor sensitive to malnutrition, and it is more reflective of inflammation.[8] The recognition and acceptance of the new definitions and characteristics behoove clinicians to abandon the use of hepatic proteins to define malnutrition since there could be a potential risk of being accused of Medicare fraud.[9]

Medications

Each medication the patient is taking should be considered for its potential nutritional impact. Medications can alter nutrient metabolism and availability. The clinician should be aware of the prescribed and over-the-counter medication that the patient is taking. Herbal and nutrition supplements should also be investigated since these can impact the nutritional status or counter the effects of prescription medications. The pharmacokinetics of medication should be evaluated when the route of providing a medication is being changed from oral to enteral or parenteral.

The following components of nutrition assessment are integral to the diagnosis of malnutrition.

Anthropometrics

Ideally, weight and height are measured and there is an opportunity to compare the current measurements to past measurements to identify the patient's usual and changes in body weight. However, a usual body weight is often obtained from the patient. As a rule, individuals tend to report being taller with a lower weight compared to the actual weight. Height and weight are used to calculate the body mass index or BMI, estimate energy and protein needs, and determine the degree of weight change over time. Therefore, a measured height and weight improves the accuracy of the equations. Arm span, summation of body parts, and knee height can be used to indirectly determine the height in a patient who is unable to stand.[10] The evaluation of both percent ideal body weight (IBW) and BMI are used to determine under- and overnutrition (Table 1.2).[11–13]

Weights can be reported as actual body weight (ABW), usual body weight (UBW), IBW, and estimated dry weight (EDW). Actual body weight is the measured weight at the time of assessment. Usual body weight is either reported by the patient or gleaned from the chart as the weight recorded during previous office visits or hospitalizations. Ideal body weight can be obtained using actuarial tables[14] or epidemiological data[15] or calculated using the Hamwi method.[16] The Hamwi method is a quick and easy way to estimate IBW in the outpatient and home care setting.

TABLE 1.2
Body Mass Index

BMI (kg/m²)	Interpretation
14–15	Associated with mortality
<18.5	Underweight, health risks are low
18.5–25	Healthy weight
>25	Overweight, health risk increased
>30	Obese, health risk is moderate
>35	Severe obese, health risk severe
>40	Morbid obesity, health risk very severe

Source: Adapted from National Institutes of Health, *Obes Res.* 1998; 6(Suppl 2):51S–209S.

- Men: 106 pounds for the first 5 ft of height and 6 lb for each additional inch.
- Women: 100 pounds for the first 5 ft of height and 5 lb for each additional inch.

When calculating IBW, subtract for any loss of body parts: 7% (hand); 5% (the entire arm); 1.5% (foot); 5.9% (foot and lower leg); and 16% (the entire leg).[17] Spinal cord injury also requires a reduction in IBW calculation with 5%–10% subtracted with paraplegia and 10%–15% subtracted with quadriplegia.[18]

The estimated dry weight is used in the dialysis population to determine the desired weight of the patient following the removal of fluid with dialysis.[19] The EDW is used in energy and protein calculations in the dialysis population or in any patient population with a propensity to retain fluid, such as liver failure with ascites and congestive heart failure.

Adjusted body weight (AdjBW) is sometimes used to take into account a higher percentage of body fat in a patient who is obese in an attempt to avoid assigning the patient to excessive energy requirements. Rather than creating an artificial weight for the patient, it may be better for the clinician to decrease the estimated needs using ABW by 10%–20%.

Functional Status

Functional status indicates the patient's ability to perform activities of daily living and interact with family and friends. It is often an indicator of the quality of life. A patient debilitated from a prolonged hospitalization may not be able to transfer from a bed to a chair or use bathroom facilities independently. Functional capacity will also be used when determining the characteristics of malnutrition. Functional capacity can be measured using a hand dynamometer, which has been shown to correlate to muscle mass and nutritional status.[6] Results are compared to standards provided by the manufacturer. Functional parameters can also include wound healing, walking endurance, and Karnofsky's scale[20] that uses activities of daily living to determine functionality (form available at http://www.hospicepatients.org/karnofsky.html) or a short physical performance battery (SPPB)[21] (instructions available at http://www.grc.nia.nih.gov/branches/leps/sppb/). In addition, the sit-to-stand assessment evaluates the ability to rise from sitting upright on a chair to a standing, erect position. Individuals who cannot rise five times from a sitting to a standing position in less than 13.6 seconds have increased the risk of disability and morbidity, often associated with muscle decline.[22] In an outpatient and home care setting, the clinician can monitor measurements overtime to look for improvement or deterioration in status.

Nutrient Intake and Nutrient Needs

Nutrient intake should be compared to the estimated energy and protein needs to determine if the patient needs to increase or decrease the intake of caloric and nutrient-dense foods. The amount of food consumed compared to the estimated needs over a period of time is part of the diagnosis of malnutrition. Review GI tract integrity when determining if nutrition intake is sufficient. Losses from diarrhea, drains, fistulae, and wounds may contribute to nutrient imbalance. The Mifflin–St Jeor equation has been reported to be the most accurate predictive equation for energy expenditure at rest (RMR) in healthy individuals [w = weight in kilograms; h = height in centimeters; and a = age in years].[23]

- Male: $RMR = 10(w) + 6.3(h) - 4.9(a) + 5$
- Female: $RMR = 10(w) + 6.3(h) - 4.9(a) - 161$

Total daily energy needs are determined by estimating the effect of disease or injury and activity on the predicted RMR. Protein needs are estimated based on metabolic demand, ongoing losses, and the disease process. Requirements range from 0.8 to 1.5 g/kg per day.[23] Requirements may be elevated with wounds, excess losses, and metabolic stress. Requirements may be reduced with renal failure without dialysis and hepatic encephalopathy responsive to protein intake. Doses >1 g/kg can contribute to hypercalciuria and the risk of a metabolic bone disease in patients on long-term parenteral nutrition.

Fluid requirements are easily determined by using 35 mL/kg for adults and 30 mL/kg for elderly adults.[24] Fluid needs for patients on tube feeding are often estimated using 1 mL/kcal of tube feeding. Regardless of how fluid needs are estimated, it is important to monitor the physical signs and symptoms of the fluid status to avoid over- or underhydration—particularly in patients who cannot express thirst. Fluid requirements may be reduced with cardiac, renal, and hepatic failure. Requirements may be increased with ongoing fluid losses through drains, fistulae, wounds, and the GI tract. Assessing signs and symptoms of the fluid status are part of the nutrition-focused physical assessment and diagnosis characteristics for malnutrition (Table 1.1). Fluid accumulation can mask the loss of weight, fat mass, and lean body mass.

Whether a patient is receiving nutrients by mouth, tube feeding, or parenteral nutrition, it is important to ensure that 100% of micronutrient needs are being provided. This can be challenging with periodic-injectable micronutrient shortages for patients reliant on parenteral nutrition. Monitoring for signs and symptoms of micronutrient deficiencies are incorporated into the nutrition-focused physical assessment (Table 1.3).[25–27]

In the outpatient setting, surgical procedures such as bariatric surgery, GI surgery/resection, a chronic disease including diabetes, renal disease, inflammatory bowel disease, as well as conditions such as heart disease, diabetes, and anorexia nervosa may cause micronutrient deficiencies and malnutrition that should be identified in a nutrition consult.

Nutrition-Focused Physical Exam

This is a head-to-toe approach for inspecting the patient. During this process, the clinician looks for signs and symptoms of micronutrient deficiencies as well as characteristics of malnutrition: muscle wasting, loss of subcutaneous fat, and fluid accumulation. Currently, there is a focus to increase the competency and confidence of RDNs in performing nutrition-focused physical assessment to diagnose malnutrition. However, RDNs should not lose sight of using inspection and light palpation to monitor for micronutrient deficiencies and the patient's overall condition. A head-to-toe approach ensures that the RDN methodically examines the skin, nails, hair, head and eyes, oral cavity, neck and chest, and the musculoskeletal system.[25–27] Table 1.3 provides a list of micronutrients and signs and symptoms associated with deficiency and toxicity. Individuals who are at risk for malnutrition and nutrient deficiencies include patients with chronic conditions and illnesses that interfere with ingestion, absorption, assimilation, or excretion of nutrients (Table 1.4).

Nutrition Diagnosis

The nutrition diagnosis focuses on the patient's primary nutrition-related problem, its signs and symptoms, and its etiology.[2,5] If a patient is malnourished, the nutrition diagnosis should clearly state the degree of malnutrition, the signs and symptoms noted, and the etiology of the development of malnutrition. A clearly written nutrition diagnosis sets the stage for the intervention. Note that the nutrition diagnosis is not a medical diagnosis. The use of NCP terminology may not be used in all outpatient and home care practices.

Nutrition Intervention

This is the primary reason for performing a nutrition assessment. The clinician must identify what can be done, if anything, to improve or stabilize the patient's nutritional status and identify the patient's nutrition education needs. The nutrition care plan should be communicated with the healthcare team,

TABLE 1.3
Micronutrient Assessment Guide (Core, Charney/Malone, and Morrison)

Nutrient	Signs and Symptoms of Deficiency	Potential Etiology (in Addition to Deficient Diet)	Signs and Symptoms of Toxicity	Potential Etiology of Toxicity	Assessment of Status	DRI (Adults)	IV Standard Dose (Adults)
Vitamin A	• Night blindness • Bitot's spots • Conjunctival xerosis • Scaling of the skin • Nasolabial seborrhea • Follicular hyperkeratosis • Blindness • Impaired mucus secretion • Depressed T-helper cell activity	• Liver disease • Critical illness • Steatorrhea	• Alopecia • Ataxia • Muscle and bone pain • Cheilitis • Headache • Conjunctivitis • Skin and vision disorders • Hepatotoxicity • Pruritis • Hyperlipidemia • Membrane dryness • Renal osteodystrophy	• Liver disease • Malnutrition • ETOH abuse • A chronic kidney disease	Serum retinol	RDA: male/female 900/700 mcg RE	3300 IU/d
Ascorbic acid, C (scurvy)	• Petechiae (perifollicular) • Swollen/bleeding gums • Purpura • Follicular hyperkeratosis • Poor wound healing • Pressure ulcers • Retracted gums • Corkscrew hair • Anorexia • Fatigue • Muscle pain	• Surgical and burn patients • Wounds/pressure ulcers • Acute inflammation/metabolic stress hinders vitamin C transport	• Nausea • Vomiting	• Renal failure • Kidney stones • Iron overload disease • Individuals on warfarin or heparin therapy should avoid high doses	Plasma ascorbic acid analysis via high-pressure liquid chromatography	RDA: male/female 90/75 mg	200 mg

(*Continued*)

TABLE 1.3 (*Continued*)
Micronutrient Assessment Guide (Core, Charney/Malone, and Morrison)

Nutrient	Signs and Symptoms of Deficiency	Potential Etiology (in Addition to Deficient Diet)	Signs and Symptoms of Toxicity	Potential Etiology of Toxicity	Assessment of Status	DRI (Adults)	IV Standard Dose (Adults)
Biotin	• Alopecia • Pallor • Glossitis • Nausea/vomiting • Depression/lethargy • Muscle pain • Erythematous seborrheic dermatitis • ↑ Cholesterol and bile pigments	• Deficiency rarely reported • Long-term PN • Alcoholism • S/p partial gastrectomy	No known toxic effects	N/A	Serum and 24-hour urine collections	AI (adequate intake): 30 mcg	60 mcg
Cyanocobalamin, B_{12}	• Atrophic lingual papillae • Dementia • Peripheral neuropathy with weakness and paresthesias • Ataxia • Poor memory • Confusion/depression • Delusions • Megaloblastic anemia with macrocytosis • Hypersegmentation of neutrophil nuclei • Bone marrow changes • Leucopenia • Thrombocytopenia • Glossitis • Constipation/diarrhea	• Malabsorption syndromes (s/p gastrectomy, gastric bypass, and ileal resection) • Vegetarianism • Impaired HCl production • Overgrowth of *Helicobacter pylori*	No known toxic effects	N/A	Serum B_{12} ↑ Methylmalonic acid and homocysteine with deficiency (homocysteine also ↑ with folic acid deficiency)	RDA: 2.4 mg	5 mcg

(Continued)

TABLE 1.3 (*Continued*)
Micronutrient Assessment Guide (Core, Charney/Malone, and Morrison)

Nutrient	Signs and Symptoms of Deficiency	Potential Etiology (in Addition to Deficient Diet)	Signs and Symptoms of Toxicity	Potential Etiology of Toxicity	Assessment of Status	DRI (Adults)	IV Standard Dose (Adults)
Vitamin D	• Tetany • Rickets or osteomalacia	• Limited sun exposure • Steatorrhea • Long-term PN • Hepatic/renal disease • Gastric resection • Antiepileptic medications (phenytoin, phenobarbital)	• Hypercalcemia • Hypercalciuria • Soft-tissue calcification	Excessive supplementation	Serum 25-hydroxyvitamin D	AI: 19–50 years 5 mcg 51–70 years 10 mcg > 70 years Male/female 15/10 mcg	200 IU
Vitamin E	• ↑ Platelet aggregation • ↓ Red blood cell survival • Hemolytic anemia • Neuronal degeneration • Creatinuria	• Steatorrhea • Fat malabsorption • Requirement for high-oxygen concentration via mechanical ventilation	• Impaired neutrophil function • Impaired coagulation • Prolonged toxicity: skeletal muscle lesions	Excessive supplementation	Plasma or serum α-tocopherol Vitamin E, plasma	RDA: 15 mg α-TE	10 IU
Folic acid	• Atrophic lingual papillae • Megaloblastic or macrocytic anemia • Diarrhea • Weight loss • ↓ Cell-mediated immunity • Dementia • Neural tube defects in infants born to mothers who are deficient	• Chronic alcoholism • Medications (phenytoin, cholestyramine, sulfasalazine, and amphotericin B) • ↑ Risk with pregnancy due to ↑ the demand for DNA synthesis for embryonic development	No known toxic effects	N/A	Stage I (early): serum folate levels Stage II (tissue depletion): RBC folate levels Stage III (erythropoiesis): neutrophil hypersegmentation and abnormal deoxyuridine suppression test Stage IV (clinical deficiency): megaloblastic anemia or macrocytic anemia	RDA: 400 mcg	600 mcg

(*Continued*)

TABLE 1.3 (*Continued*)
Micronutrient Assessment Guide (Core, Charney/Malone, and Morrison)

Nutrient	Signs and Symptoms of Deficiency	Potential Etiology (in Addition to Deficient Diet)	Signs and Symptoms of Toxicity	Potential Etiology of Toxicity	Assessment of Status	DRI (Adults)	IV Standard Dose (Adults)
Vitamin K	• Purpura • Bleeding	• Fat malabsorption • Antibiotic therapy • Oral anticoagulants • Infant hemorrhagic disease	Prolonged bleeding	Excessive supplementation	Prothrombin time: international normalized ratio	AI: male/female 120/90 mcg	150 mcg
Niacin, B_3 (pellagra)	• 3 Ds: dermatitis, diarrhea, and dementia • Pigmentation of the skin • Desquamation of sun-exposed areas • Atrophic lingual papillae • Angular stomatitis • Cheilosis	• Deficiency rare in the United States due to food fortification • Synthesized from tryptophan [60 g = 1 mg niacin equivalent (NE) or 1 mg niacin] • Alcoholism • Severe malabsorption	• Flushing of the skin • Pharmacological doses (3 g/d) cause vasodilation, itching, sensation of heat, headaches, GI irritation, and glucose intolerance	Pharmacological dosing	Urinary measurement of N-methylnicotinamide (NMN) and 2-pyridone	RDA: male/female 16/14 mcg	40 mcg
Pantothenic acid	• Listlessness • Fatigue • Irritability • Restlessness • Malaise • Sleep disturbances • Nausea/vomiting • Diarrhea/abdominal cramps • Neuromuscular imbalance—numbness, staggering gait, paresthesias, and muscle cramps • Hypoglycemia • Increased insulin sensitivity	• Occurs in conjunction with other nutrient deficiencies • ↑ Risk with diabetes, inflammatory bowel disease, and alcoholism	Rare—can cause mild GI distress	N/A	Whole blood 24-hour urinary pantothenic acid concentration	AI: 5 mg	15 mg

(*Continued*)

TABLE 1.3 (*Continued*)
Micronutrient Assessment Guide (Core, Charney/Malone, and Morrison)

Nutrient	Signs and Symptoms of Deficiency	Potential Etiology (in Addition to Deficient Diet)	Signs and Symptoms of Toxicity	Potential Etiology of Toxicity	Assessment of Status	DRI (Adults)	IV Standard Dose (Adults)
Pyridoxine, B_6	• Seborrheic dermatitis • Redness/fissuring in the corners of eyes • Scaling of the skin • Nasolabial seborrhea • Cheilosis • Angular stomatitis • Peripheral neuropathy with weakness and paresthesias • Ataxia • Microcytic anemia • Epileptiform convulsions • Confusion/depression	• Alcoholism • Dialysis • Elderly • Medications (isoniazid, penicillamine, corticosteroids, and anticonvulsants)	• Sensory neuropathy • Sensory ataxia • Areflexia • Impaired, cutaneous, and deep sensations • Dermatologic lesions	Excessive oral supplement doses	Pyridoxal 5-phosphate, combination of three tests: 1. Direct plasma PLP level 2. 24-hour urinary excretion of 4-pyridoxic acid 3. Activation of erythrocyte aspartate aminotransferase (EAST) and alanine aminotransferase (EALT)	RDA: 19–50 years 1.3 mg 51–70 years Male/female 1.7/1.5 mg	6 mg
Riboflavin, B_2	• Redness/fissuring in the corners of eyes • Magenta tongue • Photophobia • Scaling of the skin • Nasolabial seborrhea • Cheilosis • Angular stomatitis • Atrophic lingual papillae • Sore throat • Hyperemia and edema of pharyngeal and oral mucosa • Seborrheic dermatitis of the face and scrotum • Corneal vascularization	• Deficiency rarely occurs in isolation—generally it is in conjunction with other B vitamins • Diet low in dairy products and animal protein • At-risk populations: thyroid deficiency, alcoholism, and chronic malabsorption	Rare	N/A	Erythrocyte glutathione reductase activity (not valid in points with glucose 6-phosphate deficiency)	RDA: male/female 1.3/1.1 mg	3.6 mg

(Continued)

TABLE 1.3 (*Continued*)
Micronutrient Assessment Guide (Core, Charney/Malone, and Morrison)

Nutrient	Signs and Symptoms of Deficiency	Potential Etiology (in Addition to Deficient Diet)	Signs and Symptoms of Toxicity	Potential Etiology of Toxicity	Assessment of Status	DRI (Adults)	IV Standard Dose (Adults)
Thiamin, B_1 (beriberi)	Wet beriberi • Cardiac failure • Hepatomegaly • Tachycardia • Oliguria Dry beriberi • Peripheral neuropathy with weakness and paresthesias • Ataxia • Foot/wrist drop Wernicke's encephalopathy • Korsakoff's psychosis	• Alcohol abuse • Refeeding syndrome • Malabsorption • Dialysis • Hyperemesis gravidarum • PN MVI shortages	Rare	N/A	Erythrocyte transketolase activity	RDA: male/female 1.2/1.1 mg	6 mg
Chromium	• Hyperglycemia refractory to insulin • Glucosuria • Impaired amino acid utilization • ↑ LDL cholesterol • Peripheral neuropathy • Weight loss	• Trace elements omitted from PN	• Occurs with Cr^{3+} (muscle rhabdomyolysis, liver dysfunction, and renal failure)	Intake of chromium picolinate (Cr^{3+}) supplements	Deficiency is difficult to determine due to a very low concentration in the blood	AI: male/female 19–50 years 35/25 mcg >50 years 30/20 mcg	10–15 mcg

(*Continued*)

TABLE 1.3 (*Continued*)
Micronutrient Assessment Guide (Core, Charney/Malone, and Morrison)

Nutrient	Signs and Symptoms of Deficiency	Potential Etiology (in Addition to Deficient Diet)	Signs and Symptoms of Toxicity	Potential Etiology of Toxicity	Assessment of Status	DRI (Adults)	IV Standard Dose (Adults)
Copper	• Pancytopenia (hypochromic and microcytic anemia, leucopenia, and neutropenia) • Hypercholesterolemia • ↓ Ceruloplasmin and erythrocyte Cu/Zn SOD • ↑ Erythrocyte turnover • Abnormal electrocardiogram	• Omitted from PN due to hyperbilirubinemia • ↓ Absorption (intestinal surgery) • ↑ GI losses (chronic diarrhea) • Hemodialysis • Excessive zinc supplementation	Rare—liver damage	• Impaired liver function • Chronic ingestion of excessive copper • Genetic predisposition to store copper in the liver (Wilson's disease)	Serum copper and/or ceruloplasmin can be used but may not reflect liver stores and can be impacted by inflammation	RDA: 900 mcg	0.3–0.5 mg
Manganese	• Poor reproductive performance • Congenital abnormalities • Abnormal bone/cartilage formation • Ataxia • Growth retardation • Defects in CHO and lipid metabolism	• Deficiency rare unless it is totally absent from the diet or PN solution	• Central nervous system abnormalities • Hyperirritability • Hallucinations • Mn deposition in basal ganglia • Nephritis • Pancreatitis • Parkinson-like motor dysfunction	• Hepatobiliary disease • Long-term parenteral nutrition patients with biliary duct obstruction	No reliable biomarkers of status identified Toxicity: whole-blood Mn correlates best to MRI results	AI: male/female 2.3/1.8 mg	60–100 mcg

(Continued)

TABLE 1.3 (*Continued*)
Micronutrient Assessment Guide (Core, Charney/Malone, and Morrison)

Nutrient	Signs and Symptoms of Deficiency	Potential Etiology (in Addition to Deficient Diet)	Signs and Symptoms of Toxicity	Potential Etiology of Toxicity	Assessment of Status	DRI (Adults)	IV Standard Dose (Adults)
Selenium	• Oxidative injury • Altered thyroid metabolism • ↑ Plasma glutathione • Altered biotransformation enzyme activity • Keshan disease—an endemic cardiomyopathy in areas of China • Cardiomyopathy/skeletal weakness	• PN without selenium • Selenium-poor soil • Statins interfere with selenoprotein synthesis • ↓ Levels in trauma patients	• Nausea • Vomiting • Hair and nail loss • Tooth decay • Skin lesions • Irritability • Fatigue • Peripheral neuropathy	Excessive intake	Plasma/serum selenium reflects recent intake; erythrocyte concentration reflects the long-term status Measurement of functional status: plasma glutathione peroxidase	RDA: 55 mcg	20–60 mcg
Zinc	• Scaling of the skin • Nasolabial seborrhea • Poor wound healing • Pressure ulcers • Hypogeusia • Hypogonadism • Impaired night vision • Anorexia • Impaired immune function • Impaired vitamin A status • Hyposmia • Alopecia • Glucose intolerance • Impaired hepatic function	• Inhibitors of zinc absorption (calcium, vitamins, milk proteins, phytic acid, alcohol, and disease processes) • At risk—elderly, alcoholics, post-op patients, and burn patients • Malabsorption (intestinal bypass/resection) • Renal disease • Losses via wounds	• GI distress • Impaired immune function • Decreased high-density lipoprotein levels	Excessive doses of zinc	Serum or plasma zinc Interpret values cautiously with inflammation and hypoalbuminemia	RDA: 11/8 mg Excess supplementation of zinc (20–250 mg/d) can contribute to copper deficiency	2.5–5 mg

(*Continued*)

TABLE 1.3 (*Continued*)
Micronutrient Assessment Guide (Core, Charney/Malone, and Morrison)

Nutrient	Signs and Symptoms of Deficiency	Potential Etiology (in Addition to Deficient Diet)	Signs and Symptoms of Toxicity	Potential Etiology of Toxicity	Assessment of Status	DRI (Adults)	IV Standard Dose (Adults)
Iron	• Koilonychia • Pale conjunctiva • Pallor • Fatigue • Atrophic lingual papillae • Tachycardia • Poor capillary refilling • Impaired behavioral/intellectual performance • Impaired ability to maintain body temperature in a cold environment • ↓ Resistance to infections	• Blood loss • Celiac disease • Crohn's disease • Gastric/intestinal surgery • Levels ↓ with inflammation	• Damage to the liver, heart, and pancreas • Skin pigmentation	• Excessive exposure or supplementation	• Testing absorption: measure serum iron 2–4 h after 325 mg dose ferrous sulfate • ↓ Transferrin saturation and plasma iron, and ↑ plasma transferrin • Continued depletion results in ↓ serum ferritin (reflects tissue stores) • Iron deficiency anemia confirmed by ↓ mean corpuscular volume and ↓ Hgb concentration	RDA: 19–50 years Male/female 8/18 mg >50 years 8 mg	Not routinely added 25–50 mg/month (without blood loss) Provides iron dextran in lipid-free PN

TABLE 1.4
Conditions and Diseases Contribute to Malnutrition and Nutrient Deficiencies

Surgical procedures:	bariatric surgery, GI surgery
Conditions:	anorexia nervosa, substance abuse, and wound/pressure ulcers
Disease:	organ failure (heart, liver, kidney, and pancreas)
Malabsorption:	steatorrhea, short-bowel syndrome, fistula, inflammatory bowel disease, celiac disease, and cystic fibrosis

the patient, and the patient's caregivers. The plan should be directed at correcting nutrient deficits, promoting nutrition literacy, and improving the functional capacity and quality of life. The nutrition intervention should be a measurable goal that can be monitored by the healthcare team.

Monitoring and Evaluation

An intervention is not a static action. The clinical impact of the intervention as well as the patient's understanding, adherence, and tolerance to the regimen must be monitored to determine if the intervention will be effective and if not, to change the intervention to obtain the desired results. The ongoing evaluation helps to achieve outcomes that are beneficial to the patient. This requires communication among healthcare providers, the patient, the patient's caregivers, and the RDN.

Summary

When an individual requires nutrition care in the outpatient setting, running the gamete from diet instruction for weight loss to malabsorption requiring or home parenteral nutrition support, an organized approach to information gathering and problem identification and prioritization should start the process of care. Nutrition assessment is the foundation on which the nutritional care of the patient rests. A thorough review of the patient's metabolic systems, nutrient intake, physical appearance, and physical ability enables the clinician to develop a nutrition intervention to maintain or improve the patient's nutritional status and functionality. The identification of malnutrition is an integral part of the nutrition assessment. Treat a nutrition deficit with a nutrition intervention. The nutritional issues have to be identified so that the clinician knows when to institute a nutrition intervention. Communication within the healthcare team and with the patient and their caregiver is essential to monitor the plan so that it can be adjusted as needed. The nutritional well-being of the patient is the responsibility of the entire team.[28]

REFERENCES

1. Alliance to Advance Patient Nutrition. *Malnutrition Screening Tool (MST).* Available at www.malnutrition.com (accessed December 3, 2014).
2. Lacey K, Pritchett E. Nutrition care process and model ADA adopts road map to quality care and outcomes management. *J Am Diet Assoc.* 2003;103(8):1061–1072.
3. Brantley SL, Russell MK, Mogensen KM et al. American Society for Parenteral and Enteral Nutrition and Academy of Nutrition and Dietetics: Revised 2014 standards of practice and standards of professional performance for registered dietitian nutritionists (Competent, Proficient, and Expert) in nutrition support. *Nutr Clin Pract.* 2014;29(6):792–828.
4. Durfee SM, Adams SC, Arthur E et al. A.S.P.E.N. standards for nutrition support: Home and alternate site. *Nutr Clin Pract.* 2014;29(4):542–555.
5. Practice Paper of the Academy of Nutrition and Dietetics. *Critical Thinking Skills in Nutrition Assessment.* 2013. Available at www.eatright.org/members/practicepapers.
6. White JW, Guenter P, Jensen G et al. Consensus statement: Academy of Nutrition and Dietetics and American Society for Parenteral and Enteral Nutrition: Characteristics recommended for the identification and documentation of adult malnutrition (undernutrition). *JPEN J Parenter Enteral Nutr.* 2012;36(3):275–283.

7. Nicolo M, Compher CW, Still C et al. Feasibility of accessing data in hospitalized patients to support diagnosis of malnutrition by the Academy-A.S.P.E.N. malnutrition consensus recommended clinical characteristics. *JPEN J Parenter Enteral Nutr.* 2014;38(8):954–959.
8. Fuhrman MP, Charney P, Mueller C. Hepatic proteins and nutrition assessment. *J Am Diet Assoc.* 2004;104:1258–1264.
9. Charite TL. Diagnosing malnutrition: Why dietitians matter now more than ever! *Academy of Nutrition and Dietetics Food and Nutrition Conference and Expo, Georgia World Congress Center.* Atlanta, GA: October 19, 2014.
10. Fuhrman MP. Nutrition screening and assessment in home nutrition support. In: Ireton-Jones C, DeLegge MH eds. *Handbook of Home Nutrition Support.* Sudbury, MA: Jones and Bartlett Publishers, 2007:27–57.
11. National Institutes of Health. Clinical guidelines on the identification and treatment of overweight and obesity in adults—The evidence report. *Obes Res.* 1998; 6(Suppl 2):51S–209S.
12. Canada T, Crill C, Guenter P (eds.). *A.S.P.E.N. Parenteral Nutrition Handbook.* Silver Spring, MD: American Society for Parenteral and Enteral Nutrition; 2009.
13. Moore MC (ed.). *Mosby's Pocket Guide to Nutritional Care.* 4th edition. St Louis, MO: Mosby; 2001
14. Metropolitan Life Insurance Company, 1983. *Metropolitan Height and Weight Tables.* The Statistical Bulletin of the Metropolitan Life Insurance Company. 64(1):2–9. New York, 1983.
15. National Center for Health Statistics. *Plan and Operation of the Health and Nutrition Examination Survey,* United States, *1976–1980 (Part A - Development, Plan and Operation) Vital and Health Statistics.* Series 1, No. 15. DHEW Publ. No. (PHS) 81-1317. Washington, DC: US Government Printing Office, 1981.
16. Hamwi GJ. Changing dietary concepts. In: Danowski TS (ed.). *Diabetes Mellitus: Diagnosis and Treatment,* Vol. 1. New York, New York: American Diabetes Association, Inc; 1964:73–78.
17. Osterkamp LK. Current perspective on assessment of human body proportions of relevance to amputees. *J Am Diet Assoc.* 1995;95(2):215–218.
18. Peiffer SC, Blust P, Leyson JF. Nutritional assessment of the spinal cord injured patient. *J Am Diet Assoc.* 1981; 78(5):501–505.
19. McCann L (ed.). *Pocket Guide to Nutrition Assessment of the Patient with Chronic Kidney Disease.* 4th edition. New York, New York: National Kidney Foundation; 2009.
20. Karnofsky DA, Abelmann WH, Craver LF et al. The use of the nitrogen mustards in the palliative treatment of carcinoma—with particular reference to bronchogenic carcinoma. *Cancer.* 1948;1(4):634–656.
21. National Institute on Aging. *Assessing Physical Performance in the Older Patient.* Available at http://www.grc.nia.nih.gov/branches/leps/sppb/. Accessed January 27, 2015.
22. Guralnik JM, Ferrucci L et al. Lower extremity function and subsequent disability: Consistency across studies, predictive models, and value of gait speed alone compared with the short physical performance battery. *J Gerontol A Biol Sci Med Sci.* 2000;55(4):M221–M231.
23. Frankenfield D, Rowe WA, Smith JS et al. Validation of several established equations for resting metabolic rate in obese and nonobese people. *J Am Diet Assoc.* 2003;103(9):1152–1159.
24. Russell M, Malone AM. Nutrient requirements. In: Charney P, Malone AM (eds.). *ADA Pocket Guide to Nutrition Assessment.* 2nd edition. Chicago, Illinois: American Dietetic Association; 2009, pp. 167–191.
25. Fuhrman MP. Nutrition-focused physical assessment. In: Charney P, Malone AM (eds.). *ADA Pocket Guide to Nutrition Assessment.* 2nd edition. Chicago, Illinois: American Dietetic Association; 2009, pp. 40–61.
26. Morrison SG. Clinical nutrition physical examination. *Support Line.* 1997;19(2):16–18.
27. Clark SF. Vitamins and trace elements. In: Mueller CM. (ed.). *The A.S.P.E.N. Adult Nutrition Support Core Curriculum.* 2nd edition. Silver Spring, Maryland: A.S.P.E.N.; 2012:121–151.
28. Tappenden KA, Quatrara B, Parkhurst ML et al. Critical role of nutrition in improving quality of care: An interdisciplinary call to action to address adult hospital malnutrition. *JPEN J Parenter Enteral Nutr.* 2013; 37(4):482–497.

2 Nutritional Management of Diabetes Mellitus

Martha McHenry, RDN, LD, CDE

CONTENTS

OVERVIEW OF DIABETES MELLITUS

Diabetes mellitus is a chronic disease characterized by a defect in insulin secretion or insulin action that results in high blood sugar. Defects in insulin secretion can result in an absolute absence of insulin. This is often referred to as insulin deficiency and results when pancreatic beta-cells do not secret enough insulin to keep up with the demand placed by glucose in the bloodstream. Defects in insulin action result when cells involved in glucose uptake are unable to use insulin effectively resulting in a condition referred to as insulin resistance (American Diabetes Association 2009). One or both of these mechanisms are involved in the development and characterization of diabetes.

Today, diabetes afflicts approximately 9% of the world's population and by 2030, it is expected to be the seventh leading cause of death worldwide. In 2012, it was the direct cause of 1.5-million deaths appearing most frequently in low- and middle-income countries (World Health Organization 2015).

Diabetes is a broad designation for a group of all metabolic disorders that have a common characteristic of marked high blood glucose. In a clinical setting, this may be referred to as hyperglycemia or high blood glucose but in an outpatient or home care setting, the colloquial term "high blood sugar" is often used. Hyperglycemia can develop through several mechanisms that range from the autodestruction of pancreatic beta-cells resulting in zero production of insulin, to diminished production of insulin resulting in insulin deficiency or abnormalities in how cells use insulin as in insulin resistance.

The common symptoms of hyperglycemia include but are not limited to

- Increased thirst and urination as the body attempts to rid itself of glucose
- Blurred vision as the shape of the eyeball changes in response to hyperglycemia

TABLE 2.1
Classification of Diabetes Mellitus Diseases and Its Principal Distinguishing Characteristics

Classification	Type 1 Diabetes Mellitus	Type 2 Diabetes Mellitus	Gestational Diabetes Mellitus	Diabetes Due to Other Causes
Characteristics	Pancreatic beta-cell destruction resulting in complete insulin deficiency. Possibly autoimmune.	Progressive beta-cell dysfunction resulting in gradual insulin deficiency and/or insulin resistance.	Hyperglycemia detected during the second or third trimester of pregnancy.	Caused by drugs, such as steroids, monogenic syndromes such as MODY (mature onset diabetes of the young), or pancreatic diseases.
Status	Insulin dependent.	Noninsulin dependent.	Noninsulin dependent.	May or may not be insulin dependent.
Onset	Predominantly in youth but can be diagnosed at any age.	Usually after the age of 40 but can be diagnosed at any age and usually associated with obesity.	After the first trimester of pregnancy. Can be diagnosed at any age and may be associated with rapid pregnancy and weight gain.	Can be diagnosed at any age.

Source: Reprinted with permission from American Diabetes Association—A position statement, *Diabetes Care* 2015:38: S8–S16.

- Susceptibility to infection as a glucose-rich environment serves as the perfect medium for everyday bacteria
- Numbness and tingling in the hands and feet as blood vessels damaged by hyperglycemia fail to support the nerve tissue

Chronic hyperglycemia can result in neuropathy, cardio vascular disease, kidney, and vision failure, as well as sexual dysfunction. Acute hyperglycemia can be accompanied by ketoacidosis or a nonketotic hyperosmolar syndrome. This is also known as a hyperglycemic hyperosmolar syndrome/state. Patients in either one of these acute phases are often hospitalized and in-patient protocols are followed (American Diabetes Association 2015). Complications that arise from both chronic hyperglycemia and acute hyperglycemia, as well as the role played by glucose variability will be addressed in more detail later in this chapter.

There are three common classifications of diabetes mellitus that make up the preponderance of all cases of diabetes. A fourth class consists of several, uncommon types of diabetes that vary in etiology. See Table 2.1.

The classification of diabetes is typically assigned at the time of diagnosis and largely depends on the circumstances on hand at the time, such as severity of hyperglycemia, age, and other factors. An individual who exhibits signs and symptoms from more than one classification may be misdiagnosed or may be put into the fourth classification of varied etiologies (American Diabetes Association 2009).

Regardless of the classification, the end result of hyperglycemia is the same and an effective care plan for all classifications must include glycemic control as one of the goals.

DIABETES IN AMERICA

- 29.1-million people in the United States or 9.3% of the population have diabetes. 21 million have actually been diagnosed and 8.1 million are undiagnosed.
- 90%–95% of all cases of diabetes are type 2. About 5%–8% are type 1 and 2%–5% account for all other cases put together.
- Nearly 70-million Americans have prediabetes and don't know it.

- More individuals of age 45–60 were newly diagnosed in 2012 than any other age category.
  - The second-most new cases that year came from the over-65 group; so, you can expect to see more of these older individuals at home and in the outpatient setting.
- The prevalence of diabetes varies widely by race ethnicity. In the CDC report, National Diabetes Statistics Report, 2014, the ethnic groups on either end of the spectrum are non-Hispanic whites and American Indians/Alaskan natives. Non-Hispanic whites suffer from diabetes at a rate of 7.6% while American Indians and Alaska natives suffer from diabetes at a rate of 15.9%. The prevalence in the Hispanic community is nearly 13% and among non-Hispanic blacks the rate is 13.2%.
- According to the Center for Disease Control and Prevention, further stratifications of the 2014 data showed that among Hispanic adults with diabetes, the composition or subgroups were as follows:
    - 14.8% are Puerto Rican
    - 13.9% are Mexican American
    - 9.3% are Cuban
    - 8.5% are Central and South American
  - Among Asian American adults, the composition of subgroups is as follows:
    - 13.0% are Asian Indians
    - 11.3% are Filipinos
    - 4.4% are Chinese
    - 8.8% are "other" Asians
  - Among American Indian and Alaska Native adults, diagnosis by a subgroup is as follows:
    - 24.1% among Native Americans is southern Arizona
    - 6.0% is among Alaska Natives

This stratification gives an insight to the complexities of effectively treating diabetes in the United States. It's important to understand the magnitude of the diversity of persons with diabetes as it has direct implications for the dietitian. Cultural stratification can be used to drive the development of culturally relevant treatment plans that are customized to an individual's or group's:

- Beliefs about diabetes and self-efficacy
- Cultural preferences for lifestyle
- Cultural preferences for food

In turn, these culturally relevant plans may be easier to adopt by the patient with diabetes, making them more sustainable overtime, thereby matching the long-term nature of the disease.

THE FINANCIAL BURDEN OF DIABETES

Robert Ratner, MD, the chief scientific and medical officer of the American Diabetes Association (ADA) said at a press release in 2013:

> The cost of diabetes is rising at a rate higher than overall medical costs with more than one in 10 health care dollars in the country being spent directly on diabetes and its complications, and more than one in five health care dollars in the United States going to the care of people with diagnosed diabetes.

A study commissioned by the ADA, Economic Costs of Diabetes in the United States in 2012, showed that

- The total estimated costs of diabetes in 2012 were $245 billion
  - $176 billion from direct medical costs while
  - $69 billion from reduced productivity

- Dollars spent on direct medical costs were categorized as follows:
  - 43% for hospitalizations
  - 18% to treat complications of diabetes
  - 12% for drugs and supplies to treat and manage diabetes
  - 9% for physician office visits and
  - 8% on SNIFF stays
- Indirect costs were further broken down as well to show that
  - \$5 billion was attributable to increased absenteeism
  - \$23.5 billion was attributable to reduced productivity for the employed and unemployed population
  - \$21.6 billion was attributable to disease-related disability
  - \$18.5 is attributable to lost productivity due to early death

The study also looked at the burden on an individual with diabetes and found that

- Direct medical expenditures were approximately 2.3 times higher than for individuals without diabetes.
- Average annual health care costs were \$13,700, of which \$7900 were attributable to the disease.
- Individuals who do not have health insurance have 79% fewer office visits, 68% fewer medications but 55% more hospitalizations.

This is a significant financial burden on the health care system and society as a whole. Not included in these numbers are the personal costs of suffering, poor quality of life, and the additional costs incurred by those with prediabetes. Patients treated outside of hospitals, in the outpatient, or home setting may be particularly vulnerable due to poor insurance coverage increasing the chances for suboptimal care and quality of life. Dietitians in the outpatient setting must educate themselves on reimbursement rates, codes, and procedures provided by insurance companies, public, and private. *The Academy's Coding and Billing Handbook: A Guide for Program Directors and Preceptors* is one resource that can be useful for private practice, or consulting dietitians.

DIAGNOSING DIABETES

Diabetes can be diagnosed through several different tests. Usual tests used in the diagnosing of diabetes are listed as fasting plasma glucose (FPG), the 2-hour plasma glucose, the oral glucose tolerance test (OGTT), and more recently, the glycalated hemoglobin test (A1C) has been approved as a diagnostic method in addition to its historic role of just a management tool. These tests can be used for screening and diagnosing and management. Meeting one of the criteria below qualifies as a diagnosis of diabetes. See Table 2.2.

Until recently, using A1C as a diagnostic tool was quite controversial. Since tightening the standards for this test in regard to accuracy and standardization, today, A1C is a popular way to diagnose and monitor diabetes care. The following are some of the reasons why A1C is quickly becoming a routine diagnostic tool:

- Only the A1C test gives a picture of the patient's chronic glycemic status
- A1C is more tightly associated with the complications of diabetes such as retinopathy and cardiovascular disease than FPG
- No fasting needed for A1C
- Stress, eating, and exercising do not affect A1C
- Using the same biomarker for diagnosing and managing could be useful
  (Enzo Bonora and Jaakko Tuomilehto 2011)

TABLE 2.2
Diagnosing Diabetes

Test	Diagnostic Threshold	Comments
A1C	>6.5	Added to the list of diagnostic tests in 2008 after review by an expert committee. Must be standardized to the DCCT assay to assure accuracy.
Fasting plasma glucose	>126	Must fast for at least 8 h.
2-hour plasma glucose in OGTT	>/=200	A standard protocol using 75 g of anhydrous glucose dissolved in water.
Random plasma glucose	>/=200 mg/dL + symptoms of hyperglycemia	Can be done at any time.

Source: Reprinted with permission from American Diabetes Association—A position statement, *Diabetes Care*, 2015:38: S8–S16.

MONITORING A1C IN THE OUTPATIENT OR HOME SETTING

A1C can also be monitored in the home or outpatient setting. Care must be taken, however, to select an A1C monitor that meets NGSP standards for accuracy. Outpatient and consulting dietitians can easily administer this test, thereby improving their value and role in the patient's care. Today, while there is no code for reimbursement for this test when administered by dietitians, a low fee with a CLIA-waived device that involves just a finger stick for the outpatient and home-bound patient until reimbursement for dietitians is recognized, could be a low-barrier out-of-pocket, and billable service. In a study by Anna Chang, the following were demonstrated:

- Lay users found the A1CNow SELFCHECK easy to use, and both lay users and HCPs were able to measure A1C accurately.
- An A1C reading was considered accurate if it was within ±13.5% of a corresponding NGSP-certified laboratory reference value.
- The A1CNow SELFCHECK has received 2010 NGSP certification (Chang et al. 2010).

PREDIABETES

In 2003, the Expert Committee on Diagnosis and Classification of Diabetes Mellitus recognized a group of individuals who don't meet the diagnostic criteria on any of the tests above but have varying degrees of hyperglycemia. These individuals have prediabetes. They score too high on the IFG and IGT tests to be normal but not high enough to earn a diagnosis of diabetes. The diagnostic criteria for prediabetes are described in Table 2.3.

Individuals with IFG or IGT have a higher risk for future development of diabetes. As A1C is used more commonly to diagnose diabetes in individuals with risk factors, it will also identify those at a higher risk for developing diabetes in the future. In 2009, the International Expert Committee reported that those with A1C levels above the laboratory "normal" range but below the diagnostic cut point for diabetes (6 to <6.5%) are at a very high risk of developing diabetes.

Studies show that the incidence of diabetes in people with A1C levels in this range is more than 10 times that of people with lower levels and may be up to eight times higher than the incidence of diabetes found in the U.S. population (Edelman et al. 2004) (Diabetes Care-Supplement 1, 2011).

TABLE 2.3
Diagnostic Criteria for Prediabetes

Test	Diagnostic Threshold	Comments
Impaired fasting glucose (IFG)	100–125 mg/dL	WHO and other international organizations do not recognize this diagnostic threshold for prediabetes and use 110–125 mg/dL instead.
Impaired glucose tolerance (IGT)	140–199 mg/dL	
A1C	>6.0 and <6.5	Not a formal criteria. Not typically used to diagnose prediabetes.

Source: Reprinted with permission from American Diabetes Association—A position statement, *Diabetes Care*, 2015:38: S8–S16; World Health Organization, 312, 2015.

TREATING DIABETES AND PREDIABETES

The four cornerstones of a comprehensive care plan for a person with diabetes, without regard to the type, include

- Nutritional intervention
- Medication, when appropriate
- Self-monitoring of blood glucose (SMBG), when appropriate
- Physical activity

For purposes of this book, medical nutrition therapy (MNT) is the mode of nutritional intervention and is the focus of this chapter. MNT for prediabetes is very similar to MNT for diabetes. There is more focus on weight management in the care plan for prediabetes. Not all insurance plans provide MNT benefits for prediabetes.

Developing an intervention plan for diabetes and prediabetes heavily relies on the data collected for and during the assessment. Of particular importance is the data collected from the referral source, usually a primary care physician. This information may be best divided into two categories that can be helpful in organizing the intervention. One is lab values that can provide a snapshot of the patient at the time of diagnosis or referral and the second is treatment goals. An example follows:

- Lab-based data
- A1C at the time of referral
- FPG at the time of referral
- Kidney function values

Glycemic treatment goals

- A1C target
- Fasting SMBG target, when appropriate
- Postprandial target

Treatment goals may vary from referral source to referral source and while these targets do need to be individualized, there exists marked differences in targets promoted by major diabetes institutions. The table below compares the treatment goals set forth by the American Diabetes Association (ADA), the International Diabetes Federation (IDF), and the American College of Endocrinologists (ACE). All three of these targets are used and can cause quite a bit of confusion among persons with diabetes. See Table 2.4.

TABLE 2.4
Comparison of Glycemic Targets for Persons with Diabetes

Test	ADA	IDF	ACE
A1C—satisfactory control	7%	6.5%	6.5%
Fasting glucose—SMBG	70–130 mg/dL	<100 mg/dL	<110 mg/dL
2-hour postprandial—SMBG	<180 mg/dL	<140 mg/dL	<140 mg/dL

Source: Reprinted with permission from American Diabetes Association—A position statement, *Diabetes Care*, 2015:38: S8–S16; aace.com and idf.org accessed March 2015.

It's important for clinicians to appreciate the differences in these targets. The <180 mg/dL target held by the ADA for postprandial blood glucose corresponds to the upper limit that was chosen in patients who were allocated to the intensively treated group of the DCCT, the Diabetes Control, and Complications Trial. The lower value held by the IDF, the International Diabetes Federation, and ACE, American College of Endocrinology was mainly based on the fact that 140 mg/dL is the highest value for defining the impaired glucose tolerance as a part of the oral glucose tolerance test (Monnier 2009).

A patient's treatment targets are most often set by the patient in conjunction with their primary care provider. The RD's role in target achievement is twofold.

1. To deliver medical nutrition therapy that helps the patient to meet those goals within the framework of medication and/or lifestyle changes set forth by the primary care provider
2. To communicate to the primary care provider information related to nutritional changes that directly impact a patient's success or failure to reach targets

NUTRITION ASSESSMENT FOR DIABETES MELLITUS

Nutrition assessment is a crucial first step in diabetes MNT. The assessment forms the basis for developing the intervention plan and identifying potential areas of change to a client's lifestyle and habits that will help the patient to meet their goals. The main purpose of an assessment is to gather information needed to assist in the development of individual nutrition goals and establish an appropriate nutrition intervention.

Preliminary Data

Before a comprehensive nutrition assessment can be performed on a patient, preliminary data must be collected. Some of these data can be obtained from the referral source but it is likely that not all of the data will be available. At a minimum, the dietitian will need from the referral source:

- Documented diagnosis of diabetes or prediabetes, the type and date of diagnosis, or reported duration
- The type of medication and dose if applicable
- Labs that support the diagnosis(es) A1C, and FBG
- Labs/data that support related conditions such as kidney function, or hypertension

Collecting the rest of the data then becomes a part of the assessment process with this patient. Further data needed for a complete assessment include but are not limited to the points detailed in Table 2.5.

TABLE 2.5
Initial Nutrition Assessment

Data Needed	Metric
Clinical	Anthropometrics
	Energy needs (estimated or measured)
	Weight and weight history
	Lab values
	Treatment goals
Nutritional history	Usual intake, 24-hour recall
	Feeding habits
	Use of vitamins, minerals, and supplements
	Assessment of a disordered eating
	Previous nutrition intervention
Physical activity history	Type, frequency, physical limitations, and willingness to become more active
Monitoring	SMBG knowledge and skills
	Glucose levels and ranges
	Food intake journals and physical activity journals
	Benefits of monitoring
Psychosocial	Living situation
	Ethnic or religious beliefs
	Family and social support
	Level of stress
	Readiness for change
	Patient expectations for treatment
Economic	Education level
	Ability to purchase food and medicine
Knowledge	Understanding of the current disease state
	Survival skills
	Patient's self-management needs

Source: Adapted from *Practice Guidelines for Medical Nutrition Therapy Provided by Dietitians for Persons with Non-Insulin-Dependent Diabetes Mellitus*; Monk A. et al., *J Am Diet Assoc.*, 1995:95:999–1006.

The information in each of these components is used by the dietitian to formulate an appropriate care plan that includes achievable goals and interventions that are appropriate to the outpatient or home-setting patient. After an initial consultation, regular assessment is ongoing, and is continuously modified and updated throughout the diabetes MNT process. Follow-ups are needed for several reasons.

- Collecting the necessary data before the initial consultation or even during the initial consultation with a patient can be difficult, making appropriate follow-ups needed to formulate a comprehensive care plan.
- Monitoring of the care plan so that a patient is on track to meet the goals developed with the primary care provider.
- Making modifications to the care plan as needed based on goal achievement metrics and input from the patient.

The flowchart below is one guide for delivering MNT to persons with diabetes. Many variations are possible and should be guided by the needs of the patients, the dietitians time, the goals of the

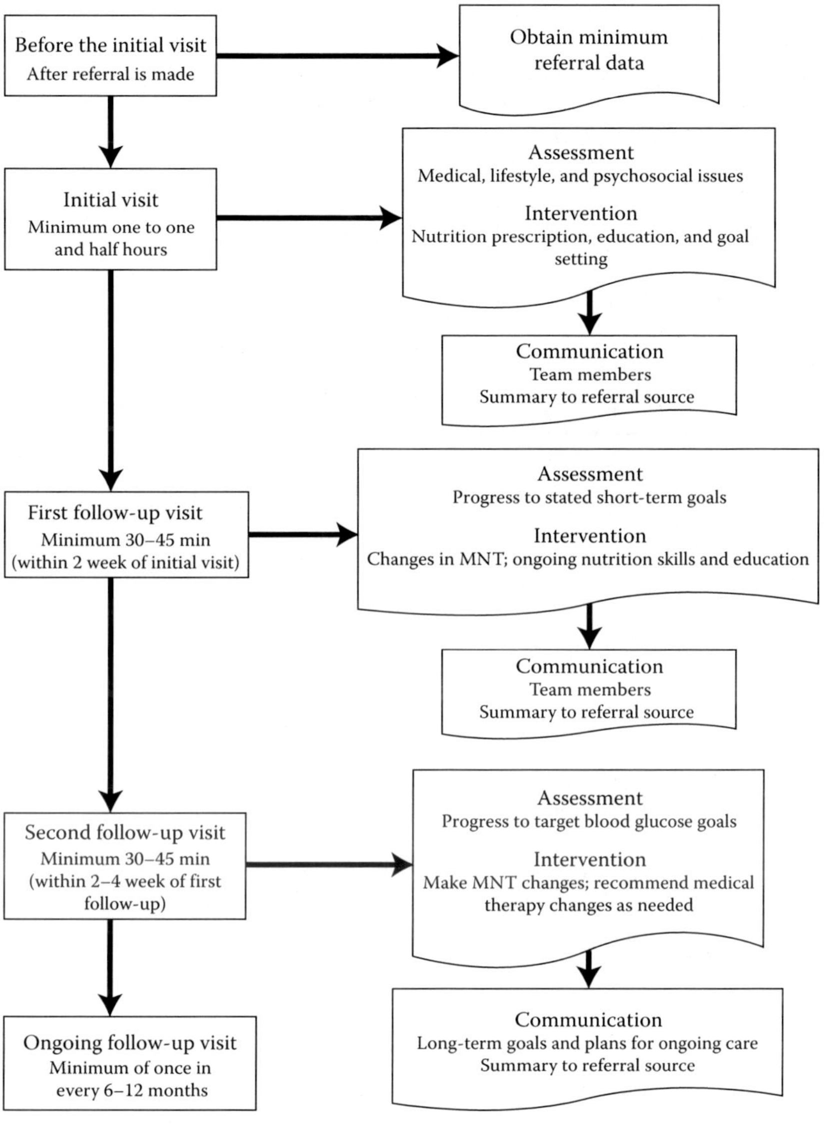

FIGURE 2.1 Flow of events in the assessment and care plan development for persons with diabetes mellitus. (Adapted from Monk A et al., *J Am Diet Assoc*, 1995:95:999–1006.)

physician, and resources at hand. While these steps originally addressed the assessment, intervention, and monitoring patients with type 2 diabetes, it is also valid and can be used with patients who have other types of diabetes and even prediabetes. Intervention and monitoring are further discussed in Figure 2.1.

NUTRITIONAL INTERVENTION FOR DIABETES

While pharmacotherapy, physical activity, and blood glucose monitoring are all components of a comprehensive care plan for diabetes, the nutritional component occupies a large portion of its overall education and nutritional management. Many patients struggle mightily with the nutritional aspect of treating diabetes (Evert et al. 2014). The ADA published a position paper that states that persons with diabetes should be referred to a registered dietitian (RD) for medical nutrition therapy or a Diabetes Self-Management Education program for nutrition counseling. The position puts forth the following goals of nutrition therapy for adults with diabetes, which are nongestational:

- To individualize nutrition needs based on personal and cultural preferences, literacy level, available resources, and willingness to make changes
- To provide practical tools for daily meal planning
- To provide positive, evidence-based information about food and the effects of foods on glycemic control
- To promote healthful eating habits that emphasize the appropriate portion size and variety so as to support
  - The prescribed A1C target
  - Blood pressure goal of 120/80
  - LDL cholesterol <100 mg/dL
  - Triglycerides <150 mg/dL
  - HDL cholesterol >50 mg/dL for women and 40 mg/dL for men
  - Body weight goal
  - The prevention or delay of the complications of diabetes (Evert et al. 2014)

The Academy of Nutrition and Dietetics recommends that these goals be met in the following way:

- A series of three to four encounters with an RD lasting from 45–90 min.
- The series of encounters should begin at diagnosis of diabetes or at first referral to an RD for MNT for diabetes and should be completed within 3–6 months.
- The RD should determine whether additional MNT encounters are needed.
- At least one follow-up encounter is recommended annually to reinforce lifestyle changes and to evaluate and monitor outcomes that indicate the need for changes in MNT or medication(s); the RD should determine whether additional MNT encounters are needed (Evert et al. 2014).

The RD needs to keep in mind that additional units of MNT can be requested and prescribed when an element of the care plan changes. For this reason, it is paramount for the patient that the RD has regular communication with the patient's primary care provider. For example, if the patient moves from a 1800-calorie meal plan to a 1500-calorie meal plan, the RD can request that the primary care provider authorizes more units of MNT so that the change can be implemented and monitored by the RD.

The following are specific, evidence-based recommendations set forth in the position statement published by the American Diabetes Association that address strategies regarding key nutrients, micronutrients, and medication and food interactions that support the goals of nutrition therapy for diabetes. These recommendations can be used as a basis for nutritional counseling during the suggested structure for MNT encounters.

- Portion control should be recommended for weight loss and maintenance.
- Carbohydrate-containing foods and beverages and endogenous insulin production are the greatest determinant of the postmeal blood glucose level; therefore, it is important to know which foods contain carbohydrates: starchy vegetables, whole grains, fruit, milk and milk products, vegetables, and sugar.
- When choosing carbohydrate-containing foods, choose nutrient-dense, high-fiber foods whenever possible instead of processed foods with added sodium, fat, and sugars.

Nutrient-dense foods and beverages provide vitamins, minerals, and other healthful substances with relatively few calories. Calories have not been added to them from solid fats, sugars, or refined starches.

- For most people, it is not necessary to subtract the amount of dietary fiber or sugar alcohols from total carbohydrates when counting the carbohydrates.
- Substitute foods higher in unsaturated fat (liquid oils) for foods higher in trans or saturated fat.
- Select leaner protein sources and meat alternatives.
- Vitamin and mineral supplements, herbal products, or cinnamon to manage diabetes are not recommended due to lack of evidence.
- Moderate alcohol consumption (one drink/day or less for adult women and two drinks or less for adult men) has minimal acute or long-term effects on blood glucose in people with diabetes. To reduce the risk of hypoglycemia for individuals using insulin or insulin secretagogues, alcohol should be consumed with food.
- Limit sodium intake to 2300 mg/day or 1500 mg/day, depending on the patient's risks for stroke.
- Priority should be given to coordinating food with the type of diabetes medications.
- For individuals who take insulin secretagogues: moderate amounts of carbohydrate at each meal and snack.
- To reduce the risk of hypoglycemia:
  - Eat a source of carbohydrates at meals.
  - Moderate amounts of carbohydrates at each meal and snacks.
  - Do not skip meals.
  - Physical activity may result in low blood glucose depending on when it is performed. Always carry a source of carbohydrates to reduce the risk of hypoglycemia.
- For individuals who take biguanides (metformin):
  - Gradually titrate to minimize gastrointestinal side effects when initiating the use.
  - Take medication with food for 15 min after a meal if symptoms persist.
  - If side effects do not resolve overtime (a few weeks), follow up with a health care provider.
  - If taking along with an insulin secretagogue or insulin, may experience hypoglycemia.
- For individuals who take a-glucosidase inhibitors:
  - Gradually titrate to minimize gastrointestinal side effects when initiating the use.
  - Take at the beginning of a meal to have maximal effect.
  - If taking along with an insulin secretagogue or insulin, may experience hypoglycemia.
  - If hypoglycemia occurs, eat something containing monosaccharides such as glucose tablets and drugs that will prevent the digestion of polysaccharides.
- For individuals who take incretin mimetics (GLP-1):
  - Gradually titrate to minimize gastrointestinal side effects when initiating the use.
  - Injection of daily or twice-daily GLP-1s should be taken premeal.
  - If side effects do not resolve overtime (a few weeks), follow up with a health care provider.
  - If taking along with an insulin secretagogue or insulin, may experience hypoglycemia.
  - Once-weekly GLP-1s can be taken at any time during the day regardless of meal times.

Nutrition and Insulin

- For individuals with type 1 diabetes and insulin-requiring type 2 diabetes:
  - Learn how to count carbohydrates or use another meal-planning approach to quantify carbohydrate intake.
  - The objective of using such a meal-planning approach is to "match" mealtime insulin to the carbohydrates consumed.

- If on a multiple-daily injection plan or on an insulin pump:
  - Take mealtime insulin before eating as directed. Some of it acts faster and lasts longer than others.
  - Meals can be consumed at different times.
  - If physical activity is performed within 1–2 h of mealtime insulin injection, this dose may need to be lowered to reduce the risk of hypoglycemia.
- If on a premixed insulin plan:
  - Insulin doses need to be taken at consistent times every day.
  - Meals need to be consumed at similar times every day.
  - Do not skip meals to reduce the risk of hypoglycemia.
- Physical activity may result in low blood glucose depending on when it is performed. Always carry a source of quick-acting carbohydrates to reduce the risk of hypoglycemia. See how to treat hypoglycemia in the section on "Complications of Diabetes."
- If on a fixed insulin plan, eat similar amounts of carbohydrates each day to match the set doses of insulin (Evert et al. 2014).

COMPLICATIONS OF DIABETES

The complications of diabetes can be categorized into two broad categories. The first category includes those that result from long-term or chronic hyperglycemia and the second category includes those that present themselves from sudden or extreme shifts in blood sugar, resulting in acute hypoglycemia or hyperglycemia that can require medical attention.

Chronic complications that result from longer-term high blood sugar can be divided into two major categories. The first category includes complications due to damage to the major arterial vessels and the second category includes complications due to damage to the small blood vessels.

- Large-vessel damage
  - Diabetic neuropathies
  - Heart disease
- Small-vessel damage
  - Kidney disease and kidney failure
  - Retinopathy resulting in blindness
  - Reproductive system dysfunction

Acute complications can include both hypoglycemia and hyperglycemia. While technically both of these can occur with any type of diabetes, acute hypoglycemia more often occurs in patients with type 1 diabetes. Care plans should include education for treatment of this condition. The typical treatment plan that is easy for the outpatient or home care dietitian to use is the rule of 15. This strategy can be found in several books about diabetes, including Dr. Alan Rubin's book, *Diabetes for Dummies*.

Diabetes ketoacidosis (DKA) and hyperglycemic hyperosmolar syndrome (HHS) are two acute, hyperglycemic conditions that can occur when blood glucose is extremely high. The most common factors that can lead to DKA or HHS are infection, inadequate insulin therapy, discontinuation of insulin therapy and other medications, pancreatitis, heart attack, stroke, and some medications. Assessing the risk of these conditions by assessing medication compliance can be included as a part of the dietitian's initial or follow-up consultation that may help in avoiding these hyperglycemic states.

- Diabetes ketoacidosis (DKA) results from a shortage of insulin and more commonly occurs in individuals with type 1 diabetes. Blood glucose of 250 or greater is a cause for concern

as the production of ketones can accelerate quickly. The outpatient and home-setting dietitian should refer the type 1 patient to their primary care as DKA can have a quick onset and can be dangerous.
- The hyperosmolar hyperglycemic syndrome or state predominantly occurs in individuals with type 2 diabetes. Very high blood sugars cause severe dehydration. It is similar to DKA but without the presence of ketones. According to Ketabchi et al., a patient with a blood sugar of 600 mg/dL or greater requires medical attention; however, practically speaking, a type 2 patient with blood sugars of over 250 can also be at risk and should be monitored.

In addition to hyperglycemia causing damage to blood vessels and thereby complications, glucose variability also plays a role in the development of complications from diabetes. In a systematic review of the literature that looked at glucose variability as an independent contributor to the development of diabetes complications, the following were found:

- In persons with type 2 diabetes, a positive association was consistent between increased variability and microvascular, or small-vessel complications, but not with large-vessel complications.
- In persons with type 1 diabetes, it appears that increased glucose variability plays a minimal role in both the large- and small-vessel complications (Smith-Palmer et al. 2014).

These associations found in 28 studies may be the basis for a case for using continuous glucose monitoring (CGM) in patients with type 2 diabetes. Historically, it is a practice largely confined to the monitoring of type 1 diabetes. Today, outpatient and home- setting dietitians can avail themselves of training, use, and in many cases, reimbursement for placing these monitors, even if just for short-term data gathering, on patients with type 2 diabetes. Medtronic is one provider of a 3-day, disposal monitors.

The life-impairing chronic complications due to diabetes are the reason that control of blood glucose is so important and why MNT care plans that treat to goal are critical. These complications can be minimized, delayed, and in some cases averted in persons with diabetes and prediabetes when nutrition therapy is integrated into the overall care plan of medication with appropriate physical activity and blood glucose monitoring.

CONCLUSION

Medical nutrition therapy in the outpatient and home care setting can offer a structured, regular intervention that can improve the outcomes and quality of life in patients with diabetes, regardless of the type. From gathering preliminary data, through the nutritional assessment and follow-up consultations, MNT must be in the context of a comprehensive plan of care that includes the goals of the primary care provider and the cultural and social aspects of the patient. MNT must be deliberate, must follow the guidelines of the best practices, and must measure and monitor the markers of progress.

HELPFUL RESOURCES FOR PROFESSIONALS

National Diabetes Information Clearinghouse (NDIC) www.diabetes.niddk.nih.gov
American Diabetes Association (ADA) www.diabetes.org
Academy of Nutrition and Dietetics (AND) www.eatright.org
International Diabetes Federation (IDF) http://www.idf.org/guidelines
Weight-Control Information Network (WIN) www.win.niddk.nih.gov
Centers for Disease Control National Diabetes Education Program (CDC-NDEP) http://www.cdc.gov/diabetes/ndep/index.htm

REFERENCES

American Diabetes Association. Classification and diagnosis of diabetes—A position statement. *Diabetes Care* (Suppl 1), 2015:38:S8–S16.

American Diabetes Association. Diagnosis and classification of diabetes mellitus. *Diabetes Care* (Suppl 1), 2009:32:S62–S67.

American Diabetes Association. *The Economic Costs of Diabetes in the US*. Alexandria: VA, 2012.

Bonora E, Tuomilehto J. Pros and cons of diagnosing diabetes with A1c. *Diabetes Care*, 2011:34 (Suppl 2):S184–90.

Center for Disease Control and Prevention. *National Diabetes Statistics Report: Estimates of Diabetes and Its Burden in the United States*. Atlanta, GA: United States Department of Health and Human Services, 2014.

Chang A, Frank J, Knaebel J. et al. Evaluation of an over-the-counter glycated hemoglobin (A1c) test kit. *Journal of Diabetes Science and Technology*. 2010:4(6):1495–1503.

Diabetes Care-Supplement 1. *Diagnosing and Classification of Diabetes Mellitus*. American Diabetes Association, 2011.

Edelman D, Olsen MK, Dudley TK, Harris AC, Oddone EZ. Utility of hemoglobin A1c in predicting diabetes risk. *J Gen Intern Med*, 2004:19:1175–1180.

Evert AB, Boucher JL, Cypress M. et al. Nutrition therapy recommendations for the management of adults with diabetes. *Diabetes Care*, 2014:37(Suppl 1):S120–43.

Franz MJ, Powers MA, Leontos C, Holzmeister LA, Kulkami K, Monk A, Wedel N, Gradwell E. The evidence for medical nutrition therapy for type 1 and type 2 diabetes in adults. *Journal of the American Dietetic Association*, 2010:110(12):1852–89.

Green Pastors J. Nutritional assessment for diabetes medical nutrition therapy. *Diabetes Spectrum*, 1996:9(2):99–103.

Monk A, Barry B, McClain K, Weaver T, Cooper N, Franz MJ. Practice guidelines for medical nutrition therapy provided by dietitians for persons with noninsulin-dependent diabetes mellitus. *Journal of the American Dietetic Association*, 1995:95:999–1006.

Monnier L, Claude C. Target for glycemic control: Concentrating on glucose. *Diabetes Care* (Suppl 2), 2009:32:S199–204.

Smith-Palmer J, Brandle M, Trevisan R. et al. Assessment of the association between glycemic variability and diabetes-related complications in type 1 and type 2 diabetes. *Diabetes Research and Clinical Practice* 2014:105(3):274–284.

World Health Organization. Diabetes fact sheet. 312:2015. Accessed November 21, 2015.

3 GI Disease Nutrition Management

Short-Bowel Syndrome, Gastroparesis, and Celiac Disease

Carol Ireton-Jones, PhD, RDN, LD, CNSC, FAND, FASPEN

CONTENTS

This chapter reviews three very different gastrointestinal (GI) disorders: short-bowel syndrome, gastroparesis (GP), and celiac disease. While all these are different, each affects nutrition through absorption of nutrients. Each also responds to nutrition intervention whether that is a diet change or provision of enteral or parenteral nutrition support. All these are very complex GI disorders and are covered in this chapter related to the required nutrition care.

SHORT-BOWEL SYNDROME

Short-bowel syndrome (SBS) is defined as an insufficient functional intestinal mass necessary to adequately digest and absorb nutrients and fluids to maintain protein, energy, and micronutrient balance [1]. In children, SBS is also associated with poor growth and development [2]. The common term for the loss of an intestinal function is intestinal failure although this relates to more than just SBS. The European Society for Parenteral and Enteral Nutrition has defined intestinal failure as "the reduction of gut function below the minimum necessary for the absorption of macronutrients and/or water and electrolytes, such that intravenous supplementation is required to maintain health and/or growth" [3]. SBS may be due to the physical loss of the intestine or due to functional impairment. Children may be born with a congenital malformation such as gastroschisis or may experience necrotizing enterocolitis or volvulus, for example, see Reference 2. Adults may experience SBS for reasons including resection from malignancies or Crohn's disease, radiation enteritis, volvulus, or trauma [4]. In adults as well as in neonates and children, the degree of malabsorption experienced and metabolic complications occurring in SBS depend on the site of intestinal resection. In neonates, intestinal growth may continue improving the absorptive capacity [2]. The length of the small intestine may be used to characterize SBS as well as to estimate the level of dependence on alternative means of nutrition support, including enteral or parenteral nutrition [4,5]. Oral or enteral intake may be inadequate because of a significant malabsorption present due to the loss of surface area of the function.

Digestion and Absorption

An understanding of GI anatomy is important in the nutrition care and management of SBS. The duodenum, jejunum, and ileum have roles in the digestion and absorption of individual nutrients (macro- and micronutrients) as well as fluids and electrolytes. In addition, the presence of the ileocecal valve and the colon effect nutrient absorption is especially related to transit time. Digestion begins in the mouth not only with mastication but also with the presence of saliva, which provides moisture for swallowing and contains amylase that begins the breakdown of starches and fats [6]. Food is swallowed and makes its way into the stomach. The stomach has been described as "pouch-like" and acts as a container not only to hold food for passage into the small intestine but begins the breakdown of food into chyme through mechanical and chemical digestion [6]. Gastric acid as well as enzymes in the stomach begin the digestion of macronutrients. The chyme or partially digested food passes through the stomach through the pyloric sphincter and into the first part of the small intestine or duodenum. The small intestine length consists of the duodenum, jejunum, and ileum (in order) and is approximately 6 m or 20 ft long [6]. In the duodenum, most chemical digestion occurs due to hormonal release of digestive enzymes from the gallbladder and pancreas. Carbohydrates, protein, and fats are broken down into monosaccharides, amino acids, and fatty acids, respectively [4]. The jejunum is where the most significant portion of absorption of nutrients happens and finally in the jejunum, vitamins (and specifically vitamin B-12), electrolytes, and any nutrients not absorbed in the jejunum occur [4,6]. The interior of the small intestine is made up of millions of villi with an absorptive surface area of approximately 30 m^2 [7]. The colon or large intestine receives any undigested food as well as water and electrolytes from the small intestine. An additional 2 m^2 of an absorptive surface area is found in the large intestine (colon). Very little nutrition absorption occurs in the colon in normal digestion and absorption although the absorption of water and electrolytes as well as compression of food contents for excretion is extremely important and can be a delicate balance in some GI disorders. Short-chain fatty acids such as butyrate may be absorbed in the colon and account for caloric intake, especially in patients with SBS [6].

Nutrition Intervention

Nutrition care for SBS is based on the length and function of the small intestine although the presence and length/function of the large intestine is important as well [1,4,5]. Various estimates have been proposed related to the type of nutrition therapy required and the length of a small bowel remaining. At least initially, parenteral nutrition (PN) is utilized to provide total nutrients for patients with SBS [4,5]. Older children and adults with less than 100–115 cm of a small bowel and a stoma (no colon), or less than 60–90 cm of a small intestine with a part of the colon present, or a small intestine less than 35 cm but not a large intestine will likely remain essentially dependent on PN for a lifetime [1,4]. Medical and surgical therapies may be utilized to improve the absorptive capacity [1,4,5].

The function of the remaining GI anatomy and an intact ileocecal valve will further influence the absorption of nutrients and the toleration of nutrition therapy [4,5]. The indication for PN in adults and children with SBS is similar, in that PN will support nutrition needs when absorption is non-existent or minimal. PN will provide carbohydrate in the form of dextrose, fat in the form of lipid and protein as amino acids plus sterile water to account for fluid needs as well as age- and need-specific vitamins, minerals, and electrolytes (see Chapters 9 and 11). Vascular access is the central venous route to allow higher concentrations of the macronutrients (see Chapter 10). In neonates and pediatric patients, calorie and protein needs are much higher than for adults [2]. In addition, higher levels of dextrose in milligrams per kilogram and specialized amino acid solutions are used in the pediatric population receiving PN [8]. Soybean oil lipid emulsion may not be well tolerated in some pediatric patients with SBS requiring PN and therefore, fish oil-based lipids have been used with success [9]. The scope of this chapter does not allow for an adequate coverage of pediatric PN requirements, monitoring, and management. Nguyen and Kerner have summarized management of home PN in pediatrics in *The Handbook of Home Nutrition Support* [8]. Management of PN and home PN in the adult is included in Chapter 9 of this book.

Adaptation in SBS is the period after resection or injury, in which the remaining small-bowel hypertrophies increase the absorptive capacity [4,10]. This adaptation phase happens over several months but usually reaches its peak level within 2 years [4,5,10]. Enteral (tube) feeding may be used in patients with SBS again, depending on the remaining GI anatomy and function (see Chapter 8). Enteral or oral nutrition is encouraged in adult SBS patients and pediatric patients because of trophic effects on the GI lumen. In pediatric patients, enteral feeding may be used even if it is in very small amounts to provide some energy and also to enhance gut function and adaptation. When an enteral (tube) feeding is used, an elemental or semielemental formula may be better tolerated due to the diminished capacity for digestion of intact nutrients and therefore the absorption of these (see Chapter 8).

For many years, people with SBS requiring PN either were told not to eat or later to eat whatever they could. Since the early work of Wilmore and colleagues, it has been shown that what is consumed can make a difference in absorption and fluid management [5,11]. The diet for SBS has become more sophisticated as management of SBS has evolved [4,5,11]. Understanding the remaining GI anatomy—length of a small bowel, presence and amount of the colon, and presence or absence of the ileocecal valve forms the basis for oral diet recommendations. In general, oral diet recommendations are [4,5,11]

- Consume small meals 5–6 times per day.
- Minimize simple carbohydrates (sugars) and maximize complex carbohydrate intake.
- Certain carbohydrates may be less well tolerated with SBS including lactose as well as FODMAP-containing foods (see Chapter 5).
- If the ileum has been removed and a full or partial colon is present, restrict oxalate intake to prevent kidney stones from forming.
- Fat should provide about 20%–30% of total calories. Fat malabsorption may be present if the ileum has been resected.
- Protein intake should be maintained at 20%–25% of total calories. Protein supplements may be necessary.
- Fiber should be provided primarily as a soluble fiber.
- A multivitamin supplement should be taken daily. Additional specific micronutrients may be required.

Adequate fluid intake should be maintained to prevent dehydration to avoid deleterious effects on kidney function. To assure fluid homeostasis, intake should equal the output. Output may be affected by ostomy output, diarrhea, vomiting or fever, and excess fluid loss should be accounted for in calculating the required intake. Because of the GI anatomy in SBS, water may not be adequately absorbed as it requires an active transporter for osmosis to occur. Therefore, fluids with added sodium and a small amount of glucose will facilitate the absorption of the fluid and prevent or treat dehydration. Beverages that are appropriate to provide this hydration are called oral rehydration solutions or ORS. An ORS should have sodium in levels of 70–90 mEq (equal to about 3/4 to 7/8 tsp NaCl or table salt, in 1 L, a small amount of glucose, or a simple sugar (28–30 g/L) to assist with the facilitation of the sodium into the lumen and should be isotonic or hypoosmolar (diluted) so that it is easily absorbed by a compromised GI tract. The WHO originated the ORS to treat the dehydration of diarrhea as seen in third-world countries. The WHO recipe for ORS and other recipes may be found at www.oley.org/resource/resmgr/ORS_Recipes/ORS_recipes_handout_2015-2.pdf. Commercial ORS beverages include Pedialyte© (requires added sodium to meet 70–90 mEq sodium content), Jianas Brothers (Amazon.com), DripDrop© (www.dripdrop.com), and Ceralyte©

(www.ceralyte.com). ORS does taste salty and can be flavored with a small amount of fruit juice (1/2 cup to 1 L of water) or a sugar-free taste enhancer. These should not be gulped but sipped over several hours.

The nutrition interventions in SBS require careful and close monitoring preferably by a team of nutrition professionals including the physician, nurse, pharmacist, and registered dietitian/nutritionist (RDN). The RDN with an expertise in SBS management can assist the patient and family whether pediatric or adult—in whatever therapy he may be receiving from PN to oral to a combination of therapies.

GASTROPARESIS

GP is a condition in which the stomach loses its contractibility and therefore, food is delayed in passing from the stomach into the small intestine for digestion and absorption [12,13,14]. This may also be called delayed gastric emptying. The most common causes of GP are neuropathic changes due to diabetes, which can affect the vagus nerve causing damage. Other causes including vagus nerve surgery, other neurological conditions, and some medications with about 30% of GP are considered as idiopathic with no known direct causative factor [14,15].

Symptoms of GP include nausea, a feeling of fullness after consuming only a small amount of food, and vomiting often-undigested food [12,15]. Individuals may also experience GI reflux, stomach pain, and abdominal bloating [12]. Because of the feeling of fullness and nausea, appetite may be depressed. There are stages or levels of GP dependent on the amount of food and the time that it takes for the food to be delivered into the small intestine [12,14]. Diagnosis of GP usually begins with an assessment of symptoms, testing for stomach or bowel obstruction, and gastric-emptying evaluation. The gastric-emptying study utilizes food treated with a radioactive material that is consumed and observed using an external camera that measures the length of time it takes for the stomach to empty over 4 h. When greater than 10% of the meal is still in the stomach after 4 h, confirmation of the diagnosis of GP can be made [12,14].

Once the diagnosis of GP is made, treatment is based on the severity of symptoms as GP is a chronic condition. Because this affects the ability for nutrients to pass into the small intestine, nutrition management is of utmost importance and a key treatment. Medications can be used to treat GP but these are limited in scope to those that stimulate muscle contractions to allow for an improvement in gastric emptying [13–15]. Metoclopramide also known as Reglan stimulates muscle contractions in the stomach; however, the side effect of tardive dyskinesia, although rare, is of concern when prescribing the medication [15]. The antibiotic erythromycin may be used to increase stomach contractions when prescribed at low doses; however, the extended use of antibiotics is not recommended [15]. Each of these also has side effects including nausea, fatigue, vomiting, and abdominal cramps.

Botulinum toxin may be used to keep the pylorus open and potentially allows for food to empty into the small intestine although this is not routinely used [16]. Gastric stimulation with an implanted gastric neurostimulator or gastric "pacemaker" is a treatment option that requires specialized expertise and management [13–15].

Nutrition Intervention

Malnutrition and weight loss may occur overtime if GP is not diagnosed and treated appropriately. Depending on the time it takes for gastric emptying, food intake may be minimally affected or severely limited requiring enteral nutrition support.

In addition, time of day may affect the severity of GP with some individuals able to tolerate more "solid" food in the mornings. Higher fat and fiber foods are poorly tolerated as these increase satiety and decrease motility [15]. Spicy and highly acidic foods as well as carbonated beverages may also be poorly tolerated.

As with any GI disease, nutrition interventions must be individualized. The fundamental components of nutrition therapy for GP include [15]:

1. Small-size meals 5–7 times per day. Include protein and carbohydrate at each "meal."
2. Avoid high-fat foods or greasy foods such as fried foods, fatty meats and sausages, and creamed products.
3. If diabetic, maintain diabetic diet restrictions by working with the health-care provider to manage blood glucose control.
4. Avoid fibrous foods such as raw fruits and vegetables and insoluble fibers. These may be associated with the development of a bezoar.
5. Chew food well. Pureed or ground foods may be better tolerated.
6. Drink fluids in-between meals and not at meals to avoid filling up the stomach.
7. Sit up while eating and at least 1–2 h after a meal to allow gravity to assist with gastric emptying.
8. Avoid dehydration by assuring an adequate fluid intake. Dehydration can occur if the fluid is limited.

Nutrition Support and GP

Some individuals with GP cannot tolerate a normal or even texture-modified intake and require an alternative method of nutrition [13]. Enteral nutrition is usually well tolerated as long as the feeding tube is placed through the pylorus and into the small intestine. A venting gastrostomy tube may also be needed to allow gastric secretions to empty [13]. This may require a specialized tube placement. Chapter 8 describes enteral nutrition for both children and adults. Occasionally, the GP is associated with further intestinal dysmotility and therefore, enteral nutrition is not tolerated and parenteral nutrition is required to maintain nutrition status (Chapter 9). Close monitoring and expert nutrition care is important for successful management of GP to avoid malnutrition and maintain health.

CELIAC DISEASE

Celiac disease is described as an immune system disorder characterized by changes in the GI lumen when gluten is ingested [17]. Gluten is the protein component of wheat, rye, and barley. When gluten is ingested, through food, and even lipstick, makeup, or other products, the villi in the small intestine may be damaged or destroyed due to an immune response triggered by gluten causing significant inflammation [17]. Because of this, foods other than gluten- containing foods may also be malabsorbed resulting in nutrient deficiencies and malnutrition.

It is estimated that one in 133 individuals has celiac disease (CD) in the United States or about 1% of the population [17,18]. This number does not include those with gluten-sensitive or nonceliac gluten sensitivity. Symptoms of CD include bloating, gas, diarrhea, constipation, stomach pain, weight loss, slow growth in children, anemia, bone and joint pain, and fatigue [17].

As many of these symptoms are also associated with other GI diseases including IBS (Chapter 5) and IBD (see Chapter 4), a diagnosis based on serum lab values for antigliadin antibodies (IgA anti-TTG) as well as intestinal biopsy is vital in making an accurate diagnosis [17–19]. Celiac disease diagnosis is confirmed with a biopsy of the small intestine using an upper endoscopy [17,20]. The biopsy is the "gold standard" for diagnosing celiac disease by observing the characteristic changes in the GI tract associated with the deleterious effects of gluten. Newer blood tests are available to evaluate the genetic predisposition of an individual for CD [21]. Those with CD have a genetic variant indicative of CD although this test alone may result in a false positive. An important caveat of the intestinal biopsy is the need for gluten intake prior to the test to cause the intestinal changes to be able to define a true diagnosis. Often, individuals will begin a gluten-free (GF) diet and see an improvement in symptoms. Their physician may want to confirm the diagnosis with the biopsy; however, if the intestinal lumen changes are not present due to the GF diet, this cannot be done. A 2-week period of gluten intake should be sufficient prior to a biopsy. Dermatitis herpetiformis may be present in up to 10% of people with CD. This skin rash triggers antibodies that cause these skin symptoms. Low serum levels of iron and folate may also be present with celiac disease [17].

The treatment for CD is to remove the irritants that cause the GI distress and damage. Therefore, a GF diet is the primary treatment. When a gluten-free diet is utilized, not only will the symptoms improve or disappear, but the GI lumen will heal and absorb nutrients normally.

Nutrition Intervention

- Avoid gluten-containing foods such as wheat, barley, and rye. Wheat is the predominant dietary component to manage. In addition, there are foods that do not appear to have gluten in them including modified food starch, some food preservatives, and stabilizers. Other names for wheat or wheat-containing grains are spelt, kamut, einkorn, emmer, triticale, durum, farina, enriched flour, wheat starch, self-rising flour, graham flour, bulgur, semolina, cake flour, pastry flour, or matzo. Wheat free does not mean GF. It still may contain rye or barley, malt, or malt flavorings (made from barley).
- Foods such as oats and oatmeal do not contain gluten but may be made in facilities where gluten-containing foods are made such that gluten becomes a contaminant, even in a very small amount. Pure, uncontaminated oat products should be used that are labeled as gluten free.
- Appliances, such as a toaster, should be designated for use only with GF products.
- Clean tools should be used for cooking, cutting, mixing, and serving GF foods. Separate containers of butter, peanut butter, and condiments should be used in households where there are non-GF users to avoid cross contamination through "double-dipping."
- Medications and nonfood products such as makeup, lipstick, vitamin and mineral supplements (especially "all natural"), as well as herbal supplements may contain gluten. These are often labeled as "contains wheat."
- Monitor key nutrients: iron, calcium, folate, B12, vitamin D, and fiber.

An excellent and comprehensive resource for understanding the gluten-free diet is *The Gluten-Free Diet: A Comprehensive Guide* by Shelley Case, RD (www.glutenfreediet.ca) as well as publications from the *Academy of Nutrition and Dietetics and Nutrition Care Manual* (www.eatright.org).

The best approach for managing the GF diet is to work with a registered dietitian nutritionist (RDN) as translating the limitations of the GF diet into good nutrition requires the expertise of the RDN. Chapter 13 provides suggestions on how to find an RDN.

REFERENCES

1. O'Keefe SJD, Buchman AL, Fishbein TM, Jeejeebhoy KN, Jeppesen PB, Shaffer J. Short bowel syndrome and intestinal failure: Consensus definitions and overview. *Clin Gastroenterol Hepatol.* 2006;4(1):6–10.
2. Abad-Sinden A, Sutphen J. Nutritional management of pediatric short bowel syndrome. *Prac Gastroenterol.* 2003;12:28–48.
3. Pironi L, Arends J, Baxter J et al. ESPEN endorsed recommendations. Definition and classification of intestinal failure in adults: Home artificial nutrition and chronic intestinal failure; Acute intestinal failure special interest groups of ESPEN. *Clin Nutr.* 2015;34(2):171–180.
4. Wall EA. An overview of short bowel syndrome management: Adherence, adaptation and practical recommendations. *J Acad Nutr Diet.* 2013;113:1200–1208.
5. Matarese LE. Short bowel syndrome. In: *Gastrointestinal and Liver Disease: Nutrition Desk Reference.* Mullin G, Matarese L, Palmer M (Eds.). Boca Raton, Florida: CRC Press; 2012:35–49.

6. van Ongen M, Mullin GE. Major components of the gastrointestinal system and their role in digestion. In: *Gastrointestinal and Liver Disease: Nutrition Desk Reference*. Mullin G, Matarese L, Palmer M (Eds.). Boca Raton, Florida: CRC Press; 2012:1–8.
7. Helander HF, Fändriks L. Surface area of the digestive tract—Revisited. *Scand J Gastroenterol*. 2014;49(6):681–689.
8. Nguyen PC, Kerner JA. Home parenteral nutrition support in pediatrics. In: *Handbook of Home Nutrition Support*. Ireton-Jones C and DeLegge M (Eds.). Sudbury, Massachusetts: Jones and Bartlett Publishers; 2007:223–252.
9. Venick RS, Calkins K. The impact of intravenous fish oil emulsions on pediatric intestinal failure-associated liver disease. *Curr Opin Organ Transplant*. 2011;16(3):306–311.
10. Jeejeebhoy K. The etiology and mechanism of intestinal failure. In: *Intestinal Failure and Rehabilitation: A Clinical Guide*. Matarese L, Steiger E, Seidner D (Eds.). Boca Raton, Florida: CRC Press; 2005:25–38.
11. Byrne T, Wilmore DW, Iyer K et al. Growth hormone, glutamine, and an optimal diet reduces parenteral nutrition with short bowel syndrome: A prospective, randomized, placebo controlled, double blind clinical trial. *Ann Surg*. 2005;242(5):655–661.
12. Mullin GE, Fischer AK. Gastrointestinal tests and procedures In: *The Health Professionals Guide to Gastrointestinal Nutrition*. Matarese L, Mullin G, Raymond J (Eds.). Chicago: Academy of Nutrition and Dietetics; 2012:9–19.
13. Camilleri M, Parkman HP, Shafi MA et al. American college of gastroenterology. Clinical guideline: Management of gastroparesis. *Am J Gastroenterol*. 2013;108(1):18–37.
14. Hasler WL. Gastroparesis: Current concepts and considerations. *Medscape J Med*. 2008;10(1):16.
15. Jones J. Gastroparesis. *Today's Dietitian*. 2014;16(7):16.
16. Bai Y, Xu MJ, Yang X et al. A systematic review on intrapyloric botulinum toxin injection for gastroparesis. *Digestion*. 2010;81(1):27–34.
17. Rampertab SD. Celiac disease. In: *The Health Professionals Guide to Gastrointestinal Nutrition*. Matarese L, Mullin G, Raymond J (Eds.). Chicago: Academy of Nutrition and Dietetics; 2012:108–128.
18. Case S, Adams PC. Celiac disease: Hidden and dangerous. *Can J Gastroenterol*. 2006; 20(9):571–573.
19. Fasano A, Catassi C. Celiac disease. *N Engl J Med*. 2012; 367(25):2419–2426.
20. Rubio-Tapia A, Hill ID, Kelly CP et al. American College of Gastroenterology clinical guidelines: Diagnosis and management of celiac disease. *Am J Gastroenterol*. 2013; 108:656–676.
21. Pietzak MM, Schofield TC, McGinniss MJ et al. Stratifying risk for celiac disease in a large at-risk United States population using HLS alleles. *Clin Gastroenterol and Hepatol*. 2009; 7(9):966–971.

4 GI Disease Nutrition Management

Inflammatory Bowel Disease

Maryann King, MPH, RDN, LD, CNSC, CSO

CONTENTS

INTRODUCTION

Inflammatory bowel disease is a term used to encompass two inflammatory bowel conditions, namely, Crohn's disease (CD) and ulcerative colitis (UC). Despite the fact that they are under the umbrella of "inflammatory bowel disease" or IBD, they are two very distinct and different diseases. The only entity that they have in common is that they are relapsing diseases of the bowel and both are affected by the environment, genetics, and the microbiome [1]. CD can cause a transmural inflammation, and affect any portion of the gastrointestinal tract, from the mouth to the anus [1]. The endoscopic appearances of CD and UC are also different. CD may present with skipped "cobblestone" mucosa, whereas UC presents as a superficial ulceration occurring only in the large intestine (colon). The most common sites of inflammation in CD are the terminal ileum, and the cecum. There are often many other manifestations of inflammation associated with CD, such as uveitis, oral ulcerations, joint pain, abscesses, fistulas, strictures, and systemic inflammation [1]. UC is typically a superficial ulceration and mucosal inflammation that is limited to the colon. UC is not associated with the nutritional deficits that can ensue with CD, although nutritional status may be compromised significantly due to the symptoms associated with UC. Approximately one-third of all patients with UC have an involvement limited to the rectum, where there may be edema, erythema, and friability [2]. The highest rates of UC are in the Scandinavian countries, Great Britain, and North America [2].

The underlying hypothesized etiologies for IBD have been felt to result from a complex interplay between susceptible genes, the environment, viruses, fungi, the host microbiome, and the immune system [3]. The exact cause of IBD is still unknown; however, new technologies have allowed researchers to quantify the different components of the microbiome [3]. The gastrointestinal tract is the most immunologic organ in the body. Some research implies that the mucosal immune system is associated with the pathogenesis of IBD; however, it is also felt that this inflammatory process can be fueled by genetics, environmental factors, intestinal microbial flora, and host immunity [3]. Other environmental factors that are considered to put one at an increased risk of developing IBD are smoking, diet, drugs, geography, social stress, and psychological stress [4]. Antibiotics, especially if given early in life, may increase the risks of developing IBD [5]. Although stress has been proposed to play a role in the pathogenesis of CD and UC, a Cochrane review shows no benefits of psychological interventions in IBD [6].

GENETICS OF IBD

Since the advances in genetic testing and analyzing technologies have allowed large genome-wide associations studies (GWAS), the number of IBD gene loci is currently up to 163 (110 are associated with CD and UC) (30 CD specific and 23 UC specific) [1,7]. The first gene was discovered in 2001 (NOD 2—nucleotide-binding oligomerization domain containing) [2]. This gene codes for a protein that is present in Gram negative and positive bacteria, and is involved in the regulation of T-cell responses [8]. Autophagy (controlled digestion of damaged organelles within a cell) has been shown to play an important role in the immune response and this has been shown through genetic analysis [9]. It is an important process for maintaining cellular homeostasis after infection [3]. Autophagy is also involved in resistance against infection and the removal of intracellular microbes [10]. Some of the genes associated with CD show defects in antibacterial autophagy [11]. The GWAS studies have also provided information between IBD and genes that encodes a subunit of receptors that are responsible for proinflammation (IL 23, Th17, and IL 12) [12]. Approximately 20%–25% of this patient population will inherit IBD [13]. The new information acquired from the exploration of gene–gene interactions, gene–pathway interactions, and gene–environment interactions will give more insight into the pathogenesis of IBD [14].

ROLE OF DIET IN IBD

Although diet is an integral part of a healthy gastrointestinal tract, there is no proven specific diet for IBD. Modifications to the diet are oftentimes recommended to decrease the symptoms; however, every person is different and the response may be different as well. Individual modifications are important to help one to maintain a "healthy and balanced" diet. A healthy and varied diet should be recommended for all patients with IBD during remission, which includes fruits, vegetables, meat, olive oil, fish, and fiber [15]. The only reason to restrict insoluble fiber is if one has intestinal stenosis, fistula(s), and/or strictures.

Patients often believe that IBD is caused by, or can be cured by diet; however, there is no clinical evidence that this is true. Many individuals receive information to follow a specific diet, which in fact; may not be beneficial, and may hinder one from eating a more balanced diet. The only reason to avoid any food would be if it worsens one's symptoms or causes an exacerbation, or pain. However, diet can influence the microbial diversity in the gastrointestinal tract. [16]. The microbiome has its own substrate preference and the type and quantity of fat and polysaccharides results in changes in the composition and function of the microbiota [16]. There is some research that suggests that the changes in diet (agriculture and animal husbandry) occurred too quickly for our human genome to adapt [17]. In recent years, there has been a question as to whether or not the lipid components of one's diet may be a trigger for IBD [15]. It has been observed that the Eskimos in Greenland, who are consumers of large amounts of n-3 polyunsaturated fatty acids, derived from fish oils, had a low prevalence of IBD [18,19]. It has been shown that n-6 PUFAs affect the arachidonic acid metabolism by increasing the production of leukotriene B4, with proinflammatory action [20]. There is still more research needed in this area, regarding dietary lipids and the effect on inflammatory processes [21].

A study was performed using twin pairs where one is a healthy twin and one with CD-demonstrated alterations in the way processed carbohydrates [17]. The enzyme pathways involved in complex carbohydrate metabolism, which results in short-chain fatty acids (SCFAs), were diminished in the twin with CD [17]. Pathways involved in mucin degradation were also decreased, which indicated that the ability to break down oligosaccharides is diminished in patients with CD [17]. One beneficial SCFA is butyrate. According to Wong et al., SCFAs are produced by fermentation of nondigestible carbohydrates via a subset of anaerobic bacteria in the human colon (primarily in the cecum and colon) [22]. Of all the SCFAs, butyrate is primarily considered to be the preferred fuel for colonocytes [22]. Butyrate enemas have shown some promise for patients with colitis [23]. Initial studies found that butyrate inhibits IL-12 production by stimulating monocytes, enhanced IL-10 production, and inhibited IL-2, which represents an anti-inflammatory profile for butyrate [24]. Work is being undertaken to determine if the IBD patient's microbiome predisposes them to butyrate deficiency [25]. In a small study of CD patients, oral butyrate did show a promise in inducing remission and improving the symptoms [26]. Butyrate has been shown to improve the intestinal defense mechanism by restoring mucosal integrity, stimulating MUC2 (mucin gene expression), in which its protein products are often altered in IBD, and modulating the expression of an antimicrobial peptide, cathelicidin (IL-37) [21,27]. Although butyrate seems to be beneficial in IBD, some studies found that nonabsorbed carbohydrates (prebiotics) such as inulin and fructooligosaccharides that enhance the proliferation of *Bifidobacterium* and *Lactobacillus* species and provide a substrate for SCFAs, may not benefit patients with IBD [28]. There are cases in a genetically susceptible host when certain carbohydrates that may seem beneficial to a "normal" gastrointestinal tract, can actually cause an immune response that causes chronic, relapsing intestinal inflammation [29]. The reinforced mucus layer helps to decrease mucosal permeability, making foreign substances impossible to pass through the defense barrier [30]. Butyrate is found in butter, whole grains, plants, and vegetables.

Mouse studies revealed that feeding mice with a high-fat and high-carbohydrate diet (Western diet) resulted in an increase in the number of *Firmicutes phylum* and a decrease in *Bacteroidetes phylum* [31,32]. With the increase in IBD throughout the world, the shift to a diet high in fat and sugar is being examined as a possible culprit in causing dysbiosis of the gut microbiome [33]. An example is a recent increase in the incidence of IBD in Asia, which has been attributed to more of a "Western" diet and lifestyle [34]. Many attempts have been made to use epidemiological data that reflect a link to dietary factors to the onset of CD, including a meta-analysis that suggested a positive association between a high intake of fat, polyunsaturated fatty acids, and omega-6 fatty acids, while a diet high in fruit and fiber intake seemed to be protective [35,36]. Children in Burkina Faso, Africa who were reared on a high-fiber, plant-based diet exhibited a vastly different gastrointestinal microbial community than children in Europe whose calories came from diets richer in sugar, fat, and protein [33]. There is a very low incidence of IBD in Africa, and a high incidence in Europe [37]. Although the cause and effect has not been proven, animal models have shown a causal role for diet-induced changes of gut microbes in the development of the disease [38].

Breast milk contains nutrients that protect against infection, including antimicrobial, anti-inflammatory, and immunomodulatory agents and there is a direct evidence that breast milk acts as a disease modifier in animal models that had colitis [39,40]. Studies that have been done in humans revealed that breast milk-fed infants develop markedly different patterns of gut colonization compared with formula-fed infants [41].

DIET MODIFICATIONS FOR IBD

As mentioned previously, there is no specific diet for IBD; however, there are diet modifications that can help to alleviate and prevent symptoms (Table 4.1). Diet recommendations should be individualized for each person based on their disease process, section of the bowel that is affected, and whether or not they have a fistula and/or stricture. It is imperative to strive for a well-balanced,

TABLE 4.1
Summary of Diet Therapy for IBD

Diet/Nutrition Therapy	Summary
Low residue	Decrease the amount of insoluble fiber, raw fruits and vegetables, nuts, seeds, popcorn, meat with gristle, watch shrimp, and lobster
Low fat	Avoid high-fat-processed foods and snacks, heavy cream (includes ice cream, whole milk, and bisque soups), fried, and fatty meats
FODMAP elimination	See Chapter 3
Low oxalate	>15 mg oxalate per 100 g (1/2 cup), specific fruits, vegetables, beer, nuts, and tea
Probiotics	VSL#3, *Saccharomyces boulardii*, and bifidobacteria may have a beneficial effect

Source: Nutrition411.com; Bibiloni R et al. *Am J Gastroenterol* 2005;100:1539–1546.

healthy diet. The following diet modifications have been recommended to help with symptoms; however, they should not be used on a continuous basis:

Low-residue diet: A low-residue diet helps to decrease the amount of insoluble fiber and waste that moves through the gastrointestinal tract. Many times, it is used if one has an exacerbation of diarrhea, or if one has a stricture (narrowing of the bowel). The diet includes the following*:

- Avoid any food made of seeds, nuts, or raw fruit
- Avoid whole grains/cereals
- Do not eat raw fruits and vegetables, and remove the skins before cooking
- Limit the amount of dairy to 2 cups per day, and use lactose-free milk or lactose enzymes if lactose intolerant
- Limit fat intake
- Avoid tough, fibrous meats with a gristle

Low-fat diet: Many patients may benefit temporarily from a low-fat diet. This is because they can have intraluminal bile salt deficiencies and have fat malabsorption because of either an inflamed ileum or removal of >100 cm of the terminal ileum. Bile acids are responsible for emulsification of fat. Unabsorbed fat acts on the mucosa of the colon, increasing motility, and decreasing water and electrolyte absorption in the colon, thus producing diarrhea (steatorrhea). Many patients do get relief of symptoms for a low-fat/low-residue diet.

Kidney stones are more prevalent in patients who have a colon and have had numerous surgical resections of their small intestine and therefore, restriction of oxalate intake may be necessary. There are numerous reasons on why this transpires. Volume depletion is the first reason due to the loss of water and salt in a diarrheal stool, which also leads to a decrease in urine output [42]. With increased malabsorption caused by an inflamed tissue or absence of the terminal ileum resulting in nonreabsorbed bile salts, the unabsorbed fat reaches the colon causing steatorrhea. Increased fat in the colon results in calcium binding with the fat rather than with oxalate for excretion in the stool. Oxalates can be reabsorbed through the colon and will bind with calcium in the kidneys to form calcium/oxalate stones.

ELIMINATION DIETS

Managing the type and amount of carbohydrates consumed by individuals with IBD may also improve the symptoms. An early elimination diet called the specific carbohydrate diet suggested removing complex carbohydrates (disaccharides) and polysaccharides (chain molecules) because

* Published with permission from nutrition411.com.

they are not easily digested and could possibly feed on harmful bacteria in the intestine [43]. The most-studied elimination diet is the FODMAPs elimination diet used for irritable bowel syndrome (see Chapter 3) but has also been evaluated for use in IBD. Foods high in short-chain poorly absorbed carbohydrates including fermentable, oligosaccharides, disaccharides, monosaccharides, and polyols (FODMAP) are replaced with lower FODMAP-containing foods or eliminated altogether for a period of time, usually 4–6 weeks. Then, higher FODMAP foods are returned to the diet based on tolerance. Symptoms were assessed in 52 patients with CD at 3–6 months after they initiated the FODMAPs elimination diet with 56% of the patients showing improvement in the symptoms experienced [44]. It has been hypothesized that the reason as to why this diet has reduced some symptoms in CD is because it reduces the osmotic load and bacterial fermentation associated with the restricted foods [45]. For a summary of the low FODMAPs diet (also called the FODMAPs elimination diet), see Chapter 3. The anti-inflammatory diet for IBD restricts certain carbohydrates, includes the ingestion of prebiotics and probiotics, and modifies fatty acid intake to decrease the inflammatory response [46]. The "diet" was based on a retrospective case series involving only 40 patients; therefore, further studies are needed to establish outcomes and recommend the application to IBD [46].

Probiotics

Probiotics are viable bacteria that can promote health benefits by influencing the composition of the microbiome [47]. These can be prescribed, bought over the counter, and found in food. Some foods that are high in probiotics are yogurt (especially Greek yogurt), sauerkraut, miso, soups (fermented soybeans), and tempeh.

For the general public, probiotics are considered to be safe; however, their use in people with CD has not been established [48]. According to Tamboli et al. (2003), patients who are immunosuppressed, have indwelling catheters with reports of bacteremia and fungemia that should not use probiotics [47]. It is also important to realize that the Food and Drug administration does not regulate probiotics; therefore, no one is overseeing quality control measures [49]. Probiotics differ in their composition, and affect IBD differently. There are numerous studies that have shown some promise as an adjunctive therapy for both CD and UC [50–52].

The most-compelling evidence for the use of probiotics for UC comes from randomized double-blind placebo-controlled trials of the probiotic called VSL#3 [53]. VSL#3 (a mixture of four species of lactobacilli, three species of bifidobacteria, and *Streptococcus thermophilus*) was given to 40 patients with pouchitis [53]. After 4 months, there were fewer relapses in the intervention group. Once the VSL#3 was stopped, patients relapsed [53]. Gionchetti et al. studied another group that was treated with VSL#3, which showed the incidence of pouchitis to be reduced, quality of life improved, and the beneficial effects were associated with colonization with probiotics [53]. In a randomized control study by Bibiloni et al., 32 patients with UC from three separate IBD referral centers orally ingested 3600-billion bacteria of VSL#3 daily in two divided doses for 6 weeks. The presence of bacteria was measured using a sigmoidoscopy with an endoscopic and histologic assessment of the mucosa at the site of the most-severe disease activity. The results of this study included remission in 53% of patients, response in 24% of patients, no response in 9% of patients, and worsening in 9% of patients [54]. The only adverse event was mild bloating [54]. According to Bibiloni et al., VSL#3 appears to be beneficial in the treatment of UC [54].

ENTERAL NUTRITION SUPPORT

Enteral nutrition (EN) is a very important treatment modality for children and adults, and is an alternative to immunomodulatory drugs [15]. It has an excellent safety record, helps to potentiate growth parameters in children [15], and has shown clear benefits in as little as 4–6 weeks [55]. Evidence has shown that patients who require long-term enteral nutrition support have done well with percutaneous gastrostomies and jejunostomies, despite the concern that they would lead to fistula formation [56]. Standard polymeric formulas are usually well tolerated and should be trialed before switching to an elemental or specific formula if not tolerated [57].

According to the European Society of Parenteral and Enteral Nutrition (ESPEN), children with an active CD should be considered for enteral nutritional support as their first-line therapy, especially since corticosteroid drugs have complications [57]. Corticosteroids (CS) (prednisone and hydrocortisone) are oftentimes considered during an acute exacerbation of UC and CD [57]. Studies that have been done on children with CD have shown that EN is an effective alternative to CS [58]. Adults with CD are typically not offered with EN as a primary alternative [59]. EN is only recommended in North America if a patient declines drug therapy, or as an adjunct therapy to nutrition [60]. These recommendations were based on a Cochrane systemic review of six randomized controlled trials that included 192 patients treated with EN and 160 patients treated with CS, concluding that CS was superior to EN in the induction of remission of the disease [61]. A polymeric formula with improved taste (orally) may improve treatment compliance, and allow for an improvement in the nutritional status [62]. EN has shown to have an anti-inflammatory effect in CD patients, with an evidence of improved intestinal permeability, and reduced inflammatory cytokine production [63].

PARENTERAL NUTRITION SUPPORT

Parenteral nutrition (PN) support is typically used for people with IBD who have lost a significant small intestinal function due to resection or disease such that they can no longer absorb adequate nutrients. PN may be used for the preoperative setting, high-output stomas or fistulas, and patients with intestinal failure [64]. PN does not offer any advantage over EN as far as disease control [64]. Patients should be allowed to continue to ingest oral foods (modified diet), despite being on PN [64]. PN can be used in patients who are severely malnourished, and unable to tolerate oral intake prior to surgery. This has been shown to improve postoperative outcomes in malnourished patients when the oral or enteral route cannot be used [63].

MALNUTRITION AND MICRONUTRIENT DEFICIENCIES IN IBD

Malnutrition is much more common in CD than in UC, mainly because of malabsorption, and the fact that most of our digestion takes place in the small intestine. The severity of the malnutrition is based on the specific segment(s) of the bowel that are involved, anorexia, fistula formation, hypertrophy of villi, blind loops, bacterial overgrowth, bile salt malabsorption, duration of the disease, severity of the disease, medications, and protein-losing enteropathy [15]. Approximately 25%–85% of IBD patients suffer from nutritional deficiencies [65]. Weight loss and nutrient deficits can also be caused by underlying inflammatory mediators involved in the physiopathology of IBD such as tumor necrosis factor (TNF-alpha), interleukin 1, and 6, which can increase catabolism and lead to anorexia [66]. Many patients will decrease their intake because they have pain. Also, the typical site for inflammation in CD is the ileum, which participates in the enterohepatic circulation (circulation of bile acids back to the liver). Therefore, the distal ileum is important for fat metabolism, fat-soluble vitamin absorption [15], and vitamin B12 synthesis [35]. Removal of greater than 100 cm of the terminal ileum can result in vitamin B12 deficiency, fat-soluble vitamin deficiency, and lipid malabsorption [15]. Iron, vitamin B12, and folic acid deficiencies should be routinely monitored and are the main cause of anemia in these patients [15]. Iron deficiency anemia is the most common mineral deficiency in IBD, with prevalence rates ranging from 36% to 88% [67]. Decreased red blood folate levels have been recorded in approximately 28% of patients with an active disease [68].

Patients with IBD have shown an increase in bone loss, which can lead to osteopenia and osteoporosis [69,70]. Vitamin D is essential for calcium and hormonal homeostasis, and is important for bone mineralization [71]. There is an increased prevalence of hypovitaminosis D in adult patients with IBD of up to 68% in one study [72,73]. It is important to monitor calcium, vitamin D, vitamin K, folate, vitamin B6, vitamin B12, iron, and zinc levels when patients are having acute exacerbations, fistula drainage, and steatorrhea [72]. Little is known regarding other micronutrient deficiencies secondary to a lack of studies in this area [65]. Maintaining good nutrition plays an essential role in the treatment of IBD in children and adults [72].

NUTRITION ASSESSMENT

Nutrition assessment should encompass a multidimensional approach that includes measurements of body composition, dietary intake, history of weight loss, lab values, measurement of vitamins and trace elements, social history, and physical assessment [74].

When assessing a patient, it is important to obtain a detailed diet history and complete a nutrition-focused physical assessment. The subjective global assessment is a good way to classify patients as generally well nourished, moderately malnourished, or severely malnourished based on the above parameters along with gastrointestinal symptoms, CD activity, functional capacity, muscle mass, subcutaneous fat, edema, and ascites [75].

Disease severity is usually associated with exudative protein losses [76]. If a patient has an increased fistula output, they may require an increased protein intake up to 1.5–2.0 g/kg: however, there are no randomized studies assessing protein needs in this patient population. Calorie needs range from 25–35 kcal/kg; however, caloric requirements should be individualized based on nutrition goals. Longitudinal studies are not available; however, a cross-sectional study showed that patients with an active disease did have an increase in the resting energy expenditure (REE), along with the disease location [77]. Medications may affect the nutritional status. The most commonly used categories of medications for IBD are aminosalicylates, corticosteroids, immunomodulators, antibiotics, and biological therapies (Table 4.2). An excellent resource for clinicians and patients is found at www.ccfa.org.

Hydration status should be monitored if patients have diarrhea or a significant ostomy output. The goal is to maintain urine output >1200 mL, and monitor for rapid weight loss [78]. Some patients may benefit from oral rehydration therapy (ORT). Monitor patients for any electrolyte anomalies.

Dual-energy x-ray absorptiometry (DXA) should be done to rule out osteopenia and/or osteoporosis. Osteoporosis is a common extraintestinal complication of IBD [79]. The prevalence of osteopenia is between 40% and 50%, and the prevalence of osteoporosis is between 5% and 36% for patients with IBD [80]. All the disease processes, vitamin D/calcium deficiencies, and corticosteroid drugs play a role in causing a metabolic bone disease in this patient population.

MICROBIOME/ENVIRONMENT

There has been an increased interest in the role of the microbiome in determining the underlying etiologies of IBD as well as other diseases that affect the GI tract [5]. The microbiome assists in the optimal breakdown of foods, uptake of nutrients (digestion and metabolism), and contributes to the development and maintenance of the intestinal epithelial barrier, and the development of the immune system [81]. The gut flora in patients with IBD has shown species diversity to be reduced and markedly distinct [82].

In a normal gut physiology, the surface of the intestine is protected by a layer of mucus that is generated by goblet cells in the epithelium. This layer is thick, firmly adherent, rich in antimicrobials, and some bacteria [83]. Some patients with CD have been found to have depletion in goblet cells and an impaired mucus layer, which allows bacteria to adhere directly to epithelial cells, and may contribute to disease progression [84]. Defects in the integrity of the epithelium may also contribute to the pathogenesis of IBD by allowing the free passage of organisms across the epithelial layer where they can cause an immune response [84].

TABLE 4.2
Medications Use in Inflammatory Bowel Disease

Drug	Side Effects May Include	Potential Metabolic and/or Nutrition Abnormalities
Sulfasalazine (oral)	Achy joints, fever, headache, sensitivity to light, skin rashes, itching	↑ Liver function tests (LFT), ↓ folic acid, neutropenia, hemolysis, fever
5 Aminosalicylic acid (ASA) oral, also available as an enema for UC (Lialda®)	Diarrhea, nausea, vomiting, dyspepsia, hair loss	Caution with hepatic or renal insufficiency, may increase lipase and amylase
Mesalamine suppositories	Headache, flatulence, diarrhea, abdominal pain	
Prednisone (oral)	Edema, electrolyte disturbance, ↑ appetite, hypertension, dyspepsia, hyperglycemia	↓ Sodium, may need ↑ vitamin K, A, calcium, vitamin D, and protein
Budesonide (oral)	Glossitis, tongue edema, dyspepsia, nausea, GI fistula, enteritis, hemorrhoids	Calcium/vitamin D supplement recommended
6 Mercaptopurine (6 MP, purinethol), imuran	Headache, nausea, vomiting, diarrhea, malaise, canker sores, hepatitis, bone marrow suppression, pancreatitis	↓ White blood cells (WBC), ↓ platelets, macrocytic anemia, ↑ mean corpuscular volume (MCV), ↑ LFTs, ↑ amylase, ↓ uric acid, ↓ albumin
Methotrexate (oral)	Stomatitis, gingivitis, nausea, vomiting, diarrhea, altered taste	↑ Homocysteine, ↑ uric acid, ↑ LFTs, ↑ blood urea nitrogen (BUN), ↓ WBC, ↓ platelets, anemia
Infliximab (Remicade®) (infusion)	Mouth ulcers, dyspepsia, vomiting, abdominal pain	Aplastic anemia, caution with congestive heart failure
Adalimumab (Humira®) (infusion)	Nausea, abdominal pain	↑ Cholesterol, ↑ alkaline phosphatase
Vedolizumab (Entyvio®) (infusion)	Cold, headache, joint pain, nausea, fever, nose and throat infection, bronchitis, flu	Need to watch LFTs (limited information)
Golimumab (Simponi®) (infusion)—for severe UC	Headache, fever, chills, difficulty breathing, low blood pressure, stomach pain, back pain, nausea, upper respiratory infection	Watch LFTs (limited information)
Natalizumab (Tysabri®)	Multifocal leukoencephalopathy, meningitis, UTI, lung infections, nausea, trouble breathing	↑ LFTs, black box warnings
Antibiotics: (oral or IV) Metronidazole (Flagyl®), Ciprofloxacin (Cipro®), Rifaximin (Xifaxan®) (oral only)	Anorexia, dry mouth, candidiasis, stomatitis, metallic taste, nausea, vomiting, epigastric distress, diarrhea, constipation	↓ WBC, ↓ platelets, ↓ false decrease in AST, ↓ ALT ↓ LDH, ↓ triglycerides

Source: Adapted and used with permission from www.ccfa.org; Pronsky ZM, Elbe D, Ayoob K, *Food Medication Interactions*, 18th Ed. Birchrunville, PA: WAZA Inc, 2015.

The intestinal microbiota plays a role in immune composition, and is most likely the most important environmental factor in IBD because of the physiological response to inflammation [85]. The microbiota is responsible for the development and differentiation of the local and systemic immune and nonimmune components [85]. The normal gut microbiome is composed of approximately 100-trillion diverse microbes, mostly bacteria, which encompass over 1100 prevalent species with at least 160 species in each individual [86]. Greater than 90% belong to two different bacteria (Bacteroidetes—Gram-negative bacteria) and (Firmicutes—Gram-positive bacteria) with the remainder belonging to rarer bacterial groups such as *Proteobacteria* (*Escherichia* and *Helicobacter*) and Actinobacteria, as well as viruses, protists (large and diverse eukaryotic microorganisms), and fungi [87]. The type of bacteria can be influenced by one's diet. For example, Bacteroides enterotype has been associated with a "western" protein- rich diet, which may be a risk factor in the development of IBD [33]. According to Eckburg et al., only approximately 20%–30% of the gut microbiome can be cultured, and the association between the changes in the microbiome and IBD has been established [88]. Many studies done in IBD patients using both inflamed and noninflamed sections, revealed a reduced biodiversity in a fecal microbiome compared to healthy controls [89]. In healthy intestines, Firmicutes and Bacteroidetes phyla predominate and contribute to the production of epithelial metabolic substrates [1]. However, in CD, the microbiota is characterized by a relative lack of Firmicutes and Bacteroidetes, and an overrepresentation of enterobacteria, while in UC, there is a reduction of *Clostridium* and an increase in *Escherichia coli* (*E. coli*) [90].

A healthy colon has a continuous mucus coating consisting of two layers of a substructure, and the outer layer is good for bacterial growth [1]. In IBD, especially in CD, there is a consistent increase in mucosa-associated *E. coli* and a reduction in Firmicutes [91,92]. There is a very strong evidence for an increase in mucosa-associated *E. coli* in both the ileum and the colon, and the fact that they are also present in the granulomas in CD implies a primary pathogenic role [93]. Also, patients with CD were found to have an alteration in bacterial carbohydrate metabolism, and bacterial–host interactions in their ileum [94]. Understanding the functional impact and physiological changes in the gut that cause this dysbiosis, will allow for help in the treatment of this disease.

The functional innate immunity physiological response is mediated by a large variety of different types of cells including epithelial cells, neutrophils, dendritic cells, monocytes, macrophages, and natural killer cells [95]. Interleukins are a group of naturally occurring proteins that mediate communication between cells. They also play a role in regulating cell growth, differentiation, and motility. Interleukins are an important aspect of stimulating an immune response such as inflammation. There are many different interleukins (IL), which contribute to the immune response in different ways, and are found in different parts of the gastrointestinal tract. Interleukins can be identified by their number; some are anti-inflammatory and some are proinflammatory. For example, IL1, IL6, IL8, IL12, IL17, IL23, and tumor necrosis factor (TNF) are the important mediators of inflammation, while IL4, IL10, IL11, and transforming growth factor (TGF) are protective and have anti-inflammatory properties [96]. Animal model studies have shown that IL 23 and IL 17 are very important in the pathogenesis of CD; antibodies that can block these proteins are now being subjected to drug development programs. Both CD and UC patients can have a defect or mutation in the IL23 receptor, and in the future can be tested for a defect in the IL23 pathway. If one has a defect in IL23 pathway, a specific drug can be selected as the treatment choice over other biological or immunosuppressive therapies (see ccfa.org). Other research is focusing on IL10, which is known for its anti-inflammatory properties. The role of IL10 is important for immune homeostasis in the gut, and mice-deficient IL10 develop chronic enterocolitis, which can be prevented by giving IL10 [97]. Millions of dollars are being spent on research to develop tests that use the composition of gut bacteria to diagnose inflammatory and liver diseases [98]. These therapies may prove to be an important adjunct or therapy for these diseases in the future.

In summary, nutrition care plays a pivotal role for this patient population. New and innovative therapies as well as diet modifications and microbiome discoveries continue to be explored.

REFERENCES

1. Yi-Zhen Zhang, Yong–Yu Li. Inflammatory bowel disease: Pathogenesis. *World J Gastroenterol* 2014;20(1):91–99.
2. www.hopkinsmedicine.org

3. Wallace KL, Zheng Li, Kanazawa, Y et al. Immunopathology of inflammatory bowel disease. *World J Gastroenterol* 2014;20(1):6–21.
4. Loftus EV. Clinical epidemiology of inflammatory bowel disease: Incidence, prevalence and environmental influences. *Gastroenterology* 2004;126:1504–1517.
5. Shaw S, Bianchard J, Berstein C. Association between the use of antibiotics and new diagnoses of Crohn's Disease and ulcerative colitis. *Am J Gastroenterol* 2011;106:2133–2142.
6. Timmer A, Preiss JC, Motschal E et al. Psychological interventions for treatment of inflammatory bowel disease. A retrospective case matched observational study. *Cochrane Database Syst Rev.* 2011;18:1232–1239.
7. Jostins L, Ripke S, Weersma R et al. Host-microbe interactions have shaped the genetic architecture of inflammatory bowel disease. *Nature* 2012;491:119–124.
8. Inohara N, Ogura Y, Fontalba A et al. Host recognition of bacterial muramyl dipeptide mediated through NOD 2. Implications for Crohn's disease. *J Biol Chem* 2003;278:5509–5512.
9. Rioux J, Xavier R, Taylor K et al. Genome-wide association study identifies new susceptibility loci for Crohn's disease and implicates autophagy in disease pathogenesis. *Nat Genet* 2007;39:596–604.
10. Khor B, Gardet A, Xavier R. Genetics and pathogenesis of inflammatory bowel disease. *Nature* 2011;474:307–317.
11. Kuballa P, Huett A, Rioux JD et al. Impaired autophagy of an intracellular pathogen induced by a Crohn's disease associated ATG 16 L1 variant. *PLos One* 2008;3:e3391.
12. Brand S. Crohn's disease: TH1,TH17 or both? The change of a paradigm: New immunological and genetic insights implicated Th17 cells in the pathogenesis of Crohn's disease. *Gut* 2009;58:1152–1167.
13. Zuk O, Hechter E, Sunyaev S, Lander E. The mystery of missing heritability: Genetic interactions create phantom heritability. *Proc Natl Acad Sci USA* 2012;109:1193–1198.
14. Yi-Zen Zhang, Yong-Yu Li, Inflammatory bowel disease: Pathogenesis. *World J Gastroenterol* 2014;20(1):91–99.
15. Lucendo A, DeRezende C. Importance of nutrition in inflammatory bowel disease. *World J Gastroenterol* 2009;15(17):2081–2088.
16. Honda K, Littman D. The microbiome in infectious disease and inflammation. *Annu Rev Immunol* 2012;30:759–795.
17. Eaton SB, Konner M, Shostak M. Stone agers in the fast lane: Chronic degenerative diseases in evolutionary perspectives. *Am J Med* 1988;84:739–749.
18. Kromann N, Green A. Epidemiological studies in the Upernavik district, Greenland. Incidence of some chronic diseases 1950–1974. *Acta Med Scan* 1980;208:401–406.
19. Bang HO, Dyerberg J, Sinclair HM. The composition of the Eskimo food in Northwestern Greenland. *Am J Clin Nutr* 1980;33:2657–2661.
20. Jeffrey NM, Newsholme EA, Calder PC. Level of polyunsaturated fatty acids and the n-6 to n-3 polyunsaturated fatty acid ratio in the rat diet alter serum lipid levels and lymphocyte functions. *Prostaglandins Leukot Essent Fatty Acids* 1997;57:149–160.
21. Willemsen LEM, Kostsier SJ, Van Deventer JH et al. Short chain fatty acids stimulate epithelial mucin 2 expression through differential effects on prostaglandin E1 and E2 production by intestinal myofibroblasts. *Gut* 2003;52:1442–1447.
22. Wong JM, de Souza R, Dendall CW et al. Colonic health: Fermentation and short chain fatty acids. *J Clin Gastroenterology* 2006;40(3):235–243.
23. Scheppach W, Sommer H, Kirchner T et al. Effect of butyrate enemas on the colonic mucosa in distal ulcerative colitis. *Gastroenterology* 1992;103(1):51–56.
24. Saemann MD, Bohmig GA, Osterreicher CH et al. Anti-inflammatory effects of sodium butyrate on human monocytes potent inhibition of IL-12 and up regulation of IL-10 production. *FASEBJ: Off Publ Fed AM Soc Exp Biol* 2000;14(15):2380–2382.
25. Frank DN, St. Amand AL, Feldman RA et al. Molecular-phylogenetic characterization of microbial community imbalances in human inflammatory bowel disease. *Proc Natl Acad Sci USA* 2007;104(34):13780–13785.
26. Di Sabatino A, Morera R, Ciccocioppo R et al. Oral butyrate for mildly to moderately active Crohn's disease. *Aliment Pharmacol Ther* 2005;22(9):789–794.
27. Moehle C, Ackerman N, Langmann T et al. Aberrant intestinal expression and allelic variants of mucin genes associated with inflammatory bowel disease. *Journal of Molecular Medicine.* 2006;84(12):1055–1066.
28. Erickson AR, Cantarel BL, Lamendella R et al. Integrated metagenomics/metaproteomics reveals human host-microbiota signatures of Crohn's disease. *PLos ONE* 2012;7:e 49138.

29. Leone V, Chang E, Devkoa S. Diet, microbes, and host genetics: The perfect storm in inflammatory bowel disease. *J Gastroenterol* 2013;48:315–321.
30. Schauber J, Svanholm C, Termen S et al. Expression of the cathelicidin IL-37 is modulated by short chain fatty acids in colonocytes: Relevance of signaling pathways. *Gut* 2003;52:735–741.
31. Turnbaugh PJ, Backhed F, Fulton L et al. Diet induced obesity is linked to marked but reversible alterations in the mouse distal gut microbiome. *Cell Host Microbe* 2008;3:213–223.
32. Zhang C, Zhang M, Wang S et al. Interactions between gut microbiota, host genetics and diet relevant to development of metabolic syndrome in mice. *ISME* 2010;4:232–241.
33. DeFilippo C, Cavalieri D, DiPaola M et al. Impact of diet in shaping gut microbiota revealed by a comparative study in children from Europe and rural Africa. *Proc Natl Acad Sci USA* 2010;107:14691–14696.
34. NG SC, Tang W, Ching JY et al. Incidence and phenotype of inflammatory bowel disease based on results from the Asia-Pacific Crohn's and colitis epidemiology study. *Gastroenterology* 2013;145(1):158–165 e2.
35. Donnellan C, Yann L, Lal S. Nutritional management of Crohn's disease. *Ther Adv Gastroenterol* 2013;6(3):231–242.
36. Hou JK, Abraham B, El-Serag H et al. Dietary intake and risk of developing inflammatory bowel disease: A systematic review of the literature. *Am J Gastrolenterol* 2011;106:563–573.
37. Lakatos PC. Changes in the epidemiology of inflammatory bowel disease. *World J Gastroenterol* 2006:12(38):6102–6108.
38. Leone V, Cham C, Chang E. Diet, gut microbes, and genetics in immune function: Can we leverage our current knowledge to achieve better outcomes in inflammatory bowel disease. *Current Opinion in Immunology* 2014;31:16–23.
39. Rodriguez-Palmero, Koletzko B, Kunz C et al. Nutritional and biochemical properties of human milk: II. Lipids, micronutrients, and bioactive factors. *Clin Perinatol* 1999;26:335–359.
40. Madsen KI, Fedork RN, Tavernini MM, Doyle JS. Normal breast milk limits the development of colitis in IL 10 deficient mice. *Inflamm Bowel Dis* 2002;8:390–398.
41. Orrhage K, Nord CE. Factors controlling the bacterial colonization of the intestine in breastfed infants. *Acia Paediatr Suppl* 1999;88:47–57.
42. Worcester, EM. Stones from bowel disease. *Endocrinol Metab Clin North AM* 2002;31(4):979–999.
43. Suskind DL, Wahbeh G, Gregory N et al. Nutritional therapy in pediatric Crohn's disease: The specific carbohydrate diet. *J Pediatr Gastroenterol Nutr* 2014;58(1):87–91.
44. Geary R, Irving P, Nathan D et al. Reduction of dietary poorly absorbed short chain carbohydrates (FODMAPs) improves abdominal symptoms in patients with inflammatory bowel disease a pilot study. *J Crohns Colitis* 2009;3:8–14.
45. Gibson P, Shepherd S. Evidence based dietary management of functional gastrointestinal symptoms: The FODMAP approach. *J Gastroenterol Hepatol* 2011;25:252–258.
46. Olendzki B, Silverstein T, Persuitte G et al. An anti-inflammatory diet as treatment for inflammatory bowel disease: A case series report running head: Diet for inflammatory bowel disease. *Nutrition Journal* 2014;13:5.
47. Tamboli CP, Caucheteux C, Cortor A. Probiotics in inflammatory bowel disease: A critical review. *Best Pract Res Clin Gastroenterol* 2003;17:805–820.
48. Cary V, Boullata J. What is the evidence for the use of probiotics in the treatment of inflammatory bowel disease? *J Nurs* 2010;19:904–916.
49. Michail S, Sylvester F, Fuchs G, Issenman R. Clinical efficacy of probiotics: Review of the evidence with focus on children. *J Pediatr Gastroenterol Nutr* 2006;43:550–557.
50. Kato K, Mizuno S, Umesaki Y et al. Randomized placebo-controlled trial assessing the effect of bifidobacteria-fermented milk on active ulcerative colitis. *Aliment Pharmacol Ther* 2004;20:1133–1141.
51. Druis W, Fric P, Lucas M et al. Maintaining remission of ulcerative colitis with the probiotic *Eschericia coli* Nissle 1917 is as effective as with standard mesalazine. *Gut* 2004;53:1617–1623.
52. Guslandi M, Mezzi G, Sorghi M et al. *Saccharomyces boulardii* in maintenance treatment of Crohn's disease. *Dig Dis Sci* 2000;45:1462–1464.
53. Gionchetti P, Rizzello F, Helwig U. Prophylaxis of pouchitis onset with probiotic therapy; a double blind, placebo-controlled trial. *Gastroenterol* 2003;124:1202–1209.
54. Bibiloni R, Fedorak RN, Tannock GW et al. VSL#3 probiotic mixture induces remission in patients with active ulcerative colitis. *Am J Gastroenterol* 2005;100:1539–1546.
55. Belli DC, Seidman E, Boutillier L et al. Chronic intermittent elemental diet improves growth failure in children with Crohn's disease. *Gastroenterol* 1988;94:603–610.
56. Anstee QM, Forbes A. The safe use of percutaneous gastrostomy for enteral nutrition in patients with Crohn's disease. *Eur J Gastroenterol Hepatol* 2000;12:1089–1093.

57. Forbes A, Goldesgeme E, Paulon E. Nutrition in inflammatory bowel disease. *JPEN* 2011;35(5):571–580.
58. Heuschkel RB. Enteral nutrition in children with Crohn's disease. *J Pediatr Gastroenterol Nutr* 2000;31:575.
59. Dignass A. Van Assche, Lindsay JO et al. The second European evidence based consensus on the diagnosis and management of Crohn's disease: Current management. *J Crohn's Colitis* 2010;4:28–62.
60. Lichtenstein GR, Hanauer SB, Sandborn WJ et al. Management of Crohn's disease in adults. *Am J Gastroenterol* 2009;104:465–483.
61. Zachos M, Tondeur M, Griffiths AM. Enteral nutritional therapy for induction of remission in Crohn's disease. *Cochrane Database Syst Rev* 2007;(1):(CD 0000541).
62. Wall C, Day A, Gearry R. Use of exclusive enteral nutrition in adults with Crohn's disease: A review. *World J Gastroenterol* 2013;19(42):7652–7660.
63. Van Gossum A, Cabre E, Hebuterne X et al. ESPEN guidelines on parenteral nutrition: Gastroenterology. *Clin Nutr* 2009;28(4):415–427.
64. Donnellan C, Yann L, Lai. Nutritional management of Crohn's disease. *Therap Adv Gastroenterol* 2013;(3):231–242.
65. Gassull MA, Cabre E. Nutrition in inflammatory bowel disease. *Curr Opin Clin Nutr Metab Care* 2001;4:561–569.
66. Cabre' E, Gassull MA. Nutrition in inflammatory bowel disease: Impact on disease and therapy. *Curr Opin Gastroenterol* 2001;17:342–349.
67. Gisbert J, Bermejo F, Pajares R et al. Oral and intravenous iron treatment in inflammatory bowel disease: Hematological response and quality of life improvement. *Inflamm Bowel Dis* 2009;15:1485–1491.
68. Elsborg L, Larsen L. Folate deficiency in chronic inflammatory bowel disease. *Scand J Gastroenterol* 1979;14:1019–1024.
69. Bjarnason I, Macpherson A, Mackintosh C et al. Reduced bone density in patients with inflammatory bowel disease. *Gut* 1997;40:228–233.
70. Jahnsen J, Falch JA, Mowinckel P et al. Bone mineral density in patients with inflammatory bowel disease: A population based prospective two-year follow up study. *Scan J Gastroenterol* 2004;39:145–153.
71. Pappa HM, Grand RJ, Gordon CM. Report on the vitamin D status of adult and pediatric patients with inflammatory bowel disease and its significance for bone health and disease. *Inflamm Bowel Dis* 2006;12:1162–1174.
72. Goh J, O'Morain CA. Review article: Nutrition and adult inflammatory bowel disease. *Aliment Pharmacol Ther* 2003;17:307–320.
73. Vogelsand H, Scofi R, Tinger W et al. 25 hydroxyvitamin D absorption in patients with Crohn's disease and pancreatic insufficiency. *Wien Klin Wochensch* 1997;109:678–682.
74. Mijac D, Jankovic G, Krstic M. Nutritional status in patients with active inflammatory bowel disease: Prevalence of malnutrition and methods for routine nutritional assessment. *Eur J Int Med* 2010;21:315–319.
75. Detsky AS, McLaughlin JR, Baker JP et al. What is subjective global assessment of nutritional status? *JPEN* 1987;11:8–13.
76. Cram-Bohbouth G, Pena AS, Biermond J. Are activity indexes helpful in assessing active intestinal inflammation in Crohn's disease? *Gut* 1989;30:1236–1241.
77. Gong J, Zuo L, Guo Z et al. Impact of disease activity on resting energy expenditure and body composition in adult Crohn's disease: A prospective longitudinal assessment. *J Parenter Enteral Nutr*, 2015;39(6):713–718.
78. Parrish CR. The clinician's guide to short bowel syndrome. *Pract Gastro-Enterol* 2005;XXIX:76–80.
79. Krok K, Lichtenstein G. Nutrition in Crohn's disease. *Curr Opin Gastroenterol* 2003;19(2):148–153.
80. Bernstein CN. Risk factors and prevalence of bone disease in IBD. In: Williams CN, Bursey DG et al. (Eds.) *Trends in IBD Therapy*. The Netherlands: Kluner Academic Publishers, 1999:147–162.
81. Honda K, Littman D. The microbiome in infectious disease and inflammation. *Annu Rev Immunol* 2010;30:759–795.
82. Sokol H, Lay C, Seksik P et al. Analysis of bacterial communities of IBD patients: What has it revealed? *Inflamm Bowel Dis* 2008;14:858–867.
83. Van der Sluis M, De Koning BA, De Bruijn AC et al. Muc 2 deficient mice spontaneously develop colitis, indicating that MUC2 is critical for colonic protection. *Gastroenterol* 2006;131:117–129.
84. Wallace K, Zheng Li-Bo, Shih D. Immunopathology of inflammatory bowel disease. *World J Gastroenterol* 2014;20(1):6–21.
85. Round JL, Mazmanian SK. The gut microbiota shapes intestinal immune responses during health and disease. *Nat Rev Immunol* 2009;9:313–323.

86. Qin J, Raes J, Arumugam M et al. A human gut microbial gene catalogue establishd by metagenomic sequencing. *Nature* 2010;464:174–180.
87. Peterson DA, Frank DN, Pace NR, Gordon JI. Metagenomic approaches for defining the pathogenesis of inflammatory bowel diseases. *Cell Host Microbe* 2008;3:417–427.
88. Eckburg PB, Bik EM, Berstein CN et al. Diversity of the human intestinal microbial flora. *Science* 2005;308:1635–1638.
89. Joossens M, Huys G, Cnockaert M et al. Dysbiosis of the fecal microbiota in patients with Crohn's disease and their unaffected relatives. *Gut* 2011;60:631–637.
90. Marinez C, Antolin M, Santos J et al. Unstable composition of the fecal microbiota in ulcerative colitis during clinical remission. *Am J Gastroenterol* 2008;103:643–648.
91. Ott SJ, Musfeldt M, Wenderoth DF et al. Reduction in diversity of the colonic mucosa associated bacterial microflora in paitents with active inflammatory bowel disease. *Gut* 2004;53:685–693.
92. Johansson ME, Phillipson M, Petersson J. The inner of the two Muc2 mucin-dependent mucus layers in the colin is devoid of bacteria. *Proc Natl Acad SCi USA* 2008;105:15064–15069.
93. Ryan P, Kelly RG, Lee G et al. Bacterial DNA wthin granulomas of patients with Crohn's disease-detection by laser capture microdissection and PCR. *Am J Gastroenterol* 2004;99:1539–1543.
94. Erickson AR, Cantarel BL, Lamendella R et al. Integrated metagenomics/metaproteomics reveals human host-microbiota signatures of Crohn's Disease. *PLosOne* 2012;7:e49138.
95. Medzhitov R, Janeway C. Innate immunity. *N Eng J Med* 2000;343:338–344.
96. Rogler G, Tilo A. Cytokines in inflammatory bowel disease. *World J Surg* 1998;22:382–389.
97. Kuhn R, Lohler J, Rennick D et al. Interleukin 10 deficient mice during chronic enterocolitis. *Cell* 1993;75:263.
98. Reardon S, Microbiome therapy gains market traction. *Nature* 2014;509:269.
99. Pronsky ZM, Elbe D, Ayoob K. *Food Medication Interactions*, 18th Ed. Birchrunville, PA: WAZA Inc, 2015.

5 GI Disease Nutrition Management

Irritable Bowel Syndrome

Carol Ireton-Jones, PhD, RDN, LD, CNSC, FAND, FASPEN and Eileen Heffernan-Swingle, MS, RDN

CONTENTS

Irritable bowel syndrome (IBS) is a disorder that involves abdominal pain and cramping, as well as changes in bowel movements. IBS is a functional bowel disorder with a prevalence of 10%–15% in Europe and North America, 15.9% in China, and 33% in Nigeria [1]. There is a greater prevalence in women. A diagnosis of IBS is based on Rome III criteria that includes abdominal pain or discomfort as well as altered bowel patterns [2]. There are three IBS subtypes that include IBS-C (constipation), IBS-D (diarrhea), and IBS-M (mixed constipation and diarrhea) [2,3]. Typically, the diagnosis is made after other diagnoses such as celiac disease and inflammatory bowel disease that have been ruled out but pain and symptoms continue [4,5].

IBS presentation of symptoms and their severity greatly varies from patient to patient. The symptoms include constipation, diarrhea, abdominal pain, bloating, gas, urgency, heartburn, and acid reflux, often without a known abnormal pathology [6,7]. Patients also report that overtime, symptoms can change and cross subgroups such as initially being IBS-C and constipation predominant to IBS-M that would also include diarrhea [4]. Bloating, defined as the sensation of abdominal fullness and distention, resulting in an increase in abdominal girth, has been reported by more than 80% of patients with IBS; however, it is not reported by all [8]. Symptoms also differ by gender with females reporting abdominal pain and constipation more often than males who report diarrhea [9]. In the United States, 5.9 million prescriptions annually are written for the treatment of IBS symptoms, with direct and indirect costs exceeding 20 billion dollars, including missed work and increased physician visits. [5,7]. Therefore, treatment requires an individualized approach.

PATHOPHYSIOLOGY OF IRRITABLE BOWEL SYNDROME

It is thought that several separate gastrointestinal disorders may be universally called IBS, which accounts for the differences observed in symptoms, etiology, and pathophysiology [5,10]. In the past, physicians treating IBS focused on abnormalities in GI motility, visceral sensation, brain–gut interactions, and psychosocial factors; however, none of these modalities accounted for symptoms in all IBS patients [11]. Additional research has shown that an altered gut immune activation, increased levels of intestinal permeability, and the intestinal and colonic microenvironment differ in patients with IBS compared to controls that may be a consideration in the treatment provided [5,10,12,13].

MANAGEMENT OF IRRITABLE BOWEL SYNDROME

Management of IBS initially may be to utilize over-the-counter medications to resolve diarrhea or constipation, although this is most often when full testing has not been done and is early in the diagnostic process [5]. This includes the use of antidiarrheals, probiotics, and antispasmodics for diarrhea, and the use of fiber supplements and laxatives for constipation [5]. If symptoms readily resolve and do not return, then, no further action is required. However, in many IBS patients, symptoms have been present from months to years and diagnosis has been hard to determine. In patients such as these, management of symptoms with a specialized nutrition program, is now being used as the first line of treatment [14].

NUTRITION INTERVENTIONS

The majority of patients with IBS report that food triggers symptoms; up to 90% restrict one or more type of food to help alleviate symptoms and symptom severity [15]. Food intolerances and food sensitivity are frequently reported in patients with IBS [5]. Through assessment of the commonly reported food intolerances, it was originally hypothesized that certain categories of foods cause an increase in susceptibility to Crohn's disease [16]. This supposition further extended into the role of these food components in functional bowel disorders such as IBS. Food that are high in fermentable oligosaccharides, disaccharides, monosaccharides, and polyols (or FODMAPs) are carbohydrates that are poorly absorbed by the small intestine, are molecularly small and osmotically active, and are rapidly fermented by bacteria [10,17]. These GI effects from consumption of high FODMAP foods result in an excessive intestinal fluid, increased gas production, bowel distention, and bloating resulting in abdominal pain and diarrhea [10,17]. The fermentation rate of these molecules is determined by the length of the carbohydrate chain, with high FODMAP foods being fermented at a faster rate [17]. Foods can be classified as those with excess fructose (like some fruits), lactose-containing oligosaccharides, and polyol-containing foods. Consuming a diet high in FODMAPs favors the production of hydrogen over other gases such as methane, which has been shown to cause gastrointestinal distress [17].

THE FODMAP ELIMINATION DIET

The FODMAP diet is an elimination of all high FODMAP foods for a specific period of time and then a gradual reintroduction of eliminated, higher FODMAP foods to determine tolerance based on symptoms [10,14,18]. Foods high in FODMAPs that are more likely to cause GI distress are listed in Table 5.1. The elimination of all high FODMAP foods followed by reintroduction of these foods allows an individual to determine what specific foods cause the most distress, allowing for an individualized approach. It is important to note that the foods noted as high FODMAP seem to "change" based on the resources used. This is because research into the FODMAP content of foods in ongoing and therefore data will change [7,10]. The Monash FODMAP app is an excellent tool for determining high FODMAP foods (http://www.med.monash.edu.au/cecs/gastro/fodmap/iphone-app.html).

OLIGOSACCHARIDES (FRUCTANS OR GALACTANS)

Fructans are linear-branched fructose polymers and naturally occurring carbohydrates that are found in onions, garlic, artichokes, some fruits, and cereals [17]. Wheat is one of the main sources of fructans in the American diet. Inulin and fructo-oligosaccharides (FOS) are commercially used

TABLE 5.1
High FODMAP-Containing Foods[a]

Food Component	Dietary Form	Food Category	Foods
Monosaccharide	Fructose	Fruits	Apples, pears, peaches, mango, watermelon, and cherries
		Vegetables	Asparagus, artichoke, and sugar snap peas
		Sweeteners	Honey, fructose, high-fructose corn syrup, and agave
		Large total fructose load	Dried fruit, fruit juice, and large servings of fruit
Disaccharides	Lactose	Milk	Cow, sheep, and goat (regular, low fat, and nonfat)
		Yogurt	Cow, sheep, and goat (regular, low fat, and nonfat)
		Cheeses (soft and fresh)	Ricotta, cottage, cream cheese, and American cheese
		Dairy desserts	Ice cream, custard, and pudding
Oligosaccharides	Fructans and galactans	Fruits	Watermelon, white peaches, and persimmon
		Vegetables	Artichokes, asparagus, Brussels sprouts, broccoli, garlic, leeks, okra, onions, onion powder, garlic powder, shallots, and peas
		Grains	Wheat, rye, and barley
		Legumes	Chickpeas, lentils, and beans
		Food additives	Inulin, soy-based products (except TOFU), and FOS (probiotic)
Polyols	Sorbitol, mannitol, xylitol, erythritol, polydextrose, and isomalt	Fruits	Apples, apricots, blackberries, cherries, lychee, pears, nectarines, peaches, plums, prunes, watermelon, and coconut milk
		Vegetables	Avocado (>1/4 cup), butternut squash, pumpkin, cauliflower, mushrooms, and snow peas
		Sweeteners	Sorbitol, mannitol, xylitol, maltitol, isomalt, and others ending in -ol

Source: Department of Gastroenterology, Central Clinical School, Monash University, Melbourne, Victoria, Australia.
[a] FODMAP composition of foods is continually being researched and updates may not be reflected on these pages.

as fiber additives [14]. Fructans, especially in patients with IBS, are not absorbed in the intestine and as a result, reach the colon undigested and are fermented into gas and short-chain fatty acids (SCFA) [15,19]. Galactans are naturally found in legumes, lentils, chickpeas, red kidney beans, and function similar to fructans [15]. Humans lack the enzyme needed to digest and absorb galactans so that they are rapidly fermented in the small intestine and produce gas [15]. In the absence of IBS or GI compromise, fructans provide a readily available source of fiber to many people and therefore, when these are eliminated, other sources of fiber should be encouraged. Soluble fibers and those derived from psyllium husk are well tolerated in IBS. In addition, the modification of the fructan intake specifically affects prebiotic foods (including FOS) and therefore changes the microbiota [19]. It is not clear if that is a negative effect.

DISACCHARIDES

Lactose is a disaccharide found in dairy products from cows, sheep, and goats [14]. For the body to completely digest a lactose molecule, the enzyme lactase is needed. The enzyme lactase breaks down the disaccharide into a monosaccharide, glucose, and galactose molecule, which can then be absorbed. Malabsorption of lactose is common and can be confirmed with a hydrogen breath test [17]. Avoidance of lactose-containing foods usually resolves symptoms if lactose intolerance is present, precluding the need for the breath hydrogen test in most cases.

MONOSACCHARIDES

Fructose is a monosaccharide found in fruit, honey, and high-fructose corn syrup [10,14]. Food manufacturing in the United States is using a more high-fructose corn syrup and it is the main ingredient in a wide variety of foods and beverages, causing the overall consumption of fructose in the American diet to be on the rise. Two pathways are involved in the absorption of fructose: GLUT-2, which cotransports fructose with glucose via facilitated diffusion (the preferred high-capacity pathway) and GLUT-5 carrier-mediated diffusion, which is used and needed when an abundance of fructose is absorbed at once [10,17,19]. Problems with digestion arise when fructose is present in excess of glucose and free fructose is in the intestinal lumen awaiting transport, causing limited absorption, and colonic fermentation [19]. The average American consumes 55 g of fructose daily; however, most healthy adults can only absorb 15–25 g [18]. To test a person's ability to completely absorb a fructose load, a hydrogen breath test is performed using a moderate high amount of fructose (35 g); however, if limiting high-fructose foods improves symptoms, a fructose malabsorption test is necessary only for confirmation [19].

POLYOLS

Polyols are a group of sugar alcohols naturally found in foods such as apples, pears, and mushrooms, and in polydextrose and isomalt [10,17]. They are also found in sugar substitutes including sorbitol, mannitol, maltitol, xylitol, and erythritol [10,17]. Only about one-third of polyols consumed are absorbed [19]. They have an osmotic effect in the small intestine and are also fermented in the colon that results in GI distress [17].

IMPLEMENTING THE FODMAP ELIMINATION DIET

There are two phases on the FODMAP elimination diet. The first phase (called the elimination phase) involves limiting or eliminating high FODMAP foods from the diet for a period of 4–8 weeks. Often, patients see an improvement in symptoms within 2 weeks but elimination for 4–6 weeks allows for improvement in understanding which foods actually cause symptoms when these are added back. When counseling on the elimination phase of the diet, it is important to provide as many low FODMAP food choices as possible. In the second phase (called the challenge phase), higher FODMAP foods in each category (fructose, lactose, etc.) are added back into the diet in a methodical and organized way to identify symptoms associated with a particular food or class of foods [10]. During the challenge phase, it is suggested to have the patient add back the foods they "missed" to determine the level of tolerance for favorite foods. It is during this "trial-and-error" time that the patient will understand the triggers of the FODMAP food and know which foods will cause symptoms. It is important to remember that although the high FODMAP foods are associated with increased symptoms that may cause pain or discomfort, these are not food allergies and therefore will not cause a reaction such as an anaphylaxis. During both phases of the FODMAP elimination diet, the expertise and support of a registered dietitian/nutritionist (RDN) to explain the diet as well as help with meal planning to avoid the potential for nutrient deficiencies is essential. The FODMAP diet is not a cure for IBS but a way of managing symptoms. The goal of the FODMAP elimination diet is to manage high FODMAP food intake to allow a variety of food and nutrient intake, as tolerated. Foods that cause symptoms can be eliminated or limited.

Evidence has repeatedly shown that the low FODMAP diet provides symptom relief for patients with IBS [20–27]. The effects on the GI tract of these foods and the relief of symptoms are reproducible and well documented. In a study of ostomy output in 12 individuals without IBS, consumption of a FODMAP diet showed increased weight and water content as well as still contained ingested FODMAP materials with high FODMAP intake in the ostomy effluent [25]. This did not occur with a low FODMAP intake demonstrating that the consumption of foods high in FODMAPs does have an osmotic effect and increases the amount of malabsorbed food particles. Following a low FODMAP diet for 21 days has been shown to decrease the total intestinal bacteria and also significantly reduce prebiotic bacteria, including Bifidobacteria, and butyrate-producing bacteria [12]. The reduction of total bacteria while following a low FODMAP diet supports a theory that IBS symptoms may be due to bacterial overgrowth of the small intestine and correction of this overgrowth can lead to symptom relief [14]. A low FODMAP does affect gut microbiota composition; however, the long-term implications of this are not yet known [12].

Overall, the current research shows that patients with IBS following a low FODMAP diet see an improvement on GI symptom severity, particularly with abdominal pain, bloating, and flatulence. To date, there is no validated and reliable tool to assess gastrointestinal symptoms in relation to the phases of the FODMAP elimination diet in IBS patients [12]. A valid and reliable tool to assess GI symptoms and their severity is needed. A new GI symptom assessment (GSS) tool specifically designed for IBS patients was used to assess symptoms prior to the low FODMAP diet initiation and after following the diet for approximately one month [28]. Although only a pilot study of 18 patients, the GSS confirmed changes in symptom severity between the two assessments as scored by the patients. The GSS not only provided feedback for the RDN but also for the patients to be able to see the magnitude of improvement they had experienced.

The FODMAP elimination diet is not the only component of the nutrition management of IBS as additional strategies should be addressed as well [7,10]. Carbonated beverages, chewing gum, and eating too may quickly result in gas and cause discomfort; so, these should be limited or avoided. Large meals may cause cramping and diarrhea; therefore, small meals, eaten more often (4–6 times per day) may improve IBS symptom management. As high-fat diet can slowdown motility, a lower-fat diet may be better tolerated. Insoluble fiber is limited in the low FODMAP diet; therefore, the importance of adding soluble fiber should be addressed to meet daily fiber needs.

Medications including antianxiety, antispasmodics, laxatives, and antidiarrheal mediations may be a part of the treatment plan. Incorporation of the low FODMAP diet with the medications may allow for discontinuation of the medications overtime. Antianxiety medications play a role in the gut–brain connection and may be a valuable concomitant therapy [10]. Herbal therapies have been used in IBS and many of them have evidence-based data to support their use [10]. For example, Iberogast and peppermint oil may help to improve global symptoms and reduce abdominal pain [10]. Relaxation training, therapy, and stress reduction are often helpful for patients experiencing IBS (and other GI disorders). Exercise has been shown to improve GI motility and adequate sleep can also improve the outcome.

IBS is considered as a diagnosis of exclusion and diagnosis may be made based on the symptoms. The evidence for improvement in symptoms and therefore the function and quality of life in IBS confirms the implementation of the FODMAP elimination diet as a primary component of treatment. The RDN has a key role in nutrition management for IBS.

RESOURCES

Patsy Catsos, MS, RDN—RDN training, recipes, cookbook, blog, website—ibsfree.net.
Kate Scarlata, RDN—RDN training, recipes, cookbook, website, blog—katescarlata.com.
Monash University—Monash FODMAP app.

REFERENCES

1. World Gastroenterology Organization. Irritable bowel syndrome: A global perspective. World Gastroenterology Organization Global Guideline. 2015, p. 7.
2. Definition of Irritable Bowel Syndrome. Rome Foundation website. http://www.romecriteria.org/criteria/ Accessed February 15, 2015.

3. Engsbro AL, Simren M, Bytzer P. Short term stability of subtypes in the irritable bowel syndrome: Prospective evaluation using the Rome III classification. *Aliment Pharmacol Ther.* 2012;35(3):350–359.
4. Spiegel BM, Farid M, Esrailian E, Talley K, Chang L. Is irritable bowel syndrome a diagnosis of exclusion? A survey of primary care providers, gastroenterologists and IBS experts. *Am J Gastroenterol.* 2010;105(4):848–858.
5. Chey WD, Kurlander J, Eswaran S. Irritable bowel syndrome: A clinical review. *JAMA* 2015;313(9):949–958.
6. Ireton-Jones C. Outcomes of nutrition intervention in IBS: Use of a symptom assessment Tool. *J Acad Nutr Diet.* 2014;114(9):A27.
7. Wolf WA, Kiraly LN, Ireton-Jones C. Incorporating FODMAP dietary restrictions: Help or hype? Current Nutrition Reports, published online July 11, 2015.
8. Ringel Y, Williams RE, Kalilani L, Cook SF. Prevalence, characteristics and impact of bloating symptoms in patients with irritable bowel syndrome. *Clin Gastroenterol Hepatol.* 2009;7(1):68–72.
9. Lovell RM, Ford AC. Effect of gender on prevalence of irritable bowel syndrome in the community: Systematic review and meta-analysis. *Am J Gastroenterol.* 2012;107(7):991–1000.
10. Matarese L, Mullin G, Roland B et al. The irritable bowel syndrome—Contemporary management strategies. *J Parenter Enteral Nutr.* 2014;38:781–799.
11. Gaman A, Bucur MC, Kuo B. Therapeutic advances in functional gastrointestinal disease: Irritable bowel syndrome. *Therap Adv Gastroenterol.* 2009;2:169–181.
12. Halmos EP, Christophersen CT, Bird AR et al. Diets that differ in their FODMAP content alter the colonic luminal microenvironment. *Gut.* 2015;64(1):93–100.
13. Staudacher HM, Lomer MC, Anderson JL et al. Fermentable carbohydrate restriction reduces luminal Bifidobacteria and gastrointestinal symptoms in patients with irritable bowel syndrome. *J Nutr.* 2012;142:1510–1518.
14. Mansueto P, Seidita A, D'Alcamo A et al. Role of FODMAPs in patients with irritable bowel syndrome: A review. *Nutr Clin Pract.* 2015;30(5):665–682.
15. Hayes PA, Fraher MH, Quigley EM. Irritable bowel syndrome: The role of food in the pathogenesis and management. *Gastroenterol Hepatol (NY)* 2014;10(3):164–174.
16. Gibson PR, Shepherd SJ. Personal view: Food for thought—Western lifestyle and susceptibility to Crohn's disease. The FODMAP hypothesis. *Aliment Pharmacol Ther.* 2005;21:1399–1409.
17. Gibson PR, Shepherd SJ. Evidence based dietary management of functional gastrointestinal symptoms: The FODMAP approach. *J Gastroenterol Hepatol.* 2010;25:252–258.
18. Gibson PR, Shepherd SJ. Food choice as a key management strategy of functional gastrointestinal symptoms. *Am J Gastroenterol.* 2012;107:657–666.
19. Khan MA, Nusrat S, Khan MI et al. Low FODMAP diet for irritable bowel syndrome: Is it ready for prime time? *Dig Dis Sci.* 2015;60(5):1169–77.
20. Shepherd SJ, Lomer MC, Gibson PR. Short-chain carbohydrates and functional gastrointestinal disorders. *Am J Gastroenterol.* 2013;108(5):707–717.
21. Staudacher HM, Whelan K, Irving PM et al. Comparison of symptom response following advice for a diet low in fermentable carbohydrates (FODMAPs) versus standard dietary advice in patients with irritable bowel syndrome. *J Hum Nutr Diet.* 2011;24L:487–495.
22. Staudacher HM, Lomer MC, Anderson JL et al. Fermentable carbohydrate restriction reduces luminal Bifidobacteria and gastrointestinal symptoms in patients with irritable bowel syndrome. *J Nutr.* 2012;142:1510–1518.
23. Ong DK, Mitchell SB, Barrett JS et al. Manipulation of dietary short chain carbohydrates alters the pattern of gas production and genesis of symptoms in irritable bowel syndrome. *J Gastroenterol Hepatol.* 2010;25:1366–1373.
24. Halmos EP, Power VA, Shepherd SJ et al. A diet low in FODMAPs reduces symptoms of irritable bowel syndrome. *Gastroenterol.* 2014;146:67–75.e5.
25. Barrett JS, Gearry RB, Muir JG et al. Dietary poorly absorbed, short chain carbohydrates increase delivery of water and fermentable substrate to the proximal colon. *Aliment Pharmacol Ther.* 2010;31:874–882.
26. De Roest RH, Dobbs BR, Chapman BA et al. The low FODMAP diet improves gastrointestinal symptoms in patients with irritable bowel syndrome: A prospective study. *Int J Clin Pract.* 2013;67:895–903.
27. Pedersen N, Vegh Z, Burisch J et al. Ehealth: Low FODMAP diet vs *Lactobacillus rhamnosus* GG in irritable bowel syndrome. *World J Gastroenterol.* 2014;20(43):16215–16226.
28. Heffernan E. Change in self reported gastrointestinal symptom severity and frequency following a registered dietitian counseling session for the management of irritable bowel syndrome. Master's thesis, Rutgers University, Newark, NJ, December 17, 2015.

6 Nutrition Management in Oncology

Assessment, Gastroenterology, Breast, Esophageal Head and Neck, Gynecologic, Lung, Prostate, and Palliative Care

Pankaj Vashi, MD, CNSC, Rachel Winston, MS, RDN, CSO, Stephanie Paver, RDN, CSO, CNSC, Kristen Trukova, MS, RDN, CSO, CNSC, LDN, Julia Fechtner, RDN, CSO, CNSC, LDN, Kamorin Samson, RDN, CSO, LDN, Renee Pieroth, RDN, CSO, LDN, Crystal Langlois, RDN, CSO, LD, Nathan Schober, MS, RDN, CNSC, Maureen Geboy, RDN, LD, Andrea Swartz, RDN, LD, Roberta Scheuer, RDN, LD, Matt Rinehart, MS, RDN, CSO, LD, Jessica Smith, MS, RDN, CSO, LD, Gabrielle Taylor, MS, RDN, LD, Kalli Castille, MS, RDN, LD, FAND, Jessica Engelbrecht, MS, RDN, CSR, LD, CNSC, Brooke McIntyre, RDN, CSO, LD, CNSC, and Jasmyn Walker, MS, RDN, LD, CSO, CNSC

CONTENTS

INTRODUCTION

The prevalence of malnutrition in people with cancer has been estimated to be up to 85%, particularly in cancers that affect the gastrointestinal (GI) tract. According to the National Cancer Institute (NCI), 20%–40% of people with cancer die from malnutrition, cachexia, or complications attributed to these conditions. Therefore, any unintended weight loss should be evaluated during cancer treatment. It has been reported that as little as a 5% weight loss can reduce tolerance to chemotherapy, increase side effects, and decrease quality of life. Weight loss can also interfere with patients' ability to complete or stay on track with their prescribed cancer therapy.

Cancer and cancer treatments can impact patients' ability to ingest, digest, absorb, and metabolize nutrients, making the management of nutritional status challenging in this population. For this reason, most evidence-based guidelines for oncology nutrition recommend that all patients being treated for cancer be screened for malnutrition and rescreened throughout treatment. Some of the main goals of nutrition therapy for those at risk are as follows:

- Prevent or treat nutrition deficiencies and problems, including preventing muscle and bone loss
- Decrease or manage symptoms that impact nutrition
- Maintain the immune system to help fight infection
- Aid recovery and healing from surgery, chemotherapy, and/or radiation therapy
- Maintain or improve the patient's strength, energy, and quality of life

Also, for patients who are well nourished, good nutrition and physical activity behaviors are important during and after treatment. All patients, especially those with excess body weight, should be counseled on eating and activity behaviors to help them achieve and maintain a healthier body weight, since obesity has been associated with poorer outcomes during treatment, as well as an increase in risk of recurrence in some cancers.

This chapter will outline approaches to nutrition screening, assessment, interventions, and monitoring in the oncology population. The chapter begins with a review of screening tools that have been validated for use in this population. After that, a review of many of the most common cancers will include a brief overview of the cancer, risk factors, and common treatments, including some nutrition interventions. Finally, the appendices in this chapter can serve as a reference to help the provider anticipate side effects of common treatments as well as offer suggestions for nutritional management of those symptoms.

NUTRITION SCREENING AND ASSESSMENT

Screening

Nutrition screening in the oncology population is used for the early identification of patients who are malnourished or at nutritional risk. A nutrition screen can be completed by any qualified health care professional, including those other than the registered dietitian (RD). The screening process enables a timely referral for nutrition assessment and intervention. Owing to the duration of cancer treatments, adjustments in regimens and modalities, and changes in an individual's tolerance to treatment over time, it is imperative that patients are screened at initial presentation and regularly rescreened at each clinic visit thereafter. There should be a process in place whereby a positive screening alerts the RD for referral. Once a patient is referred, nutrition interventions and education require continuous modification to meet the patients' dynamic needs.

A screening tool provides a valid, standardized, and efficient method to identify nutrition impact symptoms and clinical signs of malnutrition (see Chapter 1). Based on The Academy of Nutrition and Dietetics Evidence Analysis Library (EAL), there are four nutrition screening tools that have proven to be valid and reliable in the inpatient setting, two of which are appropriate in the outpatient setting (Table 6.1).

Assessment

The purpose of the oncology nutrition assessment is to perform a comprehensive evaluation of the patient's nutritional status, nutrition impact symptoms, and nutritional requirements. Furthermore, the assessment is utilized by the RD to form individualized interventions, monitoring, and continued evaluation as appropriate. As stated by the EAL Oncology Work Group, "An adult oncology nutrition assessment should characterize and document the presence of (or expected potential for) altered nutrition status and nutrition impact symptoms that may result in a measurable adverse effect on body composition, function, quality of life (QOL) or clinical outcome, and may include indicators of malnutrition."[2]

The SGA and PG–SGA nutrition assessment tools have been validated by the EAL for use among adult oncology patients in acute care and ambulatory settings.[3] Both tools include assessment of intake, weight, GI symptoms, and functional status. However, the SGA incorporates a physical examination, while the PG–SGA covers a more comprehensive review of nutrition impact symptoms.

Malnutrition is extremely prevalent in the oncology population, with incidence rates estimated to be between 40% and 80%.[4,5] Malnutrition is defined as "a state of nutrition in which a deficiency,

TABLE 6.1
Nutrition Screening Tools Validated in the Oncology Population

Screening Tool	Components Assessed	Inpatient	Outpatient
Patient generated–subjective global assessment (PG–SGA)	Weight, nutrition impact symptoms, intake, and functional status	×	×
Malnutrition screening tool (MST)	Weight and appetite	×	×
Malnutrition screening tool for cancer patients (MSTC)	Intake, weight, ECOG, and BMI	×	
Malnutrition universal screening tool (MUST)	BMI, weight, acute illness, and intake	×	
Weight loss	Percentage of lean body weight		

Source: Onc: Nutrition screening tools. 2012. Academy of Nutrition and Dietetics Evidence Analysis Library. http://www.andeal.org/topic.cfm?cat=5452&conclusion_statement_id=251796&highlight=oncology%20assessment&home=1. Updated 2012. Accessed March 2015.

excess or imbalance of energy, protein, and other nutrients causes adverse effects on body form, function and clinical outcome."[6] Complications of malnutrition include increased therapy-related toxicity, poor performance status, lower quality of life, reduced survival, increased number of hospitalizations and length of stay, and increased health care costs.[7–10]

The oncology nutrition assessment is a multifactorial approach that should be completed at every clinic visit for patients who are at risk for malnutrition or are already malnourished. Evaluation of nutrition impact symptoms that the patient is already experiencing, or is at risk for developing, is critical in helping to maintain or improve their nutritional status. Nutrition impact symptoms are defined as side effects from treatment or the cancer itself that impair intake, digestion, or absorption. Examples commonly seen in the oncology setting include nausea, vomiting, diarrhea, constipation, dysphagia, odynophagia, anorexia, mucositis, early satiety, and alterations in taste and smell.

The careful monitoring of weight status and implementation of nutritional interventions to support a healthy body weight is a key component of the nutrition assessment. Cancer-induced weight loss and more recently, lean body mass, have both been used as primary outcomes in clinical trials. Patients with significant weight loss and/or sarcopenia have been associated with greater treatment toxicity and shorter survival. Significant weight loss is defined as 1%–2% in one week, 5% in 1 month, 7.5% in 3 months, and 10% in 6 months. Computerized tomography (CT) images, bioelectrical impedance analysis (BIA), dual-energy x-ray absorptiometry (DXA), and anthropometry are used to assess changes in lean body mass.

In addition to using a validated assessment tool, the oncology nutrition assessment should encompass each component of the nutrition care process, including an in-depth diet history, medication list review, anthropometric measurements, biochemical data, nutrition-focused physical exam, and psychosocial factors.

GASTROENTEROLOGY (GENERAL)

Introduction

The GI tract refers to the route from the mouth to the anus that is responsible for digestion, absorption, and elimination. The GI tract is also host to a plethora of microorganisms that are responsible for 70% of the body's immune function, making it the largest immune tissue in the body. The GI tract is a very complex and dynamic system that is impacted by what we eat and by exposure to toxins. Chronic inflammation is linked to breakdown in this complex immune system, which triggers the formation of cancerous growth. GI cancers include organs in the upper and lower GI tract, namely, the esophagus, stomach, pancreas, liver, gallbladder, colon/rectum, and anus. GI cancers can cause alterations in anatomy and function that can affect nutritional status, quality of life, and treatment outcomes. Aberrations commonly experienced with GI cancers that make nutritional management challenging will be covered. Cancers of the head and neck and esophagus are discussed in their own section.

Statistics/Survival

Cancers of the GI tract are collectively the most lethal cancers worldwide. Lifetime risk of developing a cancer in the GI tract ranges from 0.2% to 5%, depending on location and tumor type, with anal cancer being the least common and colorectal being the most common. Survival rates depend on stage at diagnosis and tumor type, with advanced stages having much less favorable prognosis.[11]

Risk Factors

Common risk factors for GI cancers include tobacco use; alcohol consumption; history of infection, such as *Helicobacter pylori*, chronic hepatitis, Epstein–Barr virus, and human papilloma virus; and genetics and chronic inflammation.[11] Diet plays a key role in the development of several GI cancers. For example, high saturated fat and low fiber intake has been linked to colorectal cancers, and intake of smoked, salted, cured, and pickled foods are known risk factors for stomach cancer.[11,12] Furthermore, it is estimated that 15%–50% of GI cancers are preventable by diet, activity, and weight management.[13]

TABLE 6.2
Estimating Energy and Protein Requirements

Cancer Type	Energy (kcal/kg/day Actual Weight)	Protein (g/kg/day Actual Weight)	Fluid
Stomach, pancreas, gallbladder, colon, rectum, anus	30–35: repletion, weight gain 25–30: inactive, nonstressed 35: hypermetabolic 25–30: sepsis	1.0–1.5: cancer 1.5–2.5: cancer cachexia 1.0–1.5: inflammatory bowel disease 1.5–2.0: short bowel syndrome	20–40 mL/kg/day or 1 mL/kcal
Liver	25–40: based on dry weight 35–40: stable cirrhosis 25–35: without encephalopathy 35: acute encephalopathy 30–40: stable, malnourished	1.0–1.5: all except those with encephalopathy 0.6–0.8: acute encephalopathy	

Source: Adapted from Huhmann M. *Oncology Nutrition for Clinical Practice*. 3rd ed. Chicago, IL: Oncology Nutrition Dietetic Practice Group of the Academy of Nutrition and Dietetics; 2013:14.

Symptoms

Recognizing symptoms that are considered "red flags" for GI cancers is important for early detection. These include

- Unexplained weight loss
- Abdominal pain that lasts longer than 4 weeks
- Unexplained loss of appetite
- Change in bowel habits
- Nausea and vomiting lasting for more than a week
- Symptoms related to anemia (fatigue, shortness of breath, and weakness)
- New onset back pain

Early detection of GI cancers is difficult due to latent signs and symptoms and lack of routine screening tests. It is very important to recognize these warning signs so that timely referral to a gastroenterologist can be made.

Nutrition assessment should include a determination of energy and protein needs. Although predictive equations have been proposed for the outpatient and home care population, specific recommendations related to the type of cancer may lead to more accurate provision of nutrients (see Table 6.2).

Treatment Options

Surgical Management

The presence of cancer in the GI tract predisposes one to malnutrition. Patients who are malnourished preoperatively are significantly more likely to have longer length of hospital stay and postoperative morbidity and mortality.[14–17] Nutrition screening is essential for identifying patients at increased risk for perioperative morbidity, and early intervention is critical to improving outcomes.

Optimization of nutritional status preoperatively is imperative. In patients who are at severe nutritional risk, nutrition support should be implemented for 10–14 days preoperatively, and surgery should be postponed until this is achieved. Severe nutritional risk is defined as one of the following:[18]

- Weight loss of 10%–15% within 6 months
- Body mass index (BMI) <18.5 kg/m^2
- Subjective Global Assessment Grade C
- Serum albumin <3.0 g/dL (with no evidence of hepatic or renal dysfunction)

In oncology patients unable to consume above 60% of estimated intake for more than 10 days or in whom inadequate intake is anticipated for more than 7 days perioperatively, regardless of nutritional status, it is recommended that nutrition support via the enteral route (oral or tube feeding) be implemented without delay.[18] Preoperative parenteral nutrition (PN) for 7–15 days has been shown to reduce postoperative morbidity and should be considered in severely malnourished patients in whom oral or enteral nutrition (EN) is contraindicated or insufficient.[17–19]

Postoperatively, the traditional practice of holding oral or enteral feeds until return of bowel sounds is without evidence yet pervasive as a standard of care.[20] Early feeding should be initiated to promote bowel hypertrophy and anastomotic healing.[21] Feeding proximal to an anastomosis may prevent disruption or leak.[22] If feeding is started within 24 hours, dysmotility can be attenuated, even in the absence of peristalsis.[23] In patients undergoing gastrectomy, rectal pelvic surgery, pancreaticoduodenectomy, and colon resection, a normal diet should be offered on postoperative day one without restrictions, and patients should be advised caution in increasing intake according to tolerance. Early feeding reduces the risk of infection and length of hospital stay.[24–27]

Immunonutrition or pharmaconutrition refers to immune-modulating formulas containing supraphysiological doses of arginine, with or without glutamine, omega-3 fatty acids, and nucleotides, which are recommended for their effect on reducing postoperative infectious complications and hospital length of stay.[28] Results from a systematic review and meta-analysis of randomized controlled trials evaluating the effect of pharmaconutrition on postoperative clinical outcomes compared with standard nutritional provision highlight the importance of timing in the provision of immunonutrition.[28] Preoperative provision, as defined by 5–7 days prior to surgery, shows no advantage on outcomes over standard nutrition. However, perioperative and postoperative administration are associated with significantly reduced infectious complications and length of stay. Additionally, perioperative administration was associated with significant reduction in anastomic dehiscence and postoperative administration was associated with reduction in noninfectious complications. Perioperative nutrition was defined as 5–7 days before surgery plus postoperative day (POD) commencement via jejunal tube on POD 1–2 until POD7 or until oral intake was established. Postoperative nutrition was defined as pharmaconutrition commencement via jejunal tube on POD 1–2 until POD7 or until oral intake was established.[28]

Altered GI function is a common etiology for malnutrition diagnosis in the oncology population.

Dumping Syndrome

Partial or total gastrectomy and pancreaticoduodenectomy may disrupt gastric motility, resulting in delayed emptying or rapid transit of stomach contents into the small intestine, known as dumping syndrome. Removal or manipulation of the pyloric valve during surgery predisposes one to dumping syndrome. Early symptoms manifest as cramping, bloating, nausea, and diarrhea within 10–15 minutes of eating due to the influx of fluid into the small intestine in response to a concentrated sugar load. Hypotension, weakness, and faintness may follow. Late symptoms of dumping syndrome occur 2–3 hours after eating when the sugar from the intestines is absorbed and the body's response to hyperglycemia is accelerated. Elevated insulin levels cause hypoglycemia. Symptoms include high heart rate, dizziness, shakiness, sweating, fainting, and confusion.[29]

To prevent or manage the occurrence of postoperative dumping syndrome, follow these guidelines for 6–8 weeks:

- Eat slowly and chew foods thoroughly to liquefy the bolus since the digestive capability of the stomach is decreased or naught.
- Eat 6–8 small meals per day.
- Consume fluids 45 minutes before eating or 1 hour after eating, not with meals.
- Avoid raw fruits and vegetables and other fibrous foods, including whole grains, nuts, seeds, peas, and beans.
- Limit fruit to 1/2 cup cooked or canned at a time.

- Limit or avoid milk or milk products if unable to tolerate.
- Consume protein foods with each meal and snack.
- Avoid high-sugar foods such as fruit juice, sugar-sweetened beverages, honey, jam, jelly, molasses, ice cream, pudding, pastries, pies, cake, fruit ice, sherbet, and gelatin.
- Avoid foods that contain sugar, honey, corn syrup, fructose, lactose, dextrose, maltose, sorbitol, xylitol, or mannitol in the first three ingredients.

Delayed Gastric Emptying

The presence of gastric and pancreatic tumors, duodenal ulcers, subtotal gastrectomy, Whipple procedure, and narcotic use are common etiologies for gastroparesis in the oncology setting. Symptoms include protracted nausea and vomiting, decreased appetite, bloating, fullness, early satiety, and alteration in glucose control. Oral diet manipulation includes small frequent meals, use of liquid calories, and avoidance of high-fiber and high-fat foods. Prokinetic and antiemetic agents should accompany diet modification. In cases of severe gastroparesis or when symptom management is unsuccessful, jejunal feeding should be considered to prevent malnutrition. When delayed emptying occurs as a result of gastrectomy, supplementation with vitamin B12, vitamin D, calcium, and a multivitamin with minerals should be considered.[29]

Removing segments of the small intestine can alter digestion and absorption. Symptoms may include nausea, abdominal cramping, and diarrhea. Functional adaptation can occur; however, significant loss of small bowel may require PN support to maintain fluid and electrolyte balance. Diet guidelines for the first 4–6 weeks after small bowel surgery include the following:

- Eat small, frequent meals.
- Chew foods thoroughly.
- Consume protein with each meal or snack.
- Avoid high-fiber foods; limit total fiber to <20 g per day.

After 4–6 weeks, add new foods back to the diet one at a time and assess for tolerance prior to continuing transition to regular diet.[30] If short bowel syndrome (SBS) is severe, more extensive nutrition support may be required.

Ostomy Placement

Diversion of fecal transit may be required temporarily or permanently for management of bowel obstruction or removal of GI malignancy. A colostomy is performed when it is necessary to bypass or remove the distal colon, rectum, or anus. Removal of the colon typically requires minimal diet modification (except for ascending colostomy, covered below). Sufficient fiber and fluid can prevent constipation. In cases of loose stool, thickening foods may be beneficial. Similarly, reducing gaseous and odorous foods may be advised.[31]

Removal or bypass of the entire colon and rectum requires an ileostomy. High fluid output can cause dehydration and electrolyte imbalance for patients with ileostomies and ascending colostomies. Also, risk of stoma blockage exists because the ileal lumen is <1 inch in diameter. Large amounts of insoluble fibers should be avoided. Follow the below guidelines for nutritional management status post ileostomy placement[31,32]:

- Eat small frequent meals.
- Chew foods well to prevent foods from causing a blockage or obstruction as stool exits the ileostomy.
- Stay hydrated. Do not attempt to control diarrhea by restricting fluids. Monitor ostomy output and consume 1 L fluid in addition to output volume.
- Avoid fiber. Avoid stringy vegetables, foods with skins, and dried fruits. Limit foods to those with 2 g or less of fiber per serving.

- Choose low-fat foods. Avoid meats with casings.
- Avoid simple sugars (sweetened beverages and sugary foods).

After 6–8 weeks, add new foods back to the diet one at a time and assess for tolerance prior to continuing transition to regular diet.

Fat Maldigestion

Fat maldigestion can occur following GI surgeries and in the presence of GI malignancies. Following gastrectomy, accelerated transit of food into the small intestine can prevent adequate mixing of food contents with bile salts and digestive enzymes. Additionally, large food particles entering the small intestine may impair adequate degradation by enzymes. Alternatively, pancreatic exocrine insufficiency (PEI) may accompany a diagnosis of pancreatic cancer or bile duct blockage, or may occur during nonsurgical treatment and/or following whipple surgery. PEI can be ruled in by measuring pancreatic elastase. In cases of PEI, pancreatic enzyme replacement and fat-soluble vitamin supplementation may be warranted.[29]

Short Bowel Syndrome

Surgical resection of the small bowel leaving <200 cm is termed short bowel syndrome. Initially, PN and or EN will be necessary to achieve adequate nutritional provision, but over approximately 2 years, the remaining gut adapts, whereby the surface area and absorptive capacity of the small bowel increases. Loss of the terminal ileum and the ileal break mechanism results in gastric hypersecretion and accelerated transit. Without the terminal ileum, the site for bile salt reabsorption, bile salts enter the colon and cause choleric diarrhea. Cholestyramine can be helpful if <100 cm of distal ileum is resected, and the colon is intact, but should be avoided if >100 cm of terminal ileum is resected. Antimotility agents such as loperamide, diphenoxylate, and opiates can be used to slow transit and should be administered 30 minutes before meals.[29]

Patients with SBS are at risk for deficiency of fat-soluble vitamins, vitamin B12, and magnesium. Supplementation with a liquid or chewable vitamin/mineral supplement should be considered. Bowel adaptation occurs with macronutrient exposure. Whole food and/or use of a polymeric formula maximizes intestinal stimulation. Semielemental EN formulas can be considered if needed, but elemental formulas should be avoided because they are hypertonic. PN may be required to maintain electrolyte and fluid balance. Oral diet guidelines for patients with SBS include the following[29]:

- Macronutrient composition of 20%–30% carbohydrate, 20%–30% protein, and 50%–60% fat for patients with jejunostomies/ileostomies.
- Macronutrient composition of 50%–60% carbohydrate, 20%–30% protein, and 20%–30% fat for patients with intact colon.
- Avoid concentrated sweets/fluids.
- Chew foods well.
- Limit fluids with meals and drink isotonic beverages.

Obstruction

Mechanical obstruction of the small bowel can occur from adhesions from previous abdominal GI surgeries or from the presence of gastrointestinal tumors. Colonic pseudo-obstruction can develop from narcotic use and lead to significant constipation. Symptoms of obstruction include nausea, vomiting, abdominal pain, abdominal distention, and inability to pass flatus or stool.[33] Nutritional management for partial small bowel obstruction includes liquid oral nutrition drink supplements and foods that are moist and soft. For partial colonic obstruction, a very low-fiber diet and stool softeners are recommended. Complete bowel obstruction warrants nil per Os (NPO) to limit bowel distension. In the presence of weight loss and/or malnutrition, or anticipation of prolonged NPO, PN should be initiated. In some patients with chronic obstruction, PN is required long term. For patients in whom surgical intervention is appropriate, refer to "Surgical Management" section above.

Small Intestinal Bacterial Overgrowth

Small intestinal bacterial overgrowth (SIBO) is a condition in which mostly anaerobic bacteria colonize the small intestine in larger than normal quantities, causing symptoms of gas, bloating, abdominal distention, diarrhea, and weight loss. SIBO should be suspected in GI cancer patients with gastroparesis, impaired peristalsis, removal of the ileocecal valve, PEI, stricture/obstruction/adhesion of the GI tract, gastrocolic fistula, surgical bind loops, intestinal pseudo-obstruction, and/or hypochlorhydria/achlorhydria.[29,34] SIBO is diagnosed by an ileal aspirate and culture; however, the practice of empirically treating patients for SIBO without diagnostic confirmation is not uncommon.[29] Treatment includes antibiotic therapy and dietary manipulation. Since carbohydrates are fermented by bacteria and fermentation in the small bowel can contribute to symptoms, the diet should be modified to reduced carbohydrate and fiber. Fat should be substituted for carbohydrates to supply adequate calories and reduce the production of gas and bloating.[34] Nutrients of concern requiring monitoring include calcium, magnesium, iron, vitamin B12, and fat-soluble vitamins.[34]

Fistulas

A fistula is an abnormal passageway or connection between two organs or structures. Enteric fistulas are connections of the small intestine/bowel with other abdominal organs or with the chest or skin. They are named by the originating segment of bowel (gastro-, duodeno-, entero-, jejuno-, ileo-, colo-, recto-) and the point of termination (-cutaneous, -enteric, -colonic, -rectal, -vesical, -vaginal, -aortic). Etiologies include distal obstruction, radiation, and infection and can occur from the presence of tumors and from injury during surgery.[35] Malnutrition preoperatively increases the risk of fistula development. Fistulas requiring nutritional management include those that have a high output of fluid and nutrients (a high-output fistula drains more than 500 mL/day) or increased output stimulated by PO intake that prevents the fistula from closing. In either case, NPO may be indicated and PN will be necessary. Patients with high-output fistulas who are not on PN may require extra vitamin/mineral supplementation.[29] When output is <500 mL/day, enteral feeding may be possible; feeding proximal to the fistula enhances absorptive area. Fiber-free formulas or diets should be used when the fistula is distal and fiber containing products or diets can be used when the fistula is proximal to the site of feeding entry.[29]

Summary

GI cancers pose nutritional challenges that require a knowledgeable dietitian and team of providers. The functions of digestion and absorption may be altered or severely compromised; in many cases, multimodal treatment requires medical therapy and dietary modification or nutrition support to prevent or reverse malnutrition. Nutrition support or supplemental nutrition individualized by a dietitian is necessary for optimal management of GI cancer patients.

BREAST

Introduction

Statistics/Survival

Breast cancer remains the most commonly diagnosed cancer in women, and the second leading cause of cancer death in women in the United States. Between 2007 and 2011, breast cancer occurrence rates remained stable for Caucasian women, and increased by 0.3% per year in African American women.[36] Death rates from breast cancer decreased by 34% from 1990 to 2010 related to advances in early diagnosis and treatment.[37] For all women, 5 year survival is 99% for women with local disease (stages 0 and I, some stage II), 84% for regional disease (stage II and some stage III), and 24% for advanced disease (stage IIIc and stage IV).[38]

Subtypes

Subtypes of breast cancer are determined by the presence of biological markers or receptors present on tumor cells. Pathologists classify a breast tumor as estrogen receptor (ER) positive or negative, progesterone receptor (PR) positive or negative, as well as human epidermal growth factor 2 (HER2neu) positive or negative through the examination of tissue biopsied or excised.

Tumors identified as ER positive and/or PR positive are generally less aggressive and also less responsive to chemotherapy. Typically, these tumors respond to hormonal therapies. HER2 positive tumors are often more aggressive than HER2 negative tumors. Women diagnosed with triple negative tumors (no ER, PR, or HER2 receptors on the tumor cell) unfortunately have a poorer short-term prognosis, in part related to the lack of specific therapies toward this tumor type.[39] Triple negative cancers are in general more responsive to chemotherapy.

Lifestyle Risk Factors

Lifestyle factors that increase the risk of breast cancer include weight gain after age 18, being overweight or obese (related to postmenopausal breast cancer) and alcohol. Physical activity has been shown to reduce risk.[40]

Weight

Obesity has also been strongly correlated with the risk of postmenopausal breast cancer.[41] In addition, overweight and obesity status at diagnosis increases the risk of recurrence and adversely impacts breast cancer and all-cause mortality. Data have shown this obesity effect regardless of stage, treatment, and menopausal status.[42] Further, weight gain through breast cancer treatment is correlated with poor prognosis.

Unfortunately, a breast cancer event increases a woman's risk of weight gain. Recent studies have shown an average weight gain of 5–14 pounds.[43] In the HEAL study of breast cancer survivors, 68% of women gained weight, and 74% gained body fat and maintained that gain at 3 years from diagnosis.[44]

Weight gain after diagnosis is most related to chemotherapy, compared to radiation and hormonal therapy. Menopausal status and decreased activity levels appear to be the most impactful variables contributing to weight change after breast cancer.[45]

Research has suggested that it may be beneficial for women to focus on healthy weight loss during treatment, which is much different from other cancer types.[46] Clinicians are encouraged to guide women toward appropriate dietary and physical activity goals.

Physical Activity

The benefits of adequate physical activity for health cannot be understated. The Nurse's Health Study documented in a cohort of 2987 women diagnosed with breast cancer stages I–III who achieved 3–5 hours of walking per week (>3 metabolic equivalent task-hours per week, MET-h/week) reduced their risk of dying from breast cancer by half. The Collaborative Women's Longevity Study (CWLS) followed 4400 American women ages 20–79 beginning at breast cancer diagnosis for 6 years and noted that women with >2.9 MET-h/week had a reduced risk of breast cancer and all-cause mortality. Results showed that increased physical activity consistently provided a survival benefit regardless of age, stage of breast cancer, and BMI.[47]

Diet

The World Cancer Research Foundation and the American Institute for Cancer Research (WCRF/AICR) have published comprehensive reports on the evidence linking diet and lifestyle to cancer. Their general cancer recommendations are to follow a plant-based diet rich in vegetables, fruits, whole grains, beans, and limited in red and processed meats, as well as high calorie, high sugar foods and alcohol.

While no specific nutrients or foods (other than alcohol) are consistently linked to breast cancer risk, two large-scale trials reviewed diet changes and risk of breast cancer recurrence. Specifically, the Women's Healthy Eating and Living (WHEL) trial implemented a low-fat (goal 15%–20% dietary fat) and increased fruit and vegetable regimen (three fruit and five vegetable servings daily). Women in the intervention group were successful in increasing produce intake to goal and reducing dietary fat from 28% to 21% on average (did not meet target). No significant benefit of this intervention was found in relation to breast cancer recurrence after 7 years.[48]

The Women's Intervention Nutrition Study (WINS) focused specifically on reducing fat intake to 15%–20% of diet to decrease risk of breast cancer recurrence. Women were able to meet the goal of 20% dietary fat or less. This trial of nearly 2500 women, begun in 1987, did find a significant reduction in recurrent breast cancer.[49] However, a large percentage of women also experienced weight loss. Therefore, it is not possible to determine if diet change or weight loss or the combination most impacted the risk reduction noted in this study.

Alcohol

The AICR found convincing and dose–response evidence that alcohol intake is a risk factor for cancer. One standard drink per day increased breast cancer risk by 10%.[40] There are several specific mechanisms by which alcohol causes cell damage. First, alcohol influences estrogen breakdown and effects, and persons who heavily consume alcohol may have nutrient-poor diets. The detoxification of alcohol produces carcinogens and free radicals, and alcohol enhances the absorption of free radicals into cells. Finally, increased folate intake may partially reduce the risk of alcohol damage.

Omega-3 Fatty Acids

In vitro and animal studies elucidated several mechanisms by which eicosapentanoic acid and docosahexanoic acid may inhibit breast cancer.[50] Research in humans has been inconsistent but promising; more large-scale studies are needed. One report from the WHEL study noted that food intake of 73 mg EPA daily provided a 25% reduced risk of breast cancer recurrence.[51] It is appropriate to recommend two to three servings of oily fish per week. It is important to note that flax seed oil primarily contains alpha-linolenic acid (ALA), and only 5%–10% of ALA is converted to EPA and DHA by the liver, therefore limiting effective vegan options to increase intake of EPA/DHA.

Phytoestrogens

Soy foods contain phytoestrogens from isoflavone components. In the past, there was concern about phytoestrogen intake promoting ER+ breast tumor growth. Soy foods are recommended for children and adolescents to reduce breast cancer risk.[52] Further studies have shown no detriment to the intake of soy food up to three servings daily for breast cancer survivors, and potential benefit on the effectiveness of tamoxifen.[53]

It is prudent to recommend whole food sources of soy such as tofu, soy milk, soy nuts, tempeh, or miso as one serving provides 30 mg isoflavones. The isoflavone content of processed soy protein powders or soy isoflavone supplements may exceed the daily recommended limit of 100 mg. Soy foods that do not contain soy protein, such as soybean oils or soy sauce, do not contain isoflavones. Other foods such as legumes, nuts, and some fruits do contain minute amounts of isoflavones. However, the quantity is measured in micrograms (mcg), making it difficult to approach the daily limit of 100 mg.

Cruciferous Vegetables

Vegetables from the Brassica family have been investigated for their content of glucosinolates, including indole-3-carbinol. This phytochemical participates in liver detoxification and is involved in the breakdown of estrogen. *In vitro* studies have shown antiapoptotic and antiangiogenetic effects.[54] Large-scale studies have not been carried out to review the effects of increased consumption of cruciferous vegetables on breast cancer risk. However, increasing consumption is obviously part of a plant-based diet.

Lignans

Lignans are present in nearly all plant foods, but flax seeds are the most significant source. These compounds have been investigated for anticancer effects, and benefit has been seen *in vitro* and in rodent studies. Human data have been mixed, with one study of over 1200 women showing lower risk of aggressive breast tumors, and another of nearly 335,000 women not showing any relationship between dietary lignans and breast cancer risk over 11.5 years.[55,56]

Green Tea

While all tea is a source of antioxidants, green tea is specifically noted for its catechin content, specifically epigallocatechin-3-gallate (EGCG). It is known that tea catechins have antioxidant, anti-angiogenic, anti-inflammatory, and antiproliferative actions in the body. As yet, data relating green tea to breast cancer are limited to *in vitro* and epidemiological evidence only. Some observational studies have linked a higher intake of green tea to a reduced risk of breast cancer while others have shown no effect.[57]

Energy and Protein Requirements

Typical energy requirements are between 25 and 30 kcal/kg actual weight and protein requirements vary 1–1.5 g/kg for normal women.[58]

Survivorship Considerations

The cardiotoxicity of breast cancer therapies is well established, and is a concern in patients who now survive decades after completing treatment. Patnaik et al. found that in older breast cancer survivors, cardiovascular disease actually surpassed breast cancer recurrence as cause of mortality.[59]

Bone health is an important focus for this population due to the adverse effects on bone related to chemotherapy and aromatase inhibitor therapies.[60] Women should consume adequate calcium and vitamin D from food or supplements as indicated by the Dietary Reference Intakes (DRI). Although a 25-hydroxyvitamin D (25(OH)D) level of >20 ng/mL is appropriate for bone health, some researchers have suggested that the most beneficial level of 25(OH)D for breast cancer risk is between 40 and 60 ng/dL.[61,62] This topic remains controversial, but it is valuable to assess serum vitamin D status in this population.

Dietary Reference Intakes for Bone Health

Age	Calcium	Age	Vitamin D
19–50 years	1000 mg/day	19–70 years	600 IU[a]/day
51+ years	1200 mg/day	71+ years	800 IU/day

Source: Institute of Medicine (US) Committee to Review Dietary Reference Intakes for Vitamin D and Calcium; In: Ross AC et al. eds. *Dietary Reference Intakes for Calcium and Vitamin D.* Washington (DC): National Academies Press (US); 2011.

[a] International units.

Vitamin D has been investigated in the last few decades for anticancer benefits. While research is ongoing, potential mechanisms include induction of cell differentiation and apoptosis, inhibition of abnormal cell proliferation, and tumor angiogenesis. A recent meta-analysis found serum vitamin D levels at diagnosis to be strongly predictive of survival.[64]

Treatment Options

Surgery

The most common surgical interventions are lumpectomy, mastectomy, and breast reconstruction. While there are no nutrition-related side effects, it is recommended to ensure that the daily protein needs of 1–1.2 g/kg are met.

Chemotherapy

Chemotherapy was traditionally given in the breast cancer population as an adjuvant treatment, that is, after a surgical procedure to remove the tumor. However, it is increasingly employed as a neoadjuvant therapy to assess the tumor's response to the treatment, reduce the quantity of tissue resected, and target any cells outside the immediate breast region.

Side effects of chemotherapy vary based on type of drug, dose, and single- versus multiple-agent therapy; frequency of treatment; and individual differences. See Appendices 6.1 and 6.2 for specific interventions related to each drug or symptom.

Common therapeutic drugs used for breast cancer:

- Capecitabine (Xeloda)
- Carboplatin (Paraplatin)
- Cyclophosphamide (Cytoxan)
- Docetaxel (Taxotere)
- Doxorubicin (Adriamycin)
- Epirubicin (Ellence)
- Fluorouracil (5-FU)
- Gemcitabine (Gemzar)
- Ixabepilone (Ixempra)
- Methotrexate (MTX)
- Paclitaxel (Taxol)
- Paclitaxel albumin-stabilized nanoparticle formulation (Abraxane)
- Vinorelbine (Navelbine)

Common multiple-agent chemotherapy regimen acronyms used in breast cancer:

- TAC (Taxotere/Adriamycin/Cytoxan)
- A/C, then T (Adriamycin/Cytoxan, usually followed by Taxol)
- THP (Taxotere/Herceptin/Perjeta)
- TCHP (Taxotere/Cytoxan/Herceptin/Perjeta)[65]

Endocrine Therapy

Common Side Effects of Common Endocrine Therapies

Treatment	Nutrition-Related Side Effect	Nutrition Recommendations
Tamoxifen (Nolvadex)	Mild nausea	Take with a glass of water
Anastrozole (Arimidex)	Mild nausea	
Exemestane (Aromasin)	Mild nausea, abdominal pain	Take with food
Letrozole (Femara)	Nausea, weight gain	May elevate cholesterol levels
Fulvestrant (Faslodex)	Nausea, vomiting, diarrhea, constipation	
Leuprolide(Lupron)	None	
Goserelin (Zoladex)	None	

Monoclonal Antibodies

Common Side Effects of Biologic Agents

Agent	Nutrition-Related Side Effect	Nutrition Recommendations
Pertuzumab (Perjeta)	Nausea, diarrhea, mucositis	
Lapatinib (Tykerb)	Nausea, vomiting, diarrhea	Take 1 hour before, or 1 hour after eating; no grapefruit juice
Everolimus (Afinitor)	Mucositis, diarrhea	Take with water, with or without food; monitor serum lipids
Trastuzumab (Herceptin)	Diarrhea	

Radiation Therapy

Common Radiation Treatment Areas in Breast Cancer

Area of Body	Nutrition-Related Side Effect	Nutrition Recommendations
Breast/chest wall	Minimal	Protein intake 1–1.2 g/kg daily
Intraoperative radiation therapy (IORT)	None	None
Brain	Potential nausea/vomiting, hyperglycemia	Monitor blood glucose levels
Hip/spine	Minimal	None

Nutrition Intervention Summary

Dietitians are most frequently called upon in this population to manage nutrition impact symptoms during chemotherapy, provide counseling and support to guide food choices. In the survivorship phase, dietitians remain indispensable to help patients implement a plant-based, heart-healthy diet and work toward weight loss, if indicated. Finally, dietitians can encourage weight-bearing exercise and assure adequate calcium and vitamin D intake to reduce the risk of osteoporosis.

ESOPHAGEAL, HEAD AND NECK

Introduction

Cancers of the esophagus or head and neck are often very distressing due to the potential impairment of speech, swallowing and breathing and frequent effects on the patient's physical appearance and social functioning.[66] Patients with esophageal cancer (EC) and head and neck cancer (HNC) have one of the highest rates of malnutrition, with 25%–50% of these patients identified as nutritionally compromised prior to diagnosis or treatment, and nutrition status is likely to worsen with treatment initiation.[66,67] Significant weight loss and malnutrition are indicative of poor prognosis and are associated with decreased physical functioning and quality of life, and may reduce response to treatment or cause treatment delay, which may result in shorter periods of remission and increase mortality.[68,69] Early assessment and management by an RD and speech and language pathologist (SLP) along with effective symptom management are imperative to achieve best nutrition and quality of life outcomes.[70]

EC is the eighth most common cancer in the world and its prevalence continues to rise in the United States.[71] EC is commonly classified into two types: squamous cell carcinomas (SCC), and adenocarcinomas of the esophagus (AE).[71–73] In 2013, 17,990 cases of EC were diagnosed and 15,210 deaths reported. Early diagnosis, localized stage, and early treatment intervention can improve outcome and more than double survival. The 5-year survival for all cases of EC is 19%.[72–75]

Head and neck cancers (HNCs) account for 3% of all cancer cases in the United States. In 2013, 41,380 cases of HNC were diagnosed and 7890 deaths reported.[76–78] Five main types of HNC exist in the United States, including oral and oropharyngeal cancer, salivary gland cancer, laryngeal and hypopharyngeal cancer, nasopharyngeal cancer, and nasal cavity and paranasal sinus cavity.[79] Similar to EC, early detection and early stage increases the chance of survival. Five-year survival rates for HNC are approximately 90% when detected and treated while in early stages 1 and 2, but are much lower in advanced-stage disease.[79]

Risk Factors

Both EC and HNC are most commonly diagnosed in males. EC cases are three to four times more common in men than women, and the median age of diagnosis is 67 years.[72–75] The most notable and modifiable risk factors for EC, and HNC (oral cavity, oropharynx, hypopharynx, and larynx) are smoking and alcohol consumption. It has been reported that at least 75% of HNCs are caused by tobacco and alcohol use and that most cases of EC are preventable by appropriate diet and avoidance of the associated risk factors.[40] Salivary cancer is an exception; older age and exposure to radiation and toxins, particularly asbestos, in the workplace, are common risk factors. Infections from *Helicobacter pylori* and human papillomavirus (HPV) are also risk factors for SCC of the esophagus and oropharyngeal cancers.[78] The Centers of Disease Control (CDC) reported more than 2370 cases of HPV-associated oropharyngeal cancers are diagnosed in women and nearly 9360 cases in men each year in the United States.[78] Esophageal achalasia, an esophageal motility disorder, also increases risk of EC. Infection with Epstein–Barr virus has also been identified as a risk factor for nasopharynx and salivary gland cancer.[40]

Gastroesophageal reflux disease (GERD) is a primary risk factor for AE due to the damage that occurs to the esophageal tissue from the gastric acids. GERD also increases the risk of developing Barrett's esophagus, which is associated with a 30–60-fold increase in the risk of AE.[80] Recent studies have identified that obesity (classified as BMI >40 kg/m^2) elevates the risk of esophageal adenocarcinoma independent of other risk factors, especially in males, and even more prevalent when BMI >40 and GERD exist together.[80]

As mentioned, alcohol intake and tobacco usage are the greatest risk factors, although there is some evidence to support that consumption of processed meats, red meats, and certain preserved or salted foods may increase risk of HNCs and ECs.[40]

Symptoms and Support

The most common symptoms of HNCs are a nonhealing lump or sore, a sore throat that does not go away, swallowing difficulty (dysphagia), and a change or hoarseness of the voice.[77] Unfortunately, symptoms of EC do not usually occur until the disease is developing into a more advanced stage. When symptoms do occur, patients often experience dysphagia, heartburn-like symptoms, and pain, hoarseness, coughing, anorexia, and unintentional weight loss.[77]

AICR Guidelines and Diet Recommendations for Prevention

There are a few studies that show that regular consumption of nonstarchy vegetables, fruits, and carotenoid-rich foods may have the potential to protect against HNC and EC. Foods containing vitamin C, fiber, folate, pyridoxine, and vitamin E may also provide protection against EC.[40]

Estimated Energy and Nutrient Requirements

It is generally acknowledged that the energy expenditure (EE) for most cancer patients is increased, although some recent studies demonstrate that EE may vary between various cancer diagnoses. A small study estimated energy requirements of EC patients between 30 and 35 kcal/kg, which is consistent with the usual recommendations for nutrition repletion for oncology patients.[81,82] Energy needs for obese patients are recommended at 21–25 kcal/kg actual body weight.[81] Protein requirements, assuming normal renal function, range between 1 and 1.5 g/kg for stable, nonstressed patients, and 1.5 and 2.0 g/kg for stressed or nutritionally compromised patients.[81,82] Fluid needs are typical of other patients without heart failure or renal impairment at 30–35 mL/kg, although may be higher in patients experiencing GI losses or drains. It is recommended that HNC and EC patients take a vitamin and mineral supplement to meet 100% of the DRI, particularly being mindful that many of these patients' oral intakes may have been inadequate for some time related to symptoms or lifestyle that may have included excessive alcohol consumption prior to diagnosis.

Nutrition Support

Dysphagia and weight loss are the most common nutrition impact symptoms in EC and are present in over 70% of patients diagnosed worldwide.[83] Despite aggressive nutrition interventions, including diet modifications, oral nutrition supplementation, symptom management, and medication management, oral intakes may not sustain nutritional status throughout aggressive chemotherapy and/or radiation therapy, and may require EN via a percutaneous endoscopic gastrostomy (PEG) tube or jejunostomy tube (J-tube). Temporary feeding tubes will also be placed after surgical resections from glossectomy, esophagectomy, base of tongue or pharynx tumor excisions, and tracheostomy. Prophylactic feeding tubes remain controversial but have resulted in fewer hospital admissions for dehydration and malnutrition, fewer treatment interruptions, and/or delays, and maintain a higher quality of life during treatment when compared to patients solely relying on oral intakes.[84] Nutrition assessment is recommended for patients prior to treatment and frequent reassessments throughout treatment to ensure appropriate nutrition intervention are in place to prevent further nutrition decline or treatment delay. Modifications to enteral feeding formulas, schedules, water flushes, or addition of motility agents may be needed as treatment continues and requires frequent monitoring. Close follow-up after completion of therapy is essential to help avoid long-term dependence on enteral feedings and to support the transition back to an oral diet.

Treatment Options

Treatment for EC and HNC often include esophageal dilation, chemotherapy, radiation therapy, chemoradiation (CRT), targeted therapy, and surgery.[73,85] Treatment options will be determined by the patient and physician and often depends on tumor stage, size and location, primary subtype, metastasis of tumor (if present), and patient's overall health and other comorbidities.

Chemotherapy and Nutrition

Chemotherapy may be used alone or as either neoadjuvant (before) or adjuvant (after) therapy in combination with radiation or surgery. Advances in chemoradiation have led to increased survival and local and regional tumor control for patients with EC and HNC, but often cause significant toxicity to the patient.[86] Below is a list of common chemotherapeutic drugs commonly used to treat EC and HNC. See the Appendix 6.1 for specific interventions related to each drug or symptom.

Common chemotherapeutic drugs used in EC and HNC:

- Bevacizumab (Avastin®)
- Cetuximab (Erbitux®)
- Cisplatin (as single-agent or combined modality) with 5-fluorouracil (5-FU®) or capecitabine (Xeloda®)
- Capecitabine (Xeloda®)
- Oxaliplatin and either 5-FU or capecitabine
- ECF: epirubicin (Ellence®), cisplatin, and 5-FU
- DCF: docetaxel (Taxotere®), cisplatin, and 5-FU
- Carboplatin and paclitaxel (Taxol®)

Other chemotherapy or targeted therapy drugs that have been used in these cancers:

- Doxorubicin (Adriamycin®)
- Bleomycin
- Mitomycin
- Vinorelbine (Navelbine®)
- Topotecan
- Ifosafamide
- Irinotecan (Camptosar®)
- Trastuzumab (Herceptin®)[87,88]

Radiation Therapy and Nutrition

Radiation therapy acts by directing x-rays to cancerous cells or regions to cause DNA damage, inhibiting the cells' ability to replicate. Rapidly dividing cells are the most susceptible to radiation damage, such as the lining of the oral and gut mucosa and blood and hair cells.[76] Radiation may be used alone or combined with chemotherapy. It may also be given preoperatively in an attempt to shrink tumors or postoperatively to help ensure that tumor bed and surrounding margins or lymph nodes are clear of disease. The goal of therapy is to eradicate tumor cells while minimizing damage to healthy tissues. The amount of radiation a patient receives is measured in gray (Gy) and the number of treatments a person receives is referenced in fractions (fx). Radiation has a cumulative effect which means that side effects continue to worsen with each additional fraction received, with most side effects starting between 10 and 15 fractions (after 2–3 weeks of treatment) and intensifying throughout the remainder of therapy. A common treatment for EC and HNC may include CRT, 2.0 per fraction to 70 Gy in 7 weeks with single-agent Cisplatin given every 1–3 weeks.[89] Below is a list of potential side effects from radiation therapy and nutrition management. Radiation may also exacerbate tooth decay and patients may be required to have previously damaged teeth removed prior to therapy.[67,76] Late side effects may occur months or even years after completion of therapy. Owing to the rapid decline in nutritional status that can occur during radiation to the head and neck or esophagus and the potential need for alternative nutrition, close monitoring throughout the entire course of therapy and recovery is strongly recommended.

Common Side Effects of Common Radiation Treatments

Nutrition-Related Side Effect	Nutrition Recommendations
Xerostomia/thick saliva	Eat small frequent meals
	Alternate bites and sips at meals
	Add extra sauces, gravy, and broths to foods
	Maintain adequate hydration, sip throughout the day. Suck on hard candies, frozen fruits. Chew sugar-free gum
	Avoid alcohol, caffeine, acidic, or spicy foods
	Use humidifier at home to help moisten the air
Trismus	Eat slowly with small bites of food. Modify food textures to optimize intakes
	Use oral nutrition supplements
	Follow aspiration precautions
	SLP consult
Oral candidiasis	Practice good oral hygiene
	Choose soft-textured, low-acid foods
	Avoid sugar or yeast-derived foods. May try 1 tbsp yogurt held in mouth, 5 minutes daily

Surgery and Nutrition

The goal of surgery is to remove the tumor with a margin of healthy tissue. If the cancer has spread, some surrounding lymph nodes may also need to be removed. Surgeries to treat EC or HNC will commonly result in swallowing difficulties, dependent on the degree and site of the resection. Side effects of surgery may also include pain, swelling, structural deformities such as tooth loss or hemiglossectomy (partial removal of the tongue), or tracheostomy, which may make it difficult to chew or swallow after surgery and potentially limit oral intakes.[67,76] EC patients eligible for surgery commonly undergo either esophagectomy or esophagogastrectomy with jejunostomy tube placement. Data show that intensive nutrition support provided by an RD is associated with weight maintenance and fewer postoperative complications in these patients.[90] Frequent monitoring by an SLP is also recommended to assist in preservation and/or regaining of muscle function to the affected areas. Potential side effects of these surgeries are listed in the table below.

Common Side Effects of Common Surgical Procedures

Treatment	Nutrition-Related Side Effect	Enteral Nutrition	Oral Nutrition Recommendations
Esophagectomy or esophagogastrectomy	Dumping syndrome (early or late)	Temporary jejunostomy tube [a]See feeding recommendations below	Antidumping diet • Limit foods in concentrated sugars • Limit fats and fried, greasy foods • Increase soluble fiber foods • Drink liquids 30 minutes before/after meals • Eat 5–6 small frequent meals • Eat slowly
	Reflux		Eat small frequent meals Antireflux diet
	Esophagus or gastric dysmotility		Low-fat, low-fiber diet is recommended for dysmotility, and possible initiation of motility agents
	Early satiety		Eat 5–6 small frequent meals Choose carbohydrate- and protein-dense foods Use oral supplements between meals to help meet needs and prevent weight loss
Tracheostomy		Gastrostomy tube (PEG tube) with or without ability to take oral intakes [a]See feeding recommendations below	When determined to have safe swallowing function, often patients will be able to tolerate liquids and soft foods, and occasionally solids Monitor for ability to wean EN
Glossectomy—full or partial		Temporary nasogastric tube or PEG tube [a]See feeding recommendations below	SLP therapy Once safe, swallow function established, diet will start with variety of viscous liquids, then slowly advance to soft/semisolid foods as tolerated

[a] Recommended Enteral Jejunostomy Feedings Post Esophagectomy/Esophagogastectomy.

Early initiation of feedings with a full-strength isotonic polymeric formula is recommended, 1 versus 1.5 kcal/mL based on patient needs. Typically, feedings start at 24 hours continuously, and then transitions to nocturnal feedings to help optimize oral feedings once diet is advanced. If a standard formula is not tolerated, then transition to semielemental or elemental formula. These formulas are typically reserved for patients with small bowel dysfunction or malabsorption.

Recommended Enteral Feedings for Gastrostomy Tubes Post Tracheostomy, Glossectomy or Chemotherapy, and Radiation.

Use full-strength standard formula, typically 1.5–2.0 kcal/mL, but individually selected based on patients' energy needs. Bolus feeding, typically 3–4 times per day, is preferred to help simulate regular meal times and usually well tolerated. If a patient is unable to tolerate bolus feedings, then transitioning to gravity feeding bags or even a feeding pump is indicated.

Regardless of tube type, it is important to provide adequate hydration via water flushes to meet hydration needs, as many of these patients are temporarily unable to take oral intake. Use of modulars such as protein or fiber powders may be indicated to meet nutrient needs or symptom management.

Diet

Patients with EC and HNC are at increased risk for malnutrition and cachexia requiring a high-calorie, high-protein diet and frequently supplement with oral nutrition beverages. Diet modifications are often required to help support patients throughout chemotherapy and radiation therapy due to multiple nutrition impact symptoms or alterations to the GI tract as a result of surgical alteration or tumor obstruction. The RD will help direct patient toward appropriate texture modifications, nutrient-dense food and liquids, adequate hydration, and adjust timing of meals and snacks to maximize intake.

Medications and Supplements Commonly Used

Patients may require a variety of medications to achieve optimal symptom management throughout therapy, including antiemetics, acid reflux and pain medications, stool softeners, antimotility agents, and soothing mouth rinses. Ensuring appropriate medication administration and tolerance is imperative in this population as many of these patients suffer from dysphagia and may need medications modified to liquid or patch forms when available, or even administered through feeding tubes. It is important to review medications carefully as some drugs are not safe to crush and alternatives may need to be prescribed.

Glutamine is an amino acid that is used by rapidly dividing cells and has been shown to help protect the upper and lower GI tract mucosa from harmful effects of chemotherapy and radiation therapy. Multiple studies have proven the benefit in reduction of severity and duration of oral mucositis and esophagitis.[91] There are some concerns that glutamine might stimulate tumor growth, and therefore negatively impact the outcomes of anticancer treatment, although studies showing this are very limited (*in vitro*) and further evaluation is needed.[92] Typical dosing for glutamine during radiation therapy provides 10 g three times daily, mixed into 3–4 ounces of a liquid, usually juice or water, or even applesauce or yogurt. Glutamine usage should be discontinued after side effects have improved after therapy is completed.

Oral nutrition supplement packets containing β-hydroxy-β-methylbutyrate (HMB), and essential amino acids glutamine and arginine, may also be recommended during radiation and recovery. A preliminary study showed the potential for increase in weight and fat-free mass and may potentially inhibit cachexia.[81,93] Additional studies demonstrated the potential to lessen radiation-induced inflammation and mucosal atrophy and prevention of radiation dermatitis.[94,95] Consumption of one packet mixed into 8 ounces of water or juice twice daily orally or via PEG tube is recommended to try to achieve these results.

Medihoney is a medical-grade honey that has the potential to accelerate wound healing and is more commonly used topically on open wounds or burns, but can be safely consumed orally to treat mucositis and esophagitis. Recommended dosing is 1 tbsp taken orally 15 minutes prior to radiation therapy, 15 minutes after radiation therapy, and one additional dose 6 hours later.

Nutrition Intervention Summary

EC and HNC patients are a complex population with a wide range of nutritional challenges. Early nutrition intervention by an RD prior to treatment initiation and ongoing throughout treatment and recovery are crucial. Preventing decline in the patient's nutritional status by limiting weight loss and preserving lean body mass, in addition to effective symptom management, improves treatment outcomes by preventing treatment delays and unplanned hospitalizations, while also improving patients' performance status and quality of life.

GYNECOLOGIC

Gynecologic cancers are those involving female reproductive organs found in the pelvic region of the body, including endometrial, cervical, and ovarian. Treatment options depend on cancer type and stage, and include surgery, radiation, and chemotherapy either alone or in combination.

The endometrium is the lining of the uterus, with tissue that is regenerated regularly during the menstrual cycle. Because symptoms of this cancer type are exhibited early on, diagnosis can be made early.[96] In women, endometrial cancer is considered the most common of the gynecologic cancers, with nearly 53,000 new cases in the United States in 2014, most in women over the age of

60.[96,97] Eighty-two percent of women with this cancer type survive up to 5 years. Research shows that increase in overall body adipose tissue, particularly in the abdominal region, increases the risk of developing endometrial cancer.[96] Diets that are high in refined carbohydrates and sugary beverages are also believed to increase risk.[97] Regular physical activity is considered protective against developing this disease.[96]

The ovaries are organs responsible for the production of eggs, in addition to hormones such as estrogen and progesterone, in the female body.[98] Ovarian cancer afflicts about 21,000 women and is the ninth most common cancer among women in the United States, but it is considered the deadliest of the female cancers.[97] In 2014, there were 21,980 new cases and 44.6% of those with ovarian cancer survive 5 years. Overweight and obesity can increase the risk of ovarian cancer. Family history, inherited risk through BRCA 1 and BRCA 2 genes, and being the age of 55 and older are factors that increase the risk of developing this disease.[97]

The cervix is found at the base of the uterus, being the portion of tissue connecting to the vagina. It is the least common of the gynecologic cancers, with 12,360 new cases in the United States in 2014; 68% of women survive 5 years with this disease.[99] Human papilloma virus is considered a risk factor. At this time, there is no strong evidence connecting diet, amount of physical activity, or weight to increased risk. Further research is warranted.[97]

Treatment Options

Treatments include surgery, chemotherapy, or surgery/chemotherapy.[100–102] The NCCN guidelines can be referenced for specific surgeries based on stage of cancer. Note that patients may require the placement of an ostomy after surgery. Please see GI cancers for nutrition intervention guidelines, and Appendices 6.1 and 6.2 for common chemotherapy side effects and nutritional management of symptoms. Radiation treatments for cervical cancer can include external beam radiation therapy (EBRT) and brachytherapy.

Common Chemotherapy Regimens by Tumor Site
(see Appendices 6.1 and 6.2 for common side effects and nutritional management)

Uterine

Combination regimens:
- Docetaxel/gemcitabine
- Doxorubicin/ifosfamide
- Doxorubicin/dacarbazine
- Gemcitabine/decarbazine
- Gemcitabine/vinorelbine

Combination regimens:
- Docetaxel/gemcitabine
- Doxorubicin/ifosfamide
- Doxorubicin/dacarbazine
- Gemcitabine/decarbazine
- Gemcitabine/vinorelbine

Single-agent options:
- Dacarbazine
- Doxorubicin
- Epirubicin
- Gemcitabine
- Ifosfamide
- Liposomal doxorubicin
- Pazopanib
- Temozolomide
- Vinorelbine
- Docetaxel

Ovarian

- Taxanes (Paclitaxel, Docetaxel)
- Platinum (Cisplatin, Carboplatin)
- Bevacizumab (Avastin)

Cervical

- Cisplatin
- Paclitaxel
- Bevacizumab
- Carboplatin
- Topotecan
- Cisplatin/gemcitabine
- 5-FU (5-fluorouracil)
- Irinotecan
- Mitomycin
- Pemetrexed
- Vinorelbine

Nutrition Intervention Summary

Patients may initially present in good health status with no or few nutritional impact symptoms. At this point, basic nutrition guidelines are appropriate to maintaining adequate nutritional status. With initiation of treatment, nutrition-related side effect management becomes paramount. Pre- and postsurgical health complications that may hinder surgical outcomes, such as uncontrolled blood sugar levels or excessive body fatness, must be addressed. Patients may undergo chemotherapy and/or radiation treatments. Nutrition-related side effects should be mitigated with attempts in improving the patient's quality of life. Nutrition support may or may not be warranted; the goal of patient care should be the context of intervention within the interdisciplinary team.

LUNG

Introduction

Lung cancer remains the leading cause of cancer-related death and is the second most common cancer in men and women.[103] There are three main types of lung cancer: non-small cell lung cancer (85%), small cell lung cancer (10%–15%), and lung carcinoid tumor (5%).[104] Various treatments for lung cancer can pose many nutrition challenges. Patients often experience side effects that range from esophagitis, dysphagia, anorexia, nausea and vomiting, taste changes, and fatigue. Significant weight loss and malnutrition can lead to poor outcomes and may reduce response to treatment or cause delays in treatment.

Treatment Options

The primary treatments for lung cancer include chemotherapy and targeted therapy, radiation therapy, and surgery. Depending on the stage of the disease, two or more modalities may be recommended.

Surgery can be used to diagnose, stage, and treat lung cancer. Surgical options include lobectomy (removal of an entire lobe), pneumonectomy (removal of the entire lung), and wedge resection (removal of a section of the lung).[105] Depending on the histology, cytology and stage of the lung cancer, surgery can be a successful option for patients with a curative intent. The type of operation the physician recommends depends on how well a patient will tolerate the procedure, size of the tumor, and location and extent of the disease.

Surgery

Surgical intervention for lung cancer can be complex so proper caloric and protein intake is important for healing and decreasing nutrition-related complications. Often, lung cancer patients are diagnosed at later stages, which is associated with weight loss. A low BMI prior to surgery has been linked to increased mortality.[106,107] Patients with normal nutritional status had a median survival of 58 months compared to 36 months in patients with impaired nutritional status.[108]

Radiation

Radiation therapy uses beams of high energy to injure and kill cancer cells, shrink tumors, and stop the growth of cancer cells.[105] The most common types of radiation therapy delivery methods are external beam radiation and internal radiation. External beam radiation involves focusing radiation from outside the body onto the cancerous cells within the body. Radiation oncologists can use sophisticated software and imaging techniques to adjust the size and shape of the beam while maximizing the dose of radiation to the tumor. This helps to minimize the impact on healthy surrounding tissue and organs and lessen side effects from treatment. The number of external beam radiation treatments can vary from days to weeks depending on the physician's plan of care for the patient.

Internal radiation therapy, also known as high dose rate (HDR) brachytherapy, involves placing radioactive material into the tumor itself or near the cancer cells. Brachytherapy is especially helpful to shrink tumors of the bronchi, relieving symptoms of breathing difficulty.[109]

Radiation can be used at different times during the course of the treatment. Radiation can be used as the main treatment for lung cancer with or without chemotherapy, particularly if the tumor cannot be removed by surgery. It can also be used after surgery to kill any residual cancer cells that are still present. The physician may also recommend radiation before surgery in conjunction with chemotherapy to help shrink the lung tumor to make it easier to operate on.

Owing to the nature of radiation therapy and the area of treatment, patients often experience painful swallowing, dysphagia, mucus, and fatigue.

The tissues of the esophagus can become irritated and sore and patients often complain of painful swallowing or having a "lump" in the throat. Symptoms of esophagitis may not become apparent until the second or third week of radiation and can subside two to three weeks after completion of treatment. Dietary modifications include chopping foods into small pieces, avoiding acidic or spicy foods, drinking oral nutritional supplements, and eating soft or moistened foods. Another side effect of radiation can be thick mucus buildup in the esophagus. Patients often complain of thick ropey mucus that can cause them to gag or have reflux. Encouraging patients to drink at least 6–8 cups of water per day, temporarily avoiding dairy products, and drinking lemon or lime beverages can help reduce mucus. Other options to help reduce mucus include acupuncture and the use of glutamine, which has been shown to improve side effects of radiation.[92] Frequent visits to a speech therapist can also be helpful. A speech therapist can provide appropriate exercises and techniques to maintain muscle integrity and swallowing to help reduce long-term complications. In addition, the speech therapist may recommend diet texture changes or thickened liquids and may refer patients back to the dietitian for guidance. Depending on the severity of the radiation esophagitis, the physician may prescribe pain medication or swish and swallow numbing agents to reduce painful swallowing. Some patients may often require feeding tubes to provide nutrition while bypassing the esophagus.

Fatigue during radiation is one of the most common side effects. Radiation fatigue can often lead to patient inactivity and decrease of lean muscle mass. Patients with weight loss greater than 5% and fatigue correlated with a low Karnofsky performance score and quality of life.[106] Adequate protein intake and increasing physical activity as tolerated has been shown to improve visceral protein stores. Patients may benefit from seeing a physical therapist.

Chemotherapy and Targeted Therapy

Chemotherapy is a drug used to destroy cancer cells. Targeted therapies are drugs that can block the growth and spread of cancer. Depending on the agent, dose, and frequency of chemotherapy and targeted therapy, the nutritional implications vary. Appendix 6.1 is a chart that includes therapies commonly associated with lung cancer treatment and the nutritional side effects.

Prevention with Nutrition

There are certain nutrients that can increase and decrease lung cancer development risk. Items that can decrease risk include fruits, foods containing carotenoids, nonstarchy vegetables, foods containing selenium, foods containing quercetin, and physical activity.[40] While factors that can increase risk based on their current research include arsenic in drinking water (mainly in unregulated water supplies), beta-carotene supplements (not foods), red meat, processed meat, total fat, butter, retinol supplements, and low body fatness.[40]

Nutrition Intervention Summary

Patients undergoing treatment for lung cancer will have significant nutritional challenges. All patients should be assessed to determine nutritional status prior to treatment. Based on the patient plan of care, continued surveillance during treatment is warranted to help patients manage treatment related side effects, prevent weight loss, and improve outcomes.

PROSTATE

Introduction

Prostate cancer treatment depends on the stage of the cancer. If cancer is advanced, hormone therapy (or androgen deprivation therapy), chemotherapy, radiation, and/or a combination may be used for treatment. The 5-year survival rate is near 100%, with a median survival rate of 1–3 years for metastatic prostate cancer.[40] All treatments for prostate cancer have potential side effects. Side effects and nutrition recommendations to aid with side effects are listed in this chapter for chemotherapy, radiation therapy, and surgery.

Nutrition, including diet and lifestyle, play a role in prostate cancer rates worldwide.[40] A plant-based diet high in cruciferous vegetables has been linked with a reduction in prostate cancer, including metastasis and recurrence.[110] There is also evidence that suggests prostate cancer progression may be affected by diet and lifestyle choices.[111]

Nutrition Recommendations

Lycopene is a phytochemical found in red fruits and vegetables, such as tomatoes, watermelon, and grapefruit. High-lycopene foods have shown to potentially prevent prostate cancer recurrence.[112] Strive to get at least one lycopene-rich food daily.

- Adding whole soy products into the diet may have benefits for prostate cancer patients. Substituting soymilk for cow's milk or snacking on soy nuts are both good ways to get soy intake.[113]
- High intake of allium-rich foods, such as garlic and onions, may help prevent recurrence of prostate cancer and are also beneficial for your heart.[114]
- Studies show high intake of dairy is linked to prostate cancer.[115] Eat or drink low-fat dairy in moderation to reduce risk of recurrence. Substitute soymilk as mentioned previously for extra benefit.
- Studies have shown that 1 cup or 8 fl oz of 100% pomegranate juice daily may slow the progression of localized cancer. It also has been shown to potentially lengthen the time in which it took the prostate specific antigen (PSA) score to double in a research study involving prostate cancer patients.[116]
- Research has shown that ground flaxseed may help decrease prostate cancer proliferation.[117] The goal is to incorporate three tablespoons daily into foods and smoothies.
- Study showed that six cups daily of green tea for 3–8 weeks showed a decrease in PSA levels compared to the control group.[118] It also showed to help reduce the proinflammatory marker nF-Kappa B.
- Research shows turmeric may aid in stopping the formation of metastases in prostate cancer patients.[119]

Treatment Options

Chemotherapy

See Appendix 6.2 for side effect management.

- Lupron
- Firmagon
- Zoladex
- Trelstar
- Casodex
- Zytiga (Abiraterone)
- Xtandi (Enzalutamide)

Radiation Therapy

Radiation therapy (also called radiotherapy) is a prostate cancer treatment that uses targeted energy to kill cancer cells and stop them from spreading. At low doses, radiation is used as an x-ray to see inside your body and take pictures, such as x-rays of your teeth and bones. Radiation used in prostate cancer treatment works in much the same way, except that it is given in higher doses. Radiation therapy can be external beam (when a machine outside your body aims radiation at prostate cancer cells) or internal (when radiation is temporarily or permanently put inside your body, in or near the prostate cancer cells). Sometimes people get both forms of radiation therapy at different intervals. Radiation therapy is a commonly used cancer treatment option. Approximately 60% of people fighting cancer receive radiation therapy. Sometimes, radiation therapy is the only cancer treatment people need.

Common Side Effects of Common Radiation Treatments

Treatment	Nutrition-Related Side Effect
Cyberknife (typically 1–5 treatments)	Diarrhea
EBRT	Diarrhea, inflammation in GI tract, lactose intolerance
	Nausea/vomiting
	Fatigue
Radioactive injectable given IV (Xofigo) indicated for metastatic prostate cancer	Diarrhea
	Nausea/vomiting
	Fatigue
Deep tissue hyperthermia (typically given in combination with chemotherapy and/or radiation therapy)	Fatigue
Brachytherapy	Fatigue

Surgery

Surgery is a common choice to try to cure prostate cancer if it is not thought to have spread outside the gland (stage T1 or T2 cancers).

The main type of surgery for prostate cancer is known as a radical prostatectomy. Nutrition-related side effects include loss of lean body mass, nausea/vomiting, and fatigue. See Appendix 6.2 for symptom management. Other treatments include deep tissue hyperthermia (DTH) and brachytherapy. Fatigue is the most common symptom.

Nutrition Intervention Summary

Nutrition is an integral part of prostate cancer throughout all stages of treatment. Chemotherapy, radiation therapy, and surgery are all options that may cause symptoms for patients with prostate cancer. Once prostate cancer is in remission, it is recommended to follow the American Institute of Cancer Research guidelines. These guidelines encourage a diet high in plant-based proteins, fruits, and vegetables, and omega three fatty acids.[40] These guidelines also encourage decreasing simple sugars, salt, and sodium from the diet.

PALLIATIVE CARE

Overview

What is palliative care?

> Palliative care is an exercise in forward planning and prevention rather than a model of crisis intervention.
>
> **Dr. Ronald S. Schonwetter**

Palliative care is an approach that improves the quality of life of patients and their families facing the problems associated with life-threatening illness, through the prevention and relief of suffering by means of early identification and impeccable assessment and treatment of pain and other problems, physical, psychosocial and spiritual.

World Health Organization

Palliative care

- Provides relief from pain and other distressing symptoms
- Affirms life and regards dying as a normal process
- Intends neither to hasten nor postpone death
- Integrates the psychological and spiritual aspects of patient care
- Offers a support system to help patients live as actively as possible until death
- Offers a support system to help the family cope during the patients' illness and in their own bereavement
- Uses a team approach to address the needs of patients and their families, including bereavement counseling, if indicated
- Will enhance quality of life, and may also positively influence the course of illness
- Is applicable early in the course of illness, in conjunction with other therapies that are intended to prolong life, such as chemotherapy or radiation therapy, and includes those investigations needed to better understand and manage distressing clinical complications

Comparison of Palliative Care versus Hospice Care

Palliative Care	Hospice Care
Provide QOL throughout treatment	Provides QOL toward end of life
Provides care for caregivers + patient	Provides care for caregivers + patient
Prevent/treat symptoms of diagnosis	Provides medications, supplies, equipment, and hospital services related to the terminal illness
Begins at time of initial diagnosis	Begins with less than 6 months left to live
Billed through insurance as a typical treatment	Reimbursed to hospice company at a daily rate for all services

Model of Palliative Care for Oncology

Palliative care is specialized medical care for people with serious illnesses. It focuses on providing patients with relief from the symptoms and stress of a serious illness. The goal is to improve quality of life for both the patient and the family.[120]

Palliative care is provided by a specially trained team of doctors, nurses, dietitians, and other specialists who work together with a patient's other doctors to provide an extra layer of support. It is appropriate at any age and at any stage in a serious illness and can be provided along with curative treatment.[120,121]

Challenges That Occur with Oncology Patients

What role does nutrition play in oncologic palliative care?

In palliative care, nutrition has a major impact on oncology patients' quality of life. Symptoms can not only adversely affect food and fluid intake, but a patient's nutritional intake can also influence his/her symptoms and overall well-being.

Although not typically painful, anorexia and cachexia in oncology patients are unmistakable indications that the underlying disease is not under control and that death is approaching. Food and eating are some of the highest pleasures in life and often fade away in affected patients and can often lead to a condition called cachexia-related suffering (CRS).[122] CRS is defined as negative emotions associated with reduced nutritional intake and weight loss.[122] CRS affects both patients and caregivers. Patients may be embarrassed about the visibility of loss of weight or feel harassed by their caregivers. Caregivers may feel personally rejected.[122]

Oncology patients often experience a series of losses: loss of weight and the desire to eat; loss of the ability to smell, taste, chew, and swallow food; loss of the ability to digest and absorb nutrients; and loss of the ability to eliminate waste products independently.[120,123,124]

Multistep Approach to Nutritional Care of Palliative Care Patients

Step 1: Nutrition screening and assessment
Step 2: Developing a care plan
Step 3: Recognizing changes in nutritional needs
Step 4: Education: patient, family, multidisciplinary team

Palliative Care for Oncology Patients

Cancer is known to be among a long list of chronically progressive diseases that unfortunately may lose their therapeutic options. When in conjunction with other comorbidities/diseases such as HIV infection, COPD, CHF, or neurologic disorders, the challenges can be even greater. Anorexia and cachexia can cause negative emotions and may be unmistakable indications that the underlying disease is not under control and that death is approaching.

Psychosocial issues related to sustaining life with food are often times known as CRS. CRS is defined as negative emotions associated with reduced nutritional intake and weight loss. CRS is explored in advanced cancer diseases and may manifest into what is known as cancer cachexia syndrome (CCS). CRS and its relationship to CCS include aspects of distress suffered by patients, caregivers, partners, and a patient's health care professionals. CRS is more prevalent in caregivers than in patients. Emotions may be but are not limited to anxiety, anger, feeling upset, bother, concern, frustration, and guilt. Patients may even be embarrassed by their change in appearance or feel harassed by their caregivers. Conversely, caregivers may feel rejected or incompetent if they are declined by the patient.

There are constructive and adverse reactions to CRS. Recognizing the terminal nature of the disease and acceptance is the key to relief of CRS. Instead of solely focusing on food, caregivers may find other ways to care for the patient versus pressuring about food. Adverse reactions can occur if CCS is not recognized or accepted. Adversely encouraging more food intake may put more pressure on the patient verbally and nonverbally. Pushing patients may cause pain, nausea, anticipatory nausea, and even vomiting.

Palliative Care and Nutrition: Artificial Nutrition and Hydration

Artificial hydration is the provision of water or electrolyte solutions through any nonoral route. Artificial nutrition includes PN and EN by nasogastric tube (NGT), percutaneous endoscopic gastrostomy (PEG) tube, percutaneous endoscopic gastrostomy jejunostomy (PEG-J) tube, gastrostomy tube, or gastrojejunostomy tube.[125]

There is limited evidence showing increased survival and quality of life in patients receiving artificial nutrition. Current literature lacks high-quality randomized trials that might yield clear indications and guide practice. The American Gastroenterological Association (AGA) endorses PEG tube placement for prolonged tube feeding (defined as greater than 30 days) and NGT feedings when feeding is required for shorter periods. The American College of Physicians advises that the routine use of PN should be discouraged in patients undergoing chemotherapy and that, when it is used in patients with cancer with malnutrition, physicians should consider the possibility of increased risk. In other countries, PN continues to be used regularly for patients with advanced cancer.[125]

In hospice settings, parenteral hydration is not routine, but may be considered in instances where the patient is experiencing neuropsychiatric symptoms such as delirium, myoclonus, and agitation.[125] Although these symptoms are also related to the dying process and parenteral hydration may not add comfort.

It is important to consider the positive and negative when considering appropriate route of ANH for each individual patient. Consider the table below when considering EN ANH. Per the AGA,

EN is appropriate to consider when the patient cannot or will not eat, the gut is functional, and the patient can tolerate the placement of the device.[126]

Positive Considerations	Negative Considerations
Duration of survival	Pharyngeal/esophageal/bowel perforation
Improved comfort	Accidental bronchial insertion of NG/OG tube
Reduction or healing of pressure ulcer	NGTs fall out about 25% of the time or accidental removal occurs
Reduction in aspiration	Infection at insertion site
Prevents hunger and thirst	Peristomal leaks
	Sepsis
	Necrotizing fascitis
	Fluid overload
	Pain
	Possibility of restraints

Current Levels of Evidence for Artificial Nutrition in the Oncology Population

Type of Artificial Nutrition	Outcome	[a]Classification	[a]Level of Evidence
PN	During chemotherapy	III	B1
Prophylactic EN before treatment in HNC	Weight stabilization	IIa	B2
EN before surgery	GI cancer	IIa	A

[a] Description of classification based on levels of evidence:
IIa—Weight of evidence/opinion is in favor of usefulness/efficacy
III—Intervention is not useful/effective and may be harmful
B1—Limited evidence from single, randomized trial
B2—Limited evidence from other nonrandomized studies
A—Sufficient evidence from multiple randomized trials

Inconsistent results have been generated from randomized studies in patients with a variety of tumors and therapies. Because no statistical benefit from PN has been demonstrated in survival, treatment tolerance, treatment toxicity, or tumor response in patients receiving PN during chemotherapy or radiotherapy, PN has not been consistently used in advanced cancer care in the United States. Subsequent studies evaluating PN and EN remain mixed.[124,125]

PN and EN have been able to improve some nutritional indices, such as body weight, fat mass, nitrogen balance, and whole body potassium. Prealbumin and retinol-binding protein levels increase only with PN. Immune indices such as complement factors and lymphocyte number improve only with EN. PN and EN both appear to prevent further deterioration of the nutritional state and may even show some improvement which will allow for cancer treatment to continue.[124,125]

It is important to reinforce that current data regarding ANH have significant methodological weaknesses and limited evidence for current practice as described above. Providers should critically consider the patient, their wishes, and the overall potential benefits and risks before making a decision in regard to providing or not providing ANH.

Assessment

Nutrition needs will changes as the patient transitions through the palliative care spectrum. In the early phase of palliative care, the goal of nutrition treatment is to manage malnutrition risk and mitigate symptoms. Early identification and management of malnutrition risk improves and protects nutrition status and quality of life (QOL) throughout the stages of treatment and disease. Rescreening should be repeated routinely. Through the patients cancer journey, the nutrition status will change as well as the goals. The presence of cancer cachexia does not always indicate end of life or need for hospice. In the later stages of palliative care, the goal of nutrition therapy should transition to QoL including comfort, symptom relief, and food enjoyment if able. Toward the last days of life, the aim of care should provide comfort for the patient and caregiver.

The assessment should include biochemical data, medical tests, procedures, nutrition-focused physical findings, and client reported history. In the assessment, the RDN should consider the stage of the cancer cachexia.

End of Life

Nutrition care at the end of life requires a sensible, informed, and personalized approach. Helping make the right food choices and removing any anxieties about food and fluid intake often gives valuable relief and comfort to both patients and caregivers and may also provide some precious time.

Both religion and culture play an important role when end-of-life issues are at stake; therefore, it is paramount to explore and understand a patient's religious and cultural background in order to reach a consensus regarding nutrition support.

Checklist to establish religious beliefs, cultural affiliation, and family background when end-of-life decisions are necessary[125]:

- What do they think of the sanctity of life?
- What is their definition of death?
- What is their religious background and how active are they presently?
- What do they believe are causal agents in illness and how do these relate to the dying process?
- What is the patient's social support system?
- Who makes decisions about matters of importance in the family?

When nutrition support is withdrawn, it is important for the clinician to discuss with family/caregivers key points regarding end of life.

The consideration to withdraw nutrition is often not well received; therefore, factual information is necessary.

- Neither thirst nor hunger is experienced at the end of life.
- Lack of fluid and food allows for ketosis and a release of opioids in the brain, which may in fact produce a sense of euphoria.
- Physiological adaptation to lack of nourishment prevents discomfort.
- Dehydration results in azotemia, hypernatremia, and hypercalcemia, which are all assumed to produce a calming effect prior to death.
- Curtailing food and fluid can decrease oral and bronchial secretion, reduce the need to urinate, and ease coughing from pulmonary congestion.
- Withholding artificial nutrition/hydration is not painful and dehydration may actually enhance the comfort during the dying process.

Ethical Considerations[125]

- Advanced directives, living wills, and durable powers of attorney
  - Legal documents that allow individuals to express their decision about end-of-life care to family, friends, and health care providers.
  - Often, living wills or advanced directives do not stipulate whether nutrition interventions, such as ANH, are desired.

Though a patient and family may request artificial nutrition be continued once hospice is established, most insurance companies dictate whether or not PN is a covered benefit and most hospice facilities decide if they will accept the patient even if artificial nutrition and hydration is a known covered benefit.

Professional Consensus Statement on Nutritional Care in Palliative Care Patients[125]

- Nutritional care
  - Essential aspect of palliative care
  - Individualized
  - Fluid through life
    - Nutrition needs are fluid through life and person-to-person. Respect this fluidity and be ready to educate. You are the nutrition expert and you will be educating the patient/care giver/interdisciplinary team
  - Delivered safely and with compassion and dignity
  - Physical/social/cultural/emotional aspects
  - Matter for all palliative care professionals
- Staff and volunteers should receive regular training on nutrition in palliative care
- Health care organizations are responsible for delivering nutritional care

It is important to consider end of life not only in oncology but all stages of life to improve quality for both the patient and the patient's family.[120] Utilization of a specialized team of clinicians to help patients and caregivers understand the difference between palliative care and hospice care is vital for a successful transition. It can be overwhelming for everyone involved but it does not have to be with the right team by one's side.

APPENDIX 6.1

Chemotherapeutic Agent	Common Nutritional Side Effects	Notes
Abraxane	Low white blood and red blood counts, nausea, weakness/fatigue	
Afatinib (Gilotrif®)	Diarrhea, mouth sores, dry mouth	Taken on empty stomach a few hours before a meal with 8oz of water
Bevacizumab (Avastin®)	Anorexia, abdominal pain, upper respiratory infection, constipation, low white count, proteinuria, diarrhea, mouth sores, generalized weakness	*Note*: Patient has to be off Avastin four weeks prior to surgery related to wound healing issues. If needing nutrition support, consider the timeline/delays encountered.
Bleomycin (Blenoxane®)	Nausea, vomiting, mucositis, weight loss, anorexia	
Carboplatin (Paraplatin®)	Low white/red/platelet counts, nausea, vomiting, taste changes, low magnesium levels	Adequate hydration is a concern with all the platinum-based therapies
Casodex	Rapid weight gain	
Cisplatin (Platinol®)	Nausea, vomiting, kidney toxicity, low magnesium/calcium/potassium, low white/red/platelet counts	Watch for refractory low potassium related to low magnesium.
Capecitabine (Xeloda®)	Nausea, vomiting, diarrhea	
Cetuximab (Erbitux)	Nausea, vomiting, diarrhea, constipation, low magnesium	
Crizotinib (Xalkori®)	Nausea, vomiting, diarrhea, taste changes, edema	TKI mechanism; avoid grapefruit/St. John's wort
Cyclophosphamide (Cytoxan®)	Nausea, vomiting	
Dacarbazine		
Docetaxel (Taxotere®)	Low red/white counts, fluid retention, nausea, diarrhea, peripheral neuropathy, mouth sores	

(Continued)

Chemotherapeutic Agent	Common Nutritional Side Effects	Notes
Doxorubicin (Adriamycin®) (Rubex®)	Nausea, vomiting, low white/red/platelet counts, mouth sores	
Epirubicin (Ellence®)	Nausea, vomiting, diarrhea, mucositis	
Erlotinib (Tarceva®)	Diarrhea, anorexia, nausea, vomiting	Taken by mouth on empty stomach a few hours before a meal with full glass of water at the same time every day. Avoid grapefruit/St. John's wort
Etoposide (VP-16, Toposar®)	Low red/white/platelet counts, nausea, vomiting, mouth sores, anorexia, metallic taste, peripheral neuropathy	
Firmagon	Peripheral edema, fatigue, osteoporosis, decrease in lean body mass, elevated lipids, hot flashes	
Fluraeal 5-FU	Increased triamine, stomatitis, nausea, vomiting, diarrhea	
Gefitinib	HTN, dry skin, anorexia, nausea, vomiting, mucositis	
Gemcitabine (Gemzar®)	Flu symptoms, fever, nausea, vomiting, anorexia, low red/white/platelet counts	
Ifosfamide (Ifex®)	Low red/white/platelet counts, nausea, vomiting, anorexia, blood in urine	Hydration is important with this medication to help clear bladder
Irinotecan (Camptosar®)	Diarrhea, nausea, vomiting, weakness, anorexia, fever, weight loss, low red/white/platelet counts	St. John's wort is contraindicated
Ixabepilone (Ixempra®)	Diarrhea, constipation, mucositis	
Lupron	Peripheral edema, fatigue, osteoporosis, decrease in lean body mass, elevated lipids, hot flashes	
Metnutrexate (MTX®)	Mucositis, nausea	
Mitomycin (Mutamycin)	Low red/white/platelet count, mouth sores, anorexia, fatigue	
Paclitaxel (Taxol®)	Low red/white/platelets, peripheral neuropathy, nausea, vomiting, diarrhea, mouth sores	
Pazopanib		Take 1 hour before eating or 2 hours after Avoid grapefruit and grapefruit juice
Pemetrexed (Alimta®)	Low red/white/platelet counts, nausea, vomiting, constipation, anorexia, diarrhea, stomatitis, esophagitis, taste change, difficulty swallowing	Typical supplementation with Alimta to prevent severe anemia: Folic acid (350–1000 mcg) by mouth 1 week prior to first treatment and to continue daily B12 (1000 mcg) injections given 1 week prior to first treatment then every three cycles
Ramucirumab (Cyramza®)	Rare	
Sunitinib	HTN, diarrhea, stomatitis, dysgeusia, neutropenia, abdominal pain	
Topotecan	Nausea, vomiting, diarrhea, mucositis	
Trastuzumab (Herceptin®)	Nausea, vomiting, diarrhea	

(*Continued*)

Chemotherapeutic Agent	Common Nutritional Side Effects	Notes
Trelstar	Peripheral edema, fatigue, osteoporosis, decrease in lean body mass, elevated lipids, hot flashes	
Vinblastine (Velban®)	Low red/white/platelets, nausea, vomiting, constipation	Avoid St. John's wort/grapefruit. Constipation prevention is helpful as severe constipation can occur with medication
Vincristine	Neuropathy, mucositis, diarrhea	
Vinorelbine (Navelbine®)	Low red/white/platelet counts, nausea, vomiting, muscle weakness, constipation	
Xtandi (Enzulatamide)	Diarrhea, fatigue, hot flashes	
Zoladex	Peripheral edema, fatigue, osteoporosis, decrease in lean body mass, elevated lipids, hot flashes	
Zytiga (Abiraterone)	Fatigue, diarrhea, hot flashes, upset stomach, HTN, hypokalemia, edema	

APPENDIX 6.2

Chemotherapy-Related Side Effects	Management of Nutrition Impact Symptoms
Low red blood cell counts	Ensure adequate calories, protein, iron, copper, B12, folic acid intake, and adequate physical activity. Iron food examples: beef, pork, turkey, chicken, fish, enriched grains, nuts, dried beans, etc. An iron supplement may also be needed if iron saturation is low. Add vitamin C-rich foods with nonheme sources. Copper food examples: nuts, seeds, lentils. Folic acid food examples: dark leafy greens, asparagus, broccoli, beans/lentils, enriched grains. B-12 food examples: animal protein, enriched grains. Avoid caffeine with meals, which can decrease iron absorption. Physical activity: minimum of 30 minutes of moderate physical activity most days of the week. Medications that may be added could include but are not limited to Procrit and Aranesp.
Low white counts	Ensure adequate calories/protein/vitamin/minerals for recovery. If white blood cell counts are below 2.5 mcL or ANC <1.0 mcL, then special care and diet restrictions should be headed to prevent unwanted infection. See United States Department of Agriculture and Food and Drug Administration report on "Food Safety for People with Cancer." (http://www.fda.gov/downloads/Food/FoodborneIllnessContaminants/UCM312761.pdf). A low microbial diet may also be recommended: Usually what is recommended is avoiding undercooked foods and choosing cooked foods instead. Examples: cooked fruits/vegetables, cooked meat, pasteurized milks, etc. Avoid yogurt and other probiotic foods until white counts have recovered. Avoid buffets; leftovers only kept a few days and then reheated to at least 165°F. Medications that may be added could include but are not limited to Neulasta and Neupogen.
Low platelet counts	No direct causal link to help with recovery but a naturopathic doctor may have suggestions of certain supplements that may help to recover these counts. Extra care when preparing foods not to cut yourself, as the bleeding may be more difficult to stop. Medications that may be added could include but are not limited to corticosteroids, platelet transfusion, and splenectomy.

(Continued)

Chemotherapy-Related Side Effects	Management of Nutrition Impact Symptoms
Nausea/vomiting	Prevent dehydration by drinking plenty of fluids (ginger tea, water, sports drinks, water down juice, broths, popsicles, clear sodas, slushies, ice chips, etc.) Foods well tolerated: crackers, canned fruit, mashed potatoes, oatmeal, dry toast, pretzels, rice, and small frequent meals. Drink fluids in between meals instead of with meals. Avoid strong smells (cold/room-temperature foods help with this), greasy foods, acidic foods, spicy foods, caffeine. High-protein foods combined with ginger may be helpful. Ginger is a well-known antinausea tool: ginger ale (if actually formulated with ginger), ginger tea, ginger chew candies, etc. Try wearing sea bands. Medications that may be added could include but are not limited to Zofran, kytril, Compazine, Ativan, Sancuso patch, scopolamine patch, and many more.
Constipation	Ensure adequate hydration (at least 64 oz fluid daily unless specified by health care provider) and adequate fiber intake (25–35 g fiber per day) along with 30–60 minutes of moderate physical activity most days of the week if medically feasible. High-fiber foods/supplements: Wheat bran cereal, whole-grain bread/products, brown rice, raw vegetables, fruits, ground flax seed, chia seeds, Metamucil. Try 4–8 oz warm prune/prune juice or black cherry juice. Also, probiotic foods can help promote intestinal health such as yogurt/kefir/miso/etc. Medications that may be added could include but are not limited to stool softeners, laxatives, enemas, etc. Items such as vitamin C and magnesium may be added at the right dose to help with bowel movements as well.
Diarrhea	Prevention of dehydration and electrolyte disturbances is key. An easy rule of thumb is to weigh at start of day and end of day, every pound lost is close to 16 oz of fluid along with the minimum of 64 oz water. Example of oral rehydration solution from Oley.org: 3/8 tsp salt, ¼ tsp salt substitute (potassium chloride), ½ tsp baking soda, 2 tbsp + 2 tsp table sugar, add tap water to make 1 L (can add NutraSweet/Splenda for better taste). Other hydration options: Water is good but alternate with other options to maximize absorption and prevent electrolyte issues; sports drinks; juice; Pedialyte; etc. Foods recommended: BRATY diet (bananas, white rice, applesauce, white toast, and yogurt), oatmeal, barley, citrus, etc. Can add pectin powder or similar product to smoothies to help slow diarrhea. Drink/eat cold/room-temperature foods. Milk alternatives or lactaid milk. Try banatrol 1–3 packets a day or other soluble fiber supplement. Avoid lactose (regular cow milk/goat milk, cheese, etc.), hot foods, caffeine, drinking/eating at same time, insoluble fiber (uncooked fruits/vegetables, whole grains, particularly whole-wheat products), vitamin C supplements, etc. Consider sources of probiotics—yogurt, kefir, and/or supplements. Medications that may be added could include are but not limited to Imodium, Lomotil, Questran, and many more.
Anorexia	Small frequent meals with protein at all meals and snacks. Aim to eat every 2–3 hours. Add in high-calorie/high-protein foods such as avocado dips, hummus, hard-boiled eggs, cottage cheese, smoothies with whey protein powder, milk/soy milk, nuts/seeds/nut butters, etc. Supplements may include Boost/Ensure/Orgain/Boost Very High Calorie/whey protein powder, ENU, etc. In severe cases, nutrition support may be indicated if anorexia is causing significant weight loss and poor intake is intended to be for an extended period of time. Consider food and/or supplement sources of EPA. Medications that may be added could include but are not limited to corticosteroids, Marinol, Megace, Remeron, and many more.

(Continued)

Chemotherapy-Related Side Effects	Management of Nutrition Impact Symptoms
Mouth sores	Can be painful to chew and certain foods like those high in acid may be painful. Keep mouth clean by brushing and using a health-care-approved mouthwash that is alcohol free.
	Try to avoid foods high in acid such as tomatoes, oranges, lemons, etc. Also avoid spices, alcohol/alcohol-based mouth rinses, sharp foods like chips, buffalo sauce, etc.
	Try soft moist bland foods such as smoothies, mash potatoes, Boost/Ensure/Orgain/ENU supplements, puddings, room-temperature soup, eggs, soft fruit.
	Suck on hard candy, chew gum.
	Medications that may be added could include but are not limited to episeal, magic mouthwash, baking soda/salt/water mouth rinse used multiple times per day.
Taste changes	Can be bitter, metallic, salty, sweet, or just "wrong."
	Zinc supplements have been shown to help with taste changes; typical dose is usually 30 mg or more per day in split doses.
	If metallic taste, avoid red meats and switch to plastic utensils for eating and try cooking in ceramic/glass instead of metal dishes.
	If lack of taste, ensure rinsing mouth several times per day with health-care-approved mouthwash that is alcohol free and use "extra" spices (typically not salt) to flavor foods and try more gravy/sauce with foods.
	Medications that may be added could include but are not limited to zinc supplementation and alcohol-free mouthwashes multiple times per day.
Edema	Ensuring adequate protein and calories, avoiding excess salt (typically more than 2 g/day), and ensuring adequate thiamine level are first steps to nutritionally help with edema.
	If malnourished with low albumin, can cause edema or cause it to become worse. Try small frequent meals and add nutritional supplements to try and increase calories/protein; consider nutrition support if unable to increase intake to a sufficient amount.
	Excess salt can cause fluid to leak into areas of the body; avoid processed foods (frozen/canned) and eat more fresh foods, watch meat for saline additives, use other spices instead of salt when cooking, read all labels for sodium content.
	Poor intake and weight loss can also cause vitamin deficiencies and edema can be caused by a thiamine deficiency that is unrelated to cancer treatment. If poor intake is suspected along with increasing calories and protein, add a thiamine supplement that meets at a minimum 100% of the RDA.
	Medications that may be added could include but are not limited to diuretics and albumin.
Hot flashes	Foods that may trigger hot flashes: caffeine, alcohol, sugar (refined), spicy foods.

REFERENCES

1. Onc: Nutrition screening tools. 2012. Academy of Nutrition and Dietetics Evidence Analysis Library. http://www.andeal.org/topic.cfm?cat=5452&conclusion_statement_id=251796&highlight=oncology%20assessment&home=1. Updated 2012. Accessed March 2015.
2. Onc: Nutrition assessment for adult oncology patients. 2013. Academy of Nutrition and Dietetics Evidence Analysis Library. http://www.andeal.org/topic.cfm?format_tables=0&cat=5164. Updated 2013. Accessed March 2015.
3. Onc: Nutrition assessment tools. 2012. Academy of Nutrition and Dietetics Evidence Analysis Library. http://www.andeal.org/topic.cfm?cat=5453&conclusion_statement_id=251792&highlight=nutrition%20assessment%20for%20adult%20oncology%20patients&home=1. Updated 2012. Accessed March 2015.
4. Ollenschlager G, Veill B, Thomas W, Konkol K, Burger, B. Tumor anorexia: Causes, assessment, treatment. *Recent Results Cancer Res.* 1991;121:249–59.
5. Kern KA, Norton JA. Cancer cachexia. *J Parenter Enteral Nutr.* 1988 May–Jun;12(3):286–98.
6. Harris D, Haboubi N. Malnutrition screening in the elderly population. *J R Soc Med.* 2005 Sep;98(9):411–4.
7. Nutrition in cancer care (PDQ®): Nutrition screening and assessment. National Cancer Institute website. http://www.cancer.gov/cancertopics/pdq/supportivecare/nutrition/HealthProfessional/page4#_50_toc. Updated September 3, 2014. Accessed March 2015.

8. Nutrition and the adult oncology patient. Academy of Nutrition and Dietetics Evidence Analysis Library. http://www.andeal.org/files/Docs/Nutrition%20and%20the%20Adult%20Oncology%20Patient_09262013FINAL. Updated 2013. Accessed March 2015.
9. Grant M, Rivera LM. Impact of dietary counseling on quality of life in head and neck patients undergoing radiation therapy. *Qual Life Res.* 1994;3:77–8.
10. Nitenberg G, Raynard B. Nutritional support of the cancer patient: Issues and dilemmas. *Crit Rev Oncol Hematol.* 2000 Jun;34(3):137–68.
11. Cancer Types. American Cancer Society website. http://www.cancer.org/cancer/showallcancertypes/index. Accessed March 28, 2015.
12. Mehta M, Shike M. Diet and physical activity in the prevention of colorectal cancer. *J Natl Compr Canc Netw.* 2014 Dec;12(12):1721–6.
13. Cancer Prevention: By the numbers. American Institute for Cancer Research website. http://www.aicr.org/reduce-your-cancer-risk/cancer-prevention/reduce_cancer_by_numbers.html. Accessed March 28, 2015.
14. Morgan TM, Tang D, Stratton KL et al. Preoperative nutritional status is an important predictor of survival in patients undergoing surgery for renal cell carcinoma. *Eur Urol.* 2011 Jun;59(6):923–8.
15. Garth AK, Newsome CM, Simmance N, Crowe TC. Nutritional status, nutrition practices and post-operative complications in patients with gastrointestinal cancer. *J Hum Nutr Diet.* 2010 Aug;23(4):393–401.
16. Klein S, Koretz RL. Nutrition support in patients with cancer: What do the data really show? *Nutr Clin Pract.* 1994 Jun;9(3):91–100.
17. Perioperative total parenteral nutrition in surgical patients. The veterans affairs total parenteral nutrition cooperative study group. *N Engl J Med.* 1991 Aug 22;325(8):525–32.
18. Weimann A, Braga M, Harsanyi L et al. ESPEN guidelines on enteral nutrition: Surgery including organ transplantation. *Clin Nutr.* 2006 Apr;25(2):224–44.
19. Braga M, Ljungqvist O, Soeters P, Fearon K, Weimann A, Bozzetti F, ESPEN. ESPEN guidelines on parenteral nutrition: Surgery. *Clin Nutr.* 2009 Aug;28(4):378–86.
20. Martindale RG, McClave SA, Taylor B, Lawson CM. Perioperative nutrition: What is the current landscape? *J Parenter Enteral Nutr.* 2013 Sep;37(5 Suppl):5S–20S.
21. Gabor S, Renner H, Matzi V et al. Early enteral feeding compared with parenteral nutrition after oesophageal or oesophagogastric resection and reconstruction. *Br J Nutr.* 2005 Apr;93(4):509–13.
22. Osland E, Yunus RM, Khan S, Memon MA. Early versus traditional postoperative feeding in patients undergoing resectional gastrointestinal surgery: A meta-analysis. *J Parenter Enteral Nutr.* 2011 Jul;35(4):473–87.
23. Kalff JC, Türler A, Schwarz NT et al. Intra-abdominal activation of a local inflammatory response within the human muscularis externa during laparotomy. *Ann Surg.* 2003 Mar;237(3):301–15.
24. Mortensen K, Nilsson M, Slim K et al. Consensus guidelines for enhanced recovery after gastrectomy: Enhanced Recovery After Surgery (ERAS®) Society recommendations. *Br J Surg.* 2014 Sep;101(10):1209–29.
25. Gustafsson UO, Scott MJ, Schwenk W et al. Guidelines for perioperative care in elective colonic surgery: Enhanced Recovery After Surgery (ERAS®) Society recommendations. *Clin Nutr.* 2012 Dec;31(6):783–800.
26. Lassen K, Coolsen MM, Slim K et al. Guidelines for perioperative care for pancreaticoduodenectomy: Enhanced Recovery After Surgery (ERAS®) Society recommendations. *Clin Nutr.* 2012 Dec;31(6):817–30.
27. Nygren J, Thacker J, Carli F et al. Guidelines for perioperative care in elective rectal/pelvic surgery: Enhanced Recovery After Surgery (ERAS®) Society recommendations. *Clin Nutr.* 2012 Dec;31(6):801–16.
28. Osland E, Hossain MB, Khan S, Memon MA. Effect of timing of pharmaconutrition (immunonutrition) administration on outcomes of elective surgery for gastrointestinal malignancies: A systematic review and meta-analysis. *JPEN J Parenter Enteral Nutr.* 2014 Jan;38(1):53–69.
29. Frantz D, Munroe C et al. Gastrointestinal disease. In: Mueller C et al. eds. *ASPEN Adult Nutrition Support Core Curriculum.* 2nd ed. A.S.P.E.N., Silver Spring, MD; 2012:426–53.
30. Huhmann M. Nutrition management of the surgical oncology patient. In: Leser M, Ledesma N, Bergerson S, Trujillo E eds. *Oncology Nutrition for Clinical Practice.* 3rd ed. Chicago, IL: Oncology Nutrition Dietetic Practice Group of the Academy of Nutrition and Dietetics; 2013:14.
31. Doughty DB, Landmann RG. Management of patients with a colostomy or ileostomy. UpToDate.com website. http://www.uptodate.com/contents/management-of-patients-with-a-colostomy-or-ileostomy?source=search_result&search=ileostomy&selectedTitle=1%7E85#H19. Accessed April 3, 2015.

32. Gill C. Nutrition management for cancers of the gastrointestinal tract. In: Leser M, Ledesma N, Bergerson S, Trujillo E eds. *Oncology Nutrition for Clinical Practice.* 3rd ed. Chicago, IL: Oncology Nutrition Dietetic Practice Group of the Academy of Nutrition and Dietetics; 2013:20.
33. Bordeianou L, Yeh DD. Overview of management of small bowel obstruction in adults. UpToDate.com website. http://www.uptodate.com/contents/overview-of-management-of-mechanical-small-bowel-obstruction-in-adults?source=related_link. Accessed April 10, 2015.
34. Vanderhoof JA, Pauley-Hunter RJ. Treatment of small intestinal bacterial overgrowth. UpToDate.com website. http://www.uptodate.com/contents/treatment-of-small-intestinal-bacterial-overgrowth?source=search_result&search=small+bowel+bacterial+overgrowth&selectedTitle=1%7E121. Accessed April 9, 2015.
35. Stein SL. Overview of enteric fistulas. UpToDate.com website. http://www.uptodate.com/contents/overview-of-enteric-fistulas?source=search_result&search=fistula&selectedTitle=1%7E150. Accessed April 9, 2015.
36. Cancer Facts and Figures. 2015. The American Cancer Society website. www.cancer.org. Accessed February 16, 2015.
37. Breast Cancer Facts & Figures 2013–2014. The American Cancer Society website. www.cancer.org/research/cancerfactsstatistics.index. Accessed February 2015.
38. Howlader N, Noone AM, Krapcho M et al. eds. *SEER Cancer Statistics Review 1975–2010.* National Cancer Institute website. http://seer.cancer.gov/csr/1975_2010.
39. Voduc KD, Cheang MC, Tyldesley S, Gelmon K, Nielsen TO, Kennecke H. Breast cancer subtypes and the risk of local and regional relapse. *J Clin Oncol.* 2010 Apr 1;28(10):1684–91.
40. Marmot M, Atinmo T, Byers T et al. *Food, Nutrition, Physical Activity, and the Prevention of Cancer: A Global Perspective.* Washington, DC: World Cancer Research Fund/American Institute for Cancer Research (AICR) Expert Reports. AICR; 2007:289.
41. Eliassen AH, Colditz GA, Rosner B, Willett WC, Hankinson SE. Adult weight change and risk of postmenopausal breast cancer. *JAMA.* 2006;296(2):193–201.
42. Ballard-Barbash R, Friedenreich C, Slattery M, Thune I. Obesity and body composition. In: Schottenfeld D, Fraumeni JF eds. *Cancer Epidemiology and Prevention.* 3rd ed. New York, NY: Oxford University Press; 2006:422–48.
43. Knobf MT, Coviello J. Lifestyle interventions for cardiovascular risk reduction in women with breast cancer. *Curr Cardiol Rev.* 2011 Nov;7(4):250–7.
44. Irwin ML, McTiernan A, Baumgartner RN et al. Changes in body fat and weight after a breast cancer diagnosis: Influence of demographic, prognostic, and lifestyle factors. *J Clin Oncol.* 2005 Feb 1;23(4):774–82.
45. Ballard-Barbash R, Hunsberger S, Alciati MH et al. Physical activity, weight control, and breast cancer risk and survival: Clinical trial rationale and design considerations. *J Natl Cancer Inst.* 2009 May 6;101(9):640–43.
46. Majed B, Moreau T, Asselain B, Curie Institute Breast Cancer Group. Overweight, obesity and breast cancer prognosis: Optimal body size indicator cut-points. *Breast Cancer Res Treat.* 2009 May;115(1):193–203.
47. Holick CN, Newcomb PA, Trentham-Dietz A et al. Physical activity and survival after diagnosis of invasive breast cancer. *Cancer Epidemiol Biomarkers Prev.* 2008 Feb;17(2):379–86.
48. Pierce JP, Faerber S, Wright F et al. A randomized trial of the effect of a plant-based dietary pattern on additional breast cancer events and survival: The Women's Healthy Eating and Living (WHEL) Study. *Control Clin Trials.* 2002 Dec;23(6):728–56.
49. Blackburn GL, Wang KA. Dietary fat reduction and breast cancer outcome: Results from the Women's Intervention and Nutrition Study (WINS). *Am J Clin Nutr.* 2007 Sep;86(3):s878–81.
50. Spencer L, Mann C, Metcalfe M et al. The effect of omega-3 FAs on tumour angiogenesis and their therapeutic potential. *Eur J Cancer.* 2009 Aug;45(12):2077–86.
51. Patterson RE, Flatt SW, Newman VA et al. Marine fatty acid intake is associated with breast cancer prognosis. *J Nutr.* 2011 Feb;141(2):201–6.
52. Mahabir S. Association between diet during preadolescence and adolescence and the risk for breast cancer during adulthood. *J Adolesc Health.* 2013 May;52(5Suppl):S30–5.
53. Caan BJ, Natarajan L, Parker B et al. Soy food consumption and breast cancer prognosis. *Cancer Epidemiol Biomarkers Prev.* 2011 May;20(5):854–8.
54. Liu X, Lv K. Cruciferous vegetables intake is inversely associated with risk of breast cancer: A meta-analyis. *Breast.* 2013 Jun;22(3):309–13.

55. McCann SE, Hootman KC, Weaver AM et al. Dietary intakes of total and specific lignans are associated with clinical breast tumor characteristics. *J Nutr.* 2012 Jan;142(1):91–8.
56. Zamora-Ros R, Ferrari P, Gonzalez CA et al. Dietary flavonoid and lignin intake and breast cancer risk according to menopause and hormone receptor status in the European Perspective Investigation into Cancer and Nutrition (EPIC) study. *Breast Cancer Res Treat.* 2013 May;139(1):163–76.
57. Wu AH, Butler LM. Green tea and breast cancer. *Mol Nutr Food Res.* 2011 Jun;55(6):921–30.
58. Newman V. Medical nutrition therapy for breast cancer. In: Marian M, Roberts S eds. *Clinical Nutrition in Oncology Patients.* Sadbury, MA: Jones and Barlett; 2010;7:176.
59. Patnaik JL, Byers T, DiGuiseppi C, Dabelea D, Denberg TD. Cardiovascular disease competes with breast cancer as the leading cause of death for older females diagnosed with breast cancer: A retrospective cohort study. *Breast Cancer Res.* 2011 Jun 20;13(3):R64.
60. Hadji P, Body JJ, Aapro MS et al. Practical guidance for the management of aromatase inhibitor-associated bone loss. *Ann Oncol.* 2008 Aug;19(8):1407–16.
61. Ross AC, Manson JE, Abrams SA et al. The 2011 report on dietary reference intakes for calcium and vitamin D from the Institute of Medicine: What clinicians need to know. *J Clin Endocrinol Metab.* 2011 Jan;96(1):53–8.
62. Crew KD, Gammon MD, Steck SE et al. Association between plasma 25-hydroxyvitamin D and breast cancer risk. *Cancer Prev Res (Phila).* 2009;2(6):598–604.
63. Institute of Medicine (US) Committee to Review Dietary Reference Intakes for Vitamin D and Calcium; In: Ross AC, Taylor CL, Yaktine AL et al. eds. *Dietary Reference Intakes for Calcium and Vitamin D.* Washington (DC): National Academies Press (US); 2011.
64. Kim Y, Je Y. Vitamin D intake, blood 25(OH)D levels, and breast cancer risk or mortality: A meta-analysis. *Br J Cancer.* 2014 May 27;110(11):2772–84.
65. Polovich M, Olsen M, LeFebvre K eds. *Chemotherapy and Biotherapy Guidelines for Treatment and Recommendations for Practice.* 4th ed. Oncology Nursing Society, Pittsburgh, PA; 2014;27–47.
66. Terrell JE. Quality of life assessment in head and neck cancer patients. *Hematol Oncol Clin North Am.* 1999 Aug;13(4):849–65.
67. Isenring E. Esophageal and head and neck cancer. In: Marian M, Roberts S eds. *Clinical Nutrition in Oncology Patients.* Sadbury, MA: Jones and Barlett; 2010;7:165–85.
68. Lesser, M. Medical nutrition therapy for esophageal cancer. In: Leser M, Ledesma N, Bergerson S, Trujillo E eds. *Oncology Nutrition for Clinical Practice.* Chicago, IL: Oncology Nutrition Dietetic Practice Group of the Academy of Nutrition and Dietetics; 2013;19:181–6.
69. Santarpia L, Contaldo F, Pasanisi F. Nutrition screening and early treatment of malnutrition in cancer patients. *J Cachexia Sarcopenia Muscle.* 2011 Mar;2(1):27–35.
70. Riddle B, Davidson W, Elliot R, Basillie F, Porceddu S. Collaborative management of acute side effects for head and neck cancer patients receiving radiotherapy. *Asia Pac J Clin Oncol.* 2005;1(Suppl):A18.
71. Melhado RE, Alderson D, Tucker O. The changing face of esophageal cancer. *Cancers (Basel).* 2010 Jun 28;2(3):1379–404.
72. American Cancer Society: Cancer Facts and Figures 2013. American Cancer Society website. http://www.cancer.org/research/cancerfactsfigures/cancerfactsfigures/cancer-facts-figures-2013. Accessed March 4, 2015.
73. What you need to know about cancer of the esophagus. National Cancer Institute website. http://www.cancer.gov/cancertopics/wyntk/esophagus. Revised April 2013. Accessed June 4, 2013.
74. Surveillance Epidemiology and End Results. SEER Stat Fact Sheets: Esophagus Cancer. National Cancer Institute website. http://seer.cancer.gov/statfacts/html/esoph.html. Accessed March 5, 2012.
75. Esophagus Cancer. American Cancer Society website. http://www.cancer.org/Cancer/EsophagusCancer/DetailedGuide. Revised January 18, 2013. Accessed March 1, 2015.
76. Nguyyen A, Nadler E. Medical nutrition therapy for head and neck cancer. In: Leser M, Ledesma N, Bergerson S, Trujillo E eds. *Oncology Nutrition for Clinical Practice.* Chicago, IL: Oncology Nutrition Dietetic Practice Group of the Academy of Nutrition and Dietetics; 2013;21:201–8.
77. Oral Cancer Prevention PDQ. Incidence and Mortality. National Cancer Institute website. http://www.cancer.gov/cancertopics/pdq/prevention/oral/HealthProfessional/Page2#Section_159. Revised February 15, 2013. Accessed March 3, 2015.
78. Human Papillomavirus (HPV)-Associated Cancers. Centers for Disease Control and Prevention website. http://www.cdc.gov/cancer/hpv/statistics/headneck.htm. Accessed November 11, 2012.
79. Head and neck cancer. People Living with Cancer website. www.plwc.org. Accessed September 11, 2007.

80. Festi D, Scaioli E, Baldi F et al. Body weight, lifestyle, dietary habits and gastroesophageal reflux disease. *World J Gastroenterol.* 2009;15(14):1690–701.
81. Nguyen A, Nadler E. Head and neck cancer: Defining effective medical nutrition therapy for nutritional phases observed during chemoradiation. *Oncology Nutrition Connection.* 2012:20(1):3–21.
82. Hurst JD, Gallagher AL. Energy, macronutrient, micronutrient, and fluid requirements. In: Elliott L, Molseed LL, McCallum PD eds. *The Clinical Guide to Oncology Nutrition.* 2nd ed. American Dietetic Association, Chicago, IL; 2006: 54–71.
83. Lopes AB, Fagundes RB. Esophageal squamous cell carcinoma-precursor lesions and early diagnosis. *World J Gastrointest Endosc.* 2012;16;4(1):9–16.
84. Fietkau R. Principles of feeding cancer patients via enteral or parenteral nutrition during radiotherapy. *Strahlenther Onkol.* 1998:174(suppl III):47–51.
85. Esophageal Cancer Treatment; Treatment Option Overview (PDQ®). National Cancer Institute website. http://www.cancer.gov/cancertopics/pdq/treatment/esophageal/HealthProfessional/page4. Accessed November 5, 2012.
86. Forastiere A, Trotti A, Pfister D, Grandis J. Head and neck cancer: Recent advances and new standards of care. *J Clin Oncol.* 2006;24:2603–05.
87. Chemotherapy for Cancer of the Esophagus. American Cancer Society website. http://www.cancer.org/cancer/esophaguscancer/detailedguide/esophagus-cacner-treating-chemotherapy. Accessed March 13, 2015.
88. Chemotherapy Drugs and Often Used During Chemotherapy. Chemocare website. http://chemocare.com/chemotherapy/drug-info/default.aspx. Accessed March 13, 2015.
89. NCCN Guidelines for treatment of cancer by site. National Comprehensive Cancer Network (NCCN) website. http://www.nccn.org/professionals/physician_gls/pdf/head-and-neck.pdf. Accessed November 16, 2012.
90. Ligthart-Melis GC, Weijs PJ, Te Boveldt ND et al. Dietitian-delivered intensive nutritional support is associated with a decrease in severe postoperative complications after surgery in patients with esophageal cancer. *Dis Esophagus.* 2013;26(6):587–93.
91. Gaurav K, Goel RK, Shukla M, Pandey M. Glutamine: An approach to novel chemotherapy-induced toxicity. *Indian J Med Paediatr Oncol.* 2012 Jan;33(1):13–20.
92. Topkan E, Parlak C, Topuk S, Pehlivan B. Influence of oral glutamine supplementation on of survival outcomes patients treated with concurrent chemoradiotherapy for locally advanced non-small cell lung cancer. *BMC Cancer.* 2012 Oct 31;12:502.
93. Berk L, James J, Schwartz A et al. A randomized, double-blind, placebo-controlled trial of beta-hydroxyl beta-methly butyrate, glutamine, and arginine mixture for the treatment of cancer cachexia. *Support Cancer Care.* 2008;16(10):1179–88.
94. Imai T, Matsuura K, Asada Y et al. Effect of HMB/Arg/Gln on the prevention of radiation dermatitis in head and neck cancer patients treated with concurrent chemoradiotherpy. *Jpn J Clin Oncol.* 2014;44(5):422–7.
95. Yavas C, Yavas G, Acar H et al. Amelioration of radiation-induced acute inflammation and mucosal atrophy by beta-hydroxy-beta-methylbutyrate, L-glutamine, and L-arginine: Results of an experimental study. *Support Cancer Care.* 2013;21(3):883–8.
96. National Cancer Institute. Surveillance, epidemiology, and end results program (SEER) stat fact sheets: Endometrial cancer. http://seer.cancer.gov/statfacts/html/corp.html. Accessed March 13, 2015.
97. World Cancer Research Fund and American Institute for Cancer Research. *Food, Nutrition, Physical Activity, and the Prevention of Cancer: A Global Perspective.* Washington DC: AICR; 2007.
98. National Cancer Institute. Surveillance, epidemiology, and end results program (SEER) stat fact sheets: Ovary cancer. http://seer.cancer.gov/statfacts/html/ovary.html. Accessed March 13, 2015.
99. National Cancer Institute. Surveillance, epidemiology, and end results program (SEER) stat fact sheets: Cervix uteri cancer. http://seer.cancer.gov/statfacts/html/cervix.html. Accessed March 13, 2015.
100. National Comprehensive Cancer Network (NCCN). NCCN Clinical Practice Guidelines in Oncology. Ovarian Cancer. 2015. National Comprehensive Cancer Network. http://www.nccn.org/professionals/physician_gls/pdf/ovarian.pdf.
101. National Comprehensive Cancer Network (NCCN). NCCN Clinical Practice Guidelines in Oncology. Uterine Cancer. 2015. National Comprehensive Cancer Network. http://www.nccn.org/professionals/physician_gls/pdf/uterine.pdf.
102. National Comprehensive Cancer Network (NCCN). NCCN Clinical Practice Guidelines in Oncology. Cervical Cancer. 2015. National Comprehensive Cancer Network. http://www.nccn.org/professionals/physician_gls/pdf/cervical.pdf.

103. What Are the Key Statistics about Lung Cancer? American Cancer Society website. http://www.cancer.org/cancer/lungcancer-non-smallcell/detailedguide/non-small-cell-lung-cancer-key-statistics. Accessed March 19, 2015.
104. Lung Cancer. American Cancer Society website. http://www.cancer.org/cancer/lungcancer/index. Accessed March 16, 2015.
105. Non-Small Cell Lung Cancer Treatment (PDQ®). National Cancer Institute. website. http://www.cancer.gov/cancertopics/pdq/treatment/non-small-cell-lung/Patient/page4. Accessed March 16, 2015.
106. Cranganu A, Camporeale J. Nutrition aspects of lung cancer. *Nutr Clin Pract.* 2009 Dec;24(6):688–700.
107. Martin-Ucar AE, Nicum R, Oey I, Edwards JG, Waller DA. En-bloc chest wall and lung resection for non-small cell lung cancer. Predictors of 60-day non-cancer related mortality. *Eur J Cardiothorac Surg.* 2003 Jun;23(6):859–64.
108. Tewari N., Martin-Ucar AE, Black E et al. Nutritional status affects long term survival after lobectomy for lung cancer. *Lung Cancer.* 2007 Sep;57(3):389–94.
109. Scott H, McMillan DC, Brown DJ, Forrest LM, McArdle CS, Milroy R. A prospective study of the impact of weight loss and the systemic inflammatory response on quality of life in patients with inoperable non-small cell lung cancer. *Lung Cancer.* 2003 Jun;49(3):295–9.
110. National Cancer Institute (NCI) Fact Sheet. Cruciferous vegetables and cancer prevention. NCI website. http://www.cancer.gov/cancertopics/factsheet/diet.
111. Ornish D, Weidner G, Fair WR et al. Intensive lifestyle changes may affect the progression of prostate cancer. *J Urol.* 2005;174(3):1065–70.
112. Giovannucci E, Rimm EB, Liu Y, Stampfer MJ, Willett WC. A prospective study of tomato products, lycopene, and prostate cancer risk. *J Natl Cancer Inst.* 2002;94(5):391–8.
113. Hsu, A, Bray T, Helferich WG, Doerge DR, Ho E. Differential effects of whole soy extract and soy isoflavones on apoptosis in prostate cancer cells. *Exp Biol Med.* 2010 Jan;235(1):90–7.
114. Hodge AM, English DR, McCredie MR et al. Foods, nutrients and prostate cancer. *Cancer Causes Control.* 2004 Feb;15(1):11–20.
115. Chan JM, Stampfer MJ, Ma J, Gann PH, Gaziano JM, Giovannucci EL. Dairy products, calcium, and prostate cancer risk in the physicians' health study. *Am J Clin Nutr.* 2001 Oct;74(4):549–54.
116. Naiko A, Chewonarin T, Tang M et al. Ellagic acid, a component of pomegranate fruit juice, suppresses androgen-dependent prostate carcinogenesis via induction of apoptosis. *Prostate.* 2015 Feb;75(2):151–60.
117. Paddock, C. Flaxseed halts prostate cancer growth new study shows. Medical News Today website. http://www.medicalnewstoday.com/articles/72990.php. Published June 4, 2007.
118. Johnson JJ, Bailey HH, Mukhtar H. Green tea polyphenols for prostate cancer chemoprevention: A translational perspective. *Phytomedicine.* 2010 Jan;17(1):3–13.
119. Killian PH, Kronski E, Michalik K et al. Curcumin inhibits prostate cancer metastasis *in vivo* by targeting the inflammatory cytokines CXCL1 and -2. *Carcinogenesis.* 2012 Oct. doi: 10.1093/carcin/bgs312.
120. Parikh, RB. Early specialty palliative care—Translating data in oncology into practice [Sounding Board]; *N Engl J Med.* 2013;369(24):2347–51.
121. Palliative Care in Cancer. National Cancer Institute website. http://www.cancer.gov/cancertopics/factsheet/Support/palliative-care. Published 2010. Accessed January 25, 2015.
122. Oberholzer, R. The concept of cachexia-related suffering (CRS) in palliative care. In: Preedy, VR. *Diet and Nutrition in Palliative Care.* Boca Raton, FL: Taylor & Francis Group, LLC; 2011:3–16.
123. Hospice and End of Life Care. National Resource Center on Nutrition, Physical Activity & Aging website. http://nutritionandaging.fiu.edu/creative_solutions/hospice.asp. Published June 2005. Accessed January 27, 2015.
124. Fuhrman, MP. Nutrition support at the end of life: A critical decision. *Today's Dietitian.* 2008;10(9):68.
125. Berger AM, Shuster JL, Von Roenn JH. *Principles and Practice of Palliative Care and Supportive Oncology.* 4th ed. Philadelphia, PA: Lippincott Williams & Wilkins; 2013:779–89.
126. AGA medical position statement: Guidelines for the use of enteral nutrition. *Gastroenterology.* 1995;108:1280–301.

7 Nutritional Management of Osteoporosis

Nancy Robinson, RDN, LD

CONTENTS

The International Osteoporosis Foundation defines osteoporosis as "a disease in which the density and quality of bone are reduced." Bones are living tissue that undergoes an ongoing process of being broken down and then replaced. Osteoporosis is the result of the creation of new bone not keeping up with the removal of old bone, resulting in weak bones that are more prone to fracture. With severe osteoporosis, even minor trauma, from sneezing or bumping into furniture, can result in broken bones. The World Health Organization (WHO) currently bases diagnosis on the measurement of bone mineral density (BMD). A BMD equal to or more than 2.5 standard deviations below the reference measurement is considered osteoporosis. The diagnosis is osteopenia when the BMD is between 1 and 2.5 standard deviations below the reference measurement.

Worldwide, osteoporosis causes more than 8.9 million fractures annually, which translates into an osteoporotic fracture every 3 s [1]. Worldwide, 1 in 3 women over age 50 and 1 in 5 men will experience osteoporotic fractures [2–4]. By 2050, the global incidence of hip fracture is projected to increase by 310% in men and 240% in women [5]. An International Osteoporosis Foundation survey, conducted in 11 countries, found denial of personal risk by postmenopausal women, failure to discuss osteoporosis with their doctor, and restricted access to diagnosis and treatment before the first fracture, result in missed diagnosis and treatment opportunities. The report discovered that despite the significant progress made in osteoporosis research and education over the last decade, bone loss is still not being detected early enough to protect postmenopausal women from osteoporosis-related fractures [6].

A review of U.S. inpatient data from more than 1000 hospitals found that for women age 55 or older, bone fractures due to osteoporosis led to more hospitalizations and greater health care costs than heart attack, stroke, or breast cancer. Between 2000 and 2011, 4.9 million women over age 55 were hospitalized for osteoporotic fracture of the hip, pelvis, arm, leg, or spine, compared to 3 million for stroke, 2.9 million for heart attack, and 700,000 for breast cancer. Osteoporotic fractures accounted for more than 40% of the hospitalizations, and led to an estimated hospital cost of more than $5 billion per year. One of the authors of the studies noted that people often underestimate their own risk of osteoporosis and fracture. The study authors concluded that a substantial benefit could be realized by improving both primary and secondary prevention of fractures in high-risk individuals and that a greater emphasis on preventive care to prevent fractures is critical [7]. A Swiss study found that from 2000 to 2008, the burden of hospitalized osteoporotic fractures to the Swiss health care system continued to increase in both sexes. In women, the burden was significantly higher than that of major cardiovascular events [8]. Position statement 1144, of the American Academy of Orthopaedic Surgeons and the American Association of Orthopaedic Surgeons (AAOS), states they "believe that hip fractures should be a public health priority and target of health system reform given the increasing burden of disease" [9].

Bone health in men is being missed. The publication, "Osteoporosis in Men: Why Change Needs to Happen," from the International Osteoporosis Foundation, reports one-third of all hip fractures occur in men, with a mortality of 37% in the year following fracture. The coauthor of the report, Dr. Ebeling, writes that osteoporosis is "a disease that for far too long has been considered to be exclusively a problem for women. While improving management of osteoporosis for women is critical, the time has now come for a radical reappraisal of osteoporosis management in men" [10].

When osteoporosis or osteopenia are diagnosed, patients often receive inadequate nutritional counseling. Both conditions warrant proactive interventions that everyone should be concerned about. While primary osteoporosis fracture prevention is the ideal scenario, secondary prevention is critical with a need to reverse the decline often seen following fracture. Secondary prevention, as the first opportunity, to limit the damaging effects of osteoporosis is often the reality. Interventions to reduce the chance of osteoporotic fractures and pain, as well as the costs of hospital readmission and post hospital care, are consistent with ongoing efforts to transform health care systems into more preventative, cost-effective endeavors.

Age-related bone loss is asymptomatic but bone fractures can result in serious long-term pain and debilitation. Osteoporosis and osteopenia are under recognized and often missed. Regardless of age or sex, bone health should always be a part of discharge planning and outpatient nutritional assessments. Outpatient nutritional care plans should always include goals for preventing, maintaining, or improving bone health.

RISK FACTORS

There are many risk factors, diseases, and conditions that can result in osteoporosis and bone fractures. The high number of risk factors reinforces the need to always include a bone health evaluation in nutritional assessments.

TABLE 7.1
Diseases or Conditions That Increase the Risk of Osteoporosis

Autoimmune disorders such as rheumatoid arthritis (RA), lupus, multiple sclerosis, and ankylosing spondylitis are all associated with an increased risk for osteoporosis. The drugs used to treat RA and lupus can also increase the risk of osteoporosis.
Digestive and gastrointestinal disorders such as celiac disease, ulcerative colitis, and Crohn's disease as well as gastrectomy and gastrointestinal bypass procedures that can adversely affect absorption of nutrients key to bone health.
Endocrine and hormonal disorders such as diabetes, hyperparathyroidism, hyperthyroidism, Cushing's syndrome, and thyrotoxicosis can all cause bone loss.
Women with irregular periods may be at increased risk, especially if they have low estrogen levels or are too thin. Premature menopause always warrants extra attention to bone health. In men, very low levels of testosterone and estrogen can lead to bone loss.
Hematologic/blood disorders such as leukemia, lymphoma, and sickle cell disease. Many of the medications and chemotherapy used to treat these disorders can lead to bone loss and osteoporosis. Multiple myeloma, thalassemia, and any type of blood and bone marrow disorder.
Neurological/nervous system disorders such as stroke, Parkinson's disease, multiple sclerosis (MS), and spinal cord injuries generally result in significantly lower activity levels, and patients often have low vitamin D levels and a higher risk of falling.
Mental illness such as depression is associated with low bone density possibly due to medications taken and/or a lower activity level. Eating disorders such as anorexia nervosa can result in bone loss and osteoporosis.
Cancer—aromatase inhibitors, commonly used to treat women with estrogen-sensitive breast cancer, reduce the amount of estrogen in the body and can lead to bone loss and fractures. Androgen deprivation therapy, commonly used to treat prostate cancer, reduces the amount of male sex hormones in the body, which can lead to bone loss and broken bones. In addition, some chemotherapy drugs, radiation therapy to the pelvic region, steroid therapy, early menopause due to chemotherapy, radiation or surgery, long-term bed rest, and inadequate nutritional intake during therapy all increase the risk of osteoporosis.
Other diseases and conditions such as AIDS/HIV, chronic obstructive pulmonary disease (COPD), emphysema, chronic kidney disease, severe liver disease, polio and postpolio syndrome, scoliosis, organ transplantation where anti-rejection drugs are needed can all result in weakened bones and an increased risk of fractures.
Female athletes with eating disorders and who engage in excessive exercise with a loss of menstrual periods have an increased risk of osteoporosis.
A poor diet and malnutrition or a history of malnutrition can cause bone loss.
Weight loss, especially frequent and due to caloric restriction, can result in bone loss.

A normal T score or BMD in an elderly person does not translate into a low risk of fractures. According to the WHO, DXA (dual energy x-ray absorptiometry) alone for assessment of BMD is not optimal for the detection of individuals at high risk of fracture. WHO states "the risk of fracture is very high when osteoporosis is present, but by no means negligible when BMD is normal. Indeed, the majority of osteoporotic fractures will occur in individuals with a negative test. The use of the T-score alone is inappropriate since age is as great a risk factor as BMD" [11].

Risk factors for osteoporosis include age, sex, glucocorticoid use, family history, a prior fragility fracture, low body mass index, smoking and excess alcohol consumption. Many factors can contribute to the development of osteoporosis. Common issues include frequent dieting and chronic proton pump inhibitor (PPI) and anticonvulsant usage. While everyone is at risk for osteoporosis with aging, there are certain diseases and conditions that increase the risk of osteoporosis and warrant special attention.

The diseases and conditions listed in Table 7.1 may increase the risk of osteoporosis.

ARE CURRENT APPROACHES EVIDENCE BASED?

The most common, and sometimes only, nutritional advice given to individuals with osteoporosis or osteopenia is to get plenty of calcium, usually in the form of dairy products and calcium supplements. Many health care givers as well as the public believe that dairy foods and calcium supplements prevent osteoporosis and fractures. People think they need to eat lots of dairy and take calcium supplements to have strong bones because that is what they have been told by their teachers, parents, health care providers, media advertisers, and multiple government and nongovernment agencies. We know osteoporotic bone contains less calcium than healthy bone but we do not totally understand what is going on metabolically. Do we have solid evidence that milk, dairy foods, and calcium supplements give us stronger bones and reduce or prevent fractures? The whole issue is very complicated and many people are surprised to learn that it is debatable as to whether dairy and calcium prevent osteoporosis. Not all scientists support the "consume lots of dairy product to prevent osteoporosis" approach. While it is beyond the scope of this chapter, for a thorough and fascinating history of how the dairy industry has influenced the perception of milk and dairy recommendations in the United States, read Marion Nestle's books *Food Politics* and *What to Eat*.

There is no question that calcium is crucial to strong bones; the debate is over how much calcium is needed and what other nutrients need to be emphasized in the diet. Calcium myths persist despite some contradicting evidence. Presumptions in the absence of supporting scientific evidence need to be questioned and evaluated in light of what we actually know. Many, but not all, studies on the effect of calcium supplements on bone mineral content have shown that calcium supplements cause a modest increase in bone mineral content. The challenge is that this change in bone mineral content may not translate into a significant effect on the fracture rate.

A Harvard study found that men who drank one glass of milk, or less, per week were at no greater risk of breaking a hip or forearm than were those who drank two and a half or more glasses per week [12]. When data from the Harvard study were combined with data from other large prospective studies, there was still no association between calcium intake and fracture risk. Additionally, the combined results of randomized trials that compared calcium supplements with a placebo showed that calcium supplements did not protect against fractures of the hip or other bones. There was even some suggestion that calcium supplements taken without vitamin D might increase the risk of hip fractures [13]. Another study found that higher consumption of milk or other food sources of calcium by adult women did not protect against hip or forearm fractures [14]. A 2014 study found that higher milk consumption in teenagers was not associated with a lower risk of hip fracture in older adults [15]. An observational study published in the *British Medical Journal* found that a higher consumption of milk in women and men was not accompanied by a lower risk of fracture [16]. While it has not been definitely proven that calcium alone lowers fracture risk, numerous trials have reported that taking both vitamin D and calcium lowers fracture risk. It is unknown if it is the combination of calcium and vitamin D or vitamin D alone.

The Agency for Healthcare Research and Quality (AHRQ) issued a report in 2014 that found no consistent correlation between vitamin D and a variety of health outcomes, including bone health. The report summarized the evidence on the relationship between vitamin D alone or in combination with calcium on selected health outcomes, including those related to bone health. The AHRQ report concluded that the majority of the findings concerning vitamin D, alone or in combination with calcium, on the health outcomes of interest, including bone health, were inconsistent. They stated, "associations observed in prospective cohort and nested case–control studies were inconsistent, or when consistent, were rarely supported by the results of randomized controlled trials. Clear dose–response relationships between intakes of vitamin D and health outcomes were rarely observed" [17].

Western countries with the highest consumption of milk, dairy, and calcium have the world's highest fracture rates. Many developing countries with the lowest fracture rates and osteoporosis consume less calcium than Western countries (400–600 mg/day). The question as to why populations that consume low-calcium diets have fewer fractures than do Western societies, who consume high-calcium diets, is still unanswered. Explanations for this "calcium paradox" may relate to what else these populations regularly eat and the significant differences between developed and developing countries diets in intakes of processed foods, sodium, meat, dairy, fruits, and vegetables. It is possible that people who eat lots of processed foods and consume high-sodium, high-animal-protein, low-fruit-and-vegetable diets need more calcium than those eating more fruits and vegetables, less animal protein, less processed food, and less sodium.

Bones are dependent on a variety of nutrients, including but not limited to calcium. Research does not support the widely held belief that dairy products are the key to strong bones and that everyone needs to consume two to three servings of dairy per day. Counseling all patients who are trying to avoid osteoporotic bone fractures to consume two to three servings per day of dairy lacks solid evidence and does not constitute adequate or thorough dietary counseling for osteoporosis prevention and treatment.

OSTEOPOROSIS DRUGS

Drugs to prevent bone loss in people with osteoporosis and osteopenia are promoted and prescribed widely and aggressively. There is a concern among some osteoporosis experts that osteoporosis drugs are being overprescribed or prescribed before exercise and diet are given a chance to improve or stabilize bone health. Communication regarding taking osteoporosis drugs should be patient centered with a shared decision-making process that ensures patients understand all their alternatives. Informed medical decisions can only be made when a patient understands the impact of all therapies, interventions, and treatments, including nutritional interventions.

Some patients may think that taking bisphosphonates or other osteoporosis drugs will not only prevent fractures but also negate the need to worry about nutrition other than taking calcium and vitamin D supplements. It is important for patients to understand that osteoporosis drugs are not 100% effective at preventing fractures, they can have undesirable side effects and some authorities are recommending bisphosphonates not be taken for more than 3–5 years. Numerous studies on current osteoporosis drugs have found a reduced risk of fractures but the drugs vary significantly in their level of effectiveness and as to what type of fractures they actually prevent. On average, bisphosphonates impact on hip fracture reduction ranges from 40% to 50% [18]. If a patient chooses to take osteoporosis medications, they still need an appropriate exercise program and a diet that supports healthy bones. They should establish a good exercise and diet program to support current health and prepare them for when they will need to go off the drugs.

When patients are educated about the side effects and issues related to osteoporosis drugs, the decision as to whether to take the drugs may be difficult and stressful. While this is a decision that must be made by each individual based on their unique situation, both diet and exercise offer interventions patients can control without the concern for short- and long-term negative side effects. It is imperative that patients understand how significant diet and exercise are as osteoporosis treatments and that they do not mistakenly assume they are less important or effective than drug therapy. An appropriate exercise program combined with a bone-healthy diet gives patients some control and hope regarding the health of their bones.

GENERAL PRINCIPLES OF DIET FOR OSTEOPOROSIS PREVENTION AND TREATMENT

The overall goal in working with the general population is to prevent the development of low bone mass and osteoporosis. The overall goal in working with osteoporosis patients is to prevent pain and fractures. Efforts to accomplish these goals need to start early and last a lifetime. It is imperative that patients understand that nutrition for healthy bones is not just about taking a calcium and vitamin D supplement or drinking milk. A significant percent of the population, including many health care providers, lack a full understanding of how diet can affect bone health. Table 7.2 lists the key patient education goals for anyone trying to treat or prevent low bone mass.

Low-Acid Eating Theory

A popular and somewhat controversial theory related to osteoporosis and diet is that a diet high in acid-forming foods will trigger the body's ability to self-regulate and maintain a healthy blood pH

TABLE 7.2
Patient Education Goals for Treating or Preventing Low Bone Mass

Patient and/or caregivers understand calcium requirements, how to ensure adequate intake without a supplement and/or how to determine amount of supplement needed based on dietary intake as well as how to avoid oversupplementing.
Patient and/or caregivers understand the importance of consuming a variety of essential bone-healthy nutrients beyond calcium.
Patient and/or caregivers understand the importance of eating at least nine servings of vegetables and fruits per day and how to accomplish that in their eating plan.
Patient and/or caregivers understand that adequate protein is key to bone and muscle health and that inadequate protein contributes to frailty, poor balance, and an increased risk of falling, which increases the risk of fractures. They understand how to ensure adequate protein intake at all meals. If the patient is involved in strength-training, the patient understands additional protein needs for strength training and how to meet those needs.
Patient and/or caregivers are familiar with acid–alkaline food theory and concepts and are able to apply to meal planning in a practical and appropriate manner.
If needed, patient and/or caregivers have guidelines and information needed to control calorie and sodium intake while still meeting calcium, protein, and other essential nutrient needs.
Patient and/or caregivers understand how to meet their vitamin D requirement.
Patient and/or caregivers understand the role diet plays in osteoporosis prevention and treatment and that taking osteoporosis drugs does not negate the need to follow a bone-healthy diet.

and balance. The higher the acid load of the diet, the harder the body has to work to maintain a normal blood pH. The theory proposes that the body tries to defend against increasing acid by breaking down bone and muscle to obtain nutrients needed to buffer acid. Part of this balancing system is to pull the nutrients it needs from the body's mineral stores. If the imbalance is temporary, the body is thought to be able to compensate. However, if the high-acid diet is chronic and the kidneys are weakened with age, this imbalance may result in a mild but progressive metabolic acidosis that adversely affects bones and becomes a significant problem. The issue is not that the blood becomes significantly acidic or that an individual in any way significantly changes the pH of their blood. The body has several mechanisms and buffer systems that prevent your blood from becoming too acidic and you cannot live if your blood pH is not within a certain critical range (7.35–7.45). The problem is that the body's efforts to keep the body's blood pH balanced when a person consumes a high-acid, low-alkaline diet on a chronic, long-term basis may result in a loss of structural bone strength over time.

Some scientists believe dietary acid loads from Western diets may be a risk factor for osteoporosis. The acid load of a particular food is determined by what the food releases into the bloodstream upon metabolism not on the acidity of the food prior to metabolism. For instance, a lemon is acidic prior to metabolism but yields alkaline ash upon metabolism and is therefore considered to be an alkaline food when referring to the acid–alkaline theory of eating. Grains such as breads, cereals, rice, and pasta as well as meats, fish, egg yolks, and cheeses release acids into the bloodstream upon metabolism. Fruits and vegetables break down to add alkali to the bloodstream, which helps neutralize acid. Foods with higher acid loads do not have to be eliminated from the diet but they need to be eaten in moderation and adequately balanced with alkaline foods so the net effect is a more alkaline, bone-healthy diet. The best way to reduce dietary acid load is to eat lots of fruits and vegetables with modest amounts of breads, cereals, and pastas, and adequate protein, but not excessive animal protein.

There are numerous charts, food guides, and books available on the acid and alkaline values of foods but the information differs according to the source and can result in patient confusion and frustration. Trying to plan meals and eat by following these guides and charts is very difficult and often impractical. It is important that patients understand that some explanations of the dietary acid load theory are too simplistic and lack an understanding of the complexities involved in acid–base balance. Renal net acid excretion (NAE) and potential renal acid load (PRAL) calculations are more appropriate to use in estimating diet-dependent averages for groups and currently are not precise or practical enough for individual diet planning. At this point, the best approach seems to be to plan meals according to these guidelines:

Have 1 serving of fruit or vegetable
- For every ounce of meat or egg eaten
- For every cup of milk, yogurt, or beans eaten
- For every slice of bread or cup of pasta, grain, or rice eaten

Have 2 servings of fruit or vegetables
- For each ounce of cheese eaten

Since some people with life-long high-acid-eating habits may not be easily persuaded to change their eating patterns, researchers have explored the use of alkali-producing supplements. Some research administering potassium citrate in an oral form has demonstrated improvements in calcium balance and decreased markers of bone resorption [19]. Future studies should help determine if alkalinizing potassium salts can help prevent and treat osteoporosis and if there is a role for bicarbonate in reducing musculoskeletal declines in the elderly. Results of a large National Institutes of Health (NIH) trial (ClinicalTrials.gov Identifier: NCT01475214), "Musculoskeletal Effects of Bicarbonate," scheduled to end in 2015 should offer more information related to the appropriate dosing and on the study population to enroll in future bicarbonate intervention trials to determine the effects of bicarbonate on rates of bone and muscle mass loss, as well as falls and fractures. Until more data are available on the use of bicarbonate, it seems prudent to focus efforts to alkalinize the diet on consuming more fruits and vegetables and balancing acid-producing foods with alkaline foods. In addition to their alkalizing effects, fruits and vegetables offer many other bone-healthy nutrients that would not be available from a potassium bicarbonate solution. Rather than purchasing commercially available alkaline waters, encourage patients to "alkalinize" their own water by adding lemon juice. Mineral water also offers a very practical and enjoyable way to add calcium and alkalinity to the diet. The alkalizing minerals (calcium and magnesium), and the bicarbonates, in mineral water are easily absorbed by the body. Some studies have found that mineral waters can reduce calcium lost in the urine and slow bone loss [20–22]. Inhibition of bone resorption has been demonstrated with mineral waters rich in calcium and sulfate in subjects with low dietary calcium intake [20]. In subjects with relatively high calcium intake, only mineral waters, which are also rich in bicarbonate, exerted an inhibition of bone resorption. Bicarbonate-rich waters with relatively low calcium content had no measurable effect on bone metabolism [23]. The mineral and bicarbonate levels of mineral waters vary significantly from one brand to another, mainly due to the origin of the water. Select mineral waters containing calcium and with low sodium levels. The mineral content of mineral waters can usually be determined by checking the company websites or contacting the companies directly.

The pH of urine does vary; however, patients should be educated that measurement of urine pH is not a precise measurement due to volatility and solubility factors, which can result in over- or underestimation of acidity. Currently, there is inadequate evidence to support pH testing of urine to determine the efficacy of dietary interventions or osteoporosis risk in individuals. Urine pH and urine acid excretion have not been found to predict the incidence of fractures or osteoporosis [24].

More research is needed to look at the mechanisms under which potassium-rich, bicarbonate-rich foods benefit bone metabolism. Susan Lanham-New states, "The positive associations found between fruit and vegetable consumption and bone may be due to some other, yet unidentified, dietary component rather than alkali-excess effect" [25,26]. At this point, regardless of what future research on low acid load eating determines, the suggestion to eat more fruits and vegetables and less meat seems to have multiple health benefits and no adverse risks or issues.

Fruits and Vegetables

In their book, *Building Bone Vitality*, Amy Joy Lanou, PhD, and Michael Castleman reviewed 103 studies on the BMD effects of fruits and vegetables or studies of nutrients found mainly in fruits and vegetables. Eighty-four percent of the studies found that with an increase in fruit, vegetable, or antioxidant intake, BMD also increased. Nine percent of the studies were inconclusive and 7% showed no effect on BMD from fruits and vegetables [27].

Patients should be advised to eat nine or more servings per day of fruits and vegetables with two-thirds of those being vegetables. A serving size is generally half cup cooked or raw vegetables or fruit or one cup of raw greens. Encourage eating a variety of fruits and vegetables to ensure consuming a diversity of bone-healthy nutrients.

Many people are not in the habit of eating lots of fruits and vegetables and often express an aversion to vegetables. Dislike of vegetables is often based on having only eaten a limited selection of overcooked, canned, or past-their-prime vegetables. Fresh, well-prepared, high-quality vegetables are generally well accepted by most people but do require an effort to change deeply entrenched eating habits. Strategies for increasing fruit and vegetable consumption are listed in Table 7.3.

If the patient is not inclined or able to do much cooking, then preparation of smoothies by the patient or caregiver is an easy way to get lots of nutrition. Make this part of their daily routine. They can easily get five or more servings of fruits and vegetables in a smoothie. Smoothies also work well for people with little appetite, as it is much easier to drink a smoothie than to eat five servings of fruits and vegetables and one cup of yogurt. Guidelines for preparation of bone-healthy smoothies are included in Table 7.4.

TABLE 7.3
Strategies for Increasing Vegetable Consumption

Teach patients how to make delicious vegetable and fruit smoothies.
Raw vegetables are sometimes better accepted by some people than cooked vegetables, especially if served with hummus or some other tasty and nutritious dip. Raw vegetables also work well for people who cannot or do not want to cook, as they can be purchased ready-to-eat—washed and in bite-size servings.
Encourage cooking techniques, such as roasting vegetables, which yield a pleasant flavor and are easy to prepare.
Share healthy, easy-to-prepare vegetable recipes with patients.
Offer or encourage cooking classes that emphasize healthy vegetable preparation.
If practical, encourage growing some of their own vegetables as this often increases acceptance and provides some good exercise and vitamin D.

TABLE 7.4
Guidelines for High-Protein, High-Calcium, Fruit and Vegetable Smoothie

Per person, blend all of the following ingredients in a high-speed blender until smooth:
1 cup plain, nonfat Greek yogurt
1/2 cup unsweetened, plain calcium containing dairy free milk such as almond milk, skim or low-fat milk, or kefir
1 cup raw kale
1 cup raw spinach
1/2 cup raw beets
1/2 cup fruit of choice (strawberries, peaches, kiwi, blueberries, cherries, pineapple, etc.)
1 banana
1 dried plum or prune
1 tbsp. ground flaxseed
Add additional water, ice cubes, or milk if a different consistency is desired
Option: Add any extra parsley or greens that you do not expect to use before they go bad

The use of herbs should also be encouraged for the role they may play in bone health as well as for being plant foods that improve flavor. Some research, while limited to animal studies, has indicated certain herbs play a role in inhibiting bone resorption. The results of ongoing studies may provide more insight into the benefits of sage, rosemary, and thyme to bone health.

Protein

Protein is an important component of bone. Research is pointing more and more toward protein needs increasing as people age. Protein recommendations based on short-term nitrogen balance studies for young healthy men and women may not be adequate for the elderly. Aging appears to be associated with a reduced ability to stimulate skeletal muscle protein synthesis. To maximize muscle protein synthesis, it has been proposed that a dietary plan include 25–30 g of high-quality protein at three meals per day [28]. An intake of 1.0–1.3 g/kg/body weight should adequately and safely meet the needs of older adults engaged in resistance training, provided that their energy needs are met [29]. Protein recommendations should be customized to the individual depending on their age, activity level, and overall health status.

A December 2013 study in the *Nutrition* journal found a correlation between frailty and low protein intake in elderly Japanese women. Frailty in older adults is a significant risk factor for falls and broken bones, especially in men and women with low bone density. The study found that the women with a daily protein intake greater than 70 g had a significantly decreased risk of frailty. Frailty was defined by the presence of slowness and weakness, exhaustion, low physical activity, and unintentional weight loss. The women with the highest plant protein intake had a 34% decreased risk of frailty. The women with the highest animal protein intake had 27% decreased risk of frailty [30].

A 2014 study found that muscle, bone, and fat mass were significantly higher in women who had protein intake greater than 1.2 g/kg/day. A lower intake of essential amino acids in women with sarcopenia was also observed. Protein and energy intake were significant predictors of muscle mass. The study concluded "that in elderly women, an adequate protein intake in terms of quality and quantity, without need of supplementation, could have a positive impact on BMD, lean mass, and skeletal muscle mass" [31].

If the patient participates in a strength-training program to gain bone strength and improve balance, then they need to be sure they are eating enough protein to maximize muscle synthesis while still keeping a good acid–alkaline balance in their diet. In general, recreational adult exercisers need 1.1–1.6 g of protein per kilogram of body weight. Adults working to build muscle mass with strength training need 1.6–1.8 g of protein per kilogram of body weight [32]. If the patient is overweight, calculate their protein needs using their ideal body weight instead of their actual weight. Teach patients how to determine how much protein is in foods by reading the labels and looking up the nutrient content of foods using the USDA nutrient database at http://ndb.nal.usda.gov. Or they can use an online diet analysis website such as Supertracker at www.supertracker.usda.gov.

Protein is essential to healthy bones; however, when animal protein is eaten, it should be in moderate amounts and balanced out with a generous intake of fruits and vegetables. Once protein needs are determined, protein should be evenly distributed at all three meals (25–30 g protein per meal) of the day. If the individual is engaged in strength training, they can add some protein as a post workout snack within 45 min of finishing their workout. They can also include some protein in a preexercise snack and evening snack. Patients need to understand the importance of spreading out protein intake during the day and not to eat the bulk of their protein at one or two meals. Muscles need a steady supply of protein all day and in general most people cannot absorb more than 25–30 g of protein at one time. They also need to consume adequate calories from carbohydrates and healthy fats so that protein is available for optimal utilization by the body. If a patient eats only cereal, milk, and fruit for breakfast, they will probably need to add some protein at breakfast to reach 25 g. This can usually be accomplished by adding an egg (or egg whites), cottage or ricotta cheese, peanut butter or almond butter, nuts, yogurt, or lean meat.

Educate patients that in the presence of adequate carbohydrates and fats to meet energy needs, protein beyond what your body can metabolize at one meal just gets stored in the body as fat; so with protein, more is not better once you have met your needs. More research is needed to better understand the protein needs of the elderly and the optimal level for bone health.

Calcium

Studies are inconsistent as to if calcium reduces the risk of fractures. While calcium is crucial to bone health, calcium alone has not been unequivocally proven to lower the risk of fractures. Studies of calcium combined with vitamin D have found a lower risk of fractures but researchers are not sure if it is the combination of or vitamin D alone.

The report of the Joint FAO/WHO Expert Consultation on Vitamin and Mineral Requirements in Human Nutrition indicated that the requirements for calcium might vary from culture to culture for dietary, genetic, lifestyle, and geographical reasons. Therefore, two sets of allowances were recommended: one for countries with low consumption of animal protein, and another based on data from North America and Western Europe [33].

Consuming adequate calcium is key to healthy bones; however, recent studies have questioned the safety of taking large doses of calcium supplements. Calcium supplements are thought to cause blood calcium levels to increase much more abruptly than calcium-rich foods. Mark Hegsted, a long-time Harvard nutrition researcher, who died in 2009 at age 95, suggested that very high calcium intakes consumed for many years impaired the body's ability to regulate calcium, resulting in a disruption of calcium absorption and excretion [34]. The results of studies dealing with the risks and positive effects of calcium supplements have been very inconsistent. It appears that taking calcium as one or two large doses of a supplement is not the way the body is designed to absorb calcium and is not the same as obtaining calcium from food. With calcium, more is not better. Calcium from supplements may increase the risk of cardiovascular disease and kidney stones if the individual takes too much calcium from supplements or already gets enough calcium from their diet and takes supplemental calcium. The increased risk of kidney stones in women has only been observed with calcium from supplements and not with calcium from food. The theory has been proposed that giving large amounts of calcium as supplements at one time may be facilitating the development of calcifications in the arteries. The research showing an increased risk of heart disease from calcium supplements is controversial and not supported by all experts. The observed increase was seen in individuals taking calcium supplements but not with calcium from food. Some of the studies showing increased risk have been criticized for poor interpretation of the data. Other studies have not found a link. Since calcium from food is absorbed at a slower rate than from supplements and usually in smaller amounts at this point, it seems safest to recommend and help patients understand how to get calcium from food instead of supplements.

It is often stated that it is very difficult to get enough calcium from food alone; however, detailed diet histories often discover people consuming typical Western diets, high in cheese and other dairy products, can easily consume 1200 mg or more of calcium per day. Individuals on calorie-restricted diets are more likely to have low calcium intakes but are by no means precluded from obtaining enough calcium. Careful menu planning and a knowledge of good calcium food sources can ensure adequate calcium from diet alone. It may be healthier to get calcium from a variety of plant foods because they contain other important bone-building nutrients. While calcium is necessary to good bone health, the strength of bones depends more on everything eaten and how active the individual is than just how much calcium is consumed.

The absorption of calcium is highest when the meal or snack contains 500 mg or less of calcium, so it is a good idea to consume calcium in increments of 500 mg or less throughout the day. If a patient has a very high dietary sodium intake and is resistant to advice to lower their salt intake, then it may be even more crucial that they consume the recommended amounts of calcium. Calcium is lost daily from the body and if calcium from the diet is inadequate the body takes calcium from bone. Recommend getting calcium from food not supplements.

To determine the amount of calcium in a food without a label, patients can use the online USDA Nutrient Database at http://ndb.nal.usda.gov or go to www.supertracker.usda.gov to access a variety of helpful nutritional tools, including "Food-A-Pedia," "Food Tracker," and "My Recipe."

The American Association of Clinical Endocrinologists (AACE) recommends the measurement of 24-hour urine calcium be strongly considered to determine the calcium balance in any given patient if this will make a difference in patient management [35].

A June 2014 study published in the medical journal *Menopause* concludes that high calcium levels in urine and blood commonly occur with calcium and vitamin D supplementation. The study investigators were able to predict which women would have a problem by looking at their prestudy 24-hour urine calcium level. The authors noted, "Even a modest calcium supplementation of 500 mg per day may be too high for some women." The authors recommended measuring blood and urine calcium levels before starting women on supplements. It was unclear whether the high levels were caused by calcium, vitamin D, or a combination of the two. The authors of the study indicated that due to the widely recommended use of 1200 mg calcium and 800 IU vitamin D in postmenopausal women, further studies as to the wisdom of this recommendation are warranted [36]. Based on this study, it is recommended that women have their urine and blood calcium levels evaluated before they take calcium supplements. This problem can be avoided by obtaining calcium from food, which requires dietary planning and guidance but can be accomplished.

In some patients, overconsumption of calcium supplements could potentially be a significant problem. The common recommendation by many health care providers to take a 1200 mg calcium supplement, without considering the calcium being consumed in the diet, results in patients getting too much calcium. The patient should first try to get all their calcium from food. If that is not possible, then the patient should only supplement at the level they need to meet their calcium requirement beyond what they do not get from food. For example, if the patient consumes 800 mg calcium per day and their recommended amount is 1200 mg, then they only need to take a 400 mg calcium supplement.

Vitamin D

Vitamin D is essential for the absorption of calcium and phosphate into bone. It also plays a key role in muscle strength and therefore affects the risk of falling. Vitamin D blood levels less than 30 ng/mL have been associated with balance problems [37], impaired lower extremity function [38], high fall rates [39,40], and muscle weakness [41–43]. A meta-analysis of clinical trials to estimate the effectiveness of vitamin D supplementation in preventing hip and nonvertebral fractures in older persons found 700–800 IUs of vitamin D per day decreases the risk of hip and nonvertebral fractures [44]. A second meta-analysis suggested that oral vitamin D appears to reduce the risk of hip fractures only when calcium supplementation is added [45]. A third meta-analysis concluded vitamin D supplementation appears to reduce the risk of falls among ambulatory or institutionalized older individuals with stable health by more than 20% [46]. The impact from vitamin D on fractures is most likely due to a measurable reduction in falls, as the impact of vitamin D on bone density appears very limited. Research presented at the American Society for Bone and Mineral Research (ASBMR) 2014 annual meeting reported that women with a mean age at the time of 25(OH)D measure of 48.5 years, with 25(OH)D levels of greater than 20 ng/mL had as much as a 45% lower risk of fracture, compared with women with lower levels [47].

The diet is not rich in vitamin D and low blood levels are not uncommon. However, some people do get enough vitamin D from the sun and the foods they eat. Fatty fish and mushrooms exposed to ultraviolet light are some of the best food sources. Fortified foods can also be a significant source of vitamin D. Without sun exposure, it can be difficult to get enough vitamin D from diet alone. There are a variety of formulas and recommendations for determining how much time is needed in the sun to make enough vitamin D. A general recommendation is 15–20 min to the face, arms, legs or back, two to three times per week without sunscreen with the sun at least 45° above the horizon. Vitamin D production by the body depends on the following:

- Age—After age 50, the body's ability to make vitamin D seems to decline.
- The time of year and where the person lives.
- Skin pigmentation—Darker skin may mean less vitamin D production; however, some research suggests that people who are black may have lower vitamin D levels than whites and these lower levels may be sufficient for blacks.
- Sunscreen use can interfere with vitamin D synthesis, depending on the extent and frequency of use.

Some recent research has indicated that it is healthiest for vitamin D levels to not be too low or too high [48]. Body levels of vitamin D can be determined with a blood test. If the level is below 20 ng/L, then if possible and not contraindicated, it may be appropriate to suggest getting a little more sun as well as trying to consume more vitamin D-fortified foods. If a vitamin D deficiency cannot be corrected with diet and sun exposure, then supplementation should be discussed and recommended as appropriate. Assist patients and caregivers in choosing a vitamin D supplementation schedule they are most likely to follow. D3 as a supplement is preferable to D1 or D2 as D3 may raise levels more effectively and is less likely to cause erroneously low vitamin D blood test results. To increase absorption by as much as 50% suggest taking the supplement with meals that contain some healthy fat. A rule of thumb for raising serum levels of 25-hydroxyvitamin D is that about 100 IU of vitamin D3 daily will raise serum levels by about 1 ng/dL; however, more (up to twice) may be required in obese individuals [49]. The ConsumerLab.com® website at www.consumerlab.com is a good resource for learning which vitamin D supplements ConsumerLab.com has approved (service does require an annual subscription). ConsumerLab.com also includes information on which supplements are the best buy. The Institute of Medicine provides reference values and information on vitamin D at http://www.iom.edu/Reports/2010/Dietary-Reference-Intakes-for-Calcium-and-Vitamin-D.aspx (The Institute of Medicine November 30 2010 Dietary Reference Intakes for Calcium and Vitamin D). The Endocrine Society provides vitamin D supplementation guidelines in their "Evaluation, Treatment, and Prevention of Vitamin D Deficiency: an Endocrine Society Clinical Practice Guideline" [50].

As with many supplements, it is important that patients understand more is not better and that they can get too much vitamin D in the form of a supplement. Excessive vitamin D can cause high blood levels of calcium and increase the risk of kidney stones. Some evidence has even suggested too much vitamin D might increase the risk of falls [51]. Vitamin D recommendations should be made in conjunction with medical judgment on an individual patient basis.

Based on the Institute of Medicines report, ConsumerLab.com recommends maintaining blood levels of vitamin D above 20 ng/mL, but not much higher than 30 ng/mL. If the vitamin D blood level rises above 35 ng/L on a supplement, they recommend cutting back on the supplement to avoid possibly doing more harm than good [49]. Bess Dawson-Hughes, MD, Director of Tufts HNRCA Bone Metabolism Laboratory, indicates that research at Tufts and other laboratories suggests 30 ng/mL of vitamin D is the optimum blood level for bone health [52]. The Clinician's Guide to Prevention and Treatment of Osteoporosis Position Paper published in 2014 states, "Vitamin D supplements should be recommended in amounts sufficient to bring the serum 25(OH)D level to approximately 30 ng/mL (75 nmol/L) and a maintenance dose recommended to maintain this level, particularly for individuals with osteoporosis [18]. The American Geriatrics Society (AGS) Consensus report, "Vitamin D for the Prevention of Falls and Their Consequences in Older Adults" provides clinical guidance on vitamin D supplementation for older adults. The report is a result of concerns about falls and fall-related injuries in older adults. The committee responsible for the report was composed of experts on vitamin D and geriatricians with clinical research and clinical experience related to falls and/or vitamin D. Key points from the report include the following:

- Vitamin D levels of approximately 30 ng/mL appear to protect against fall-related injuries.
- A total average daily intake of vitamin D from all sources (dietary, sunlight, and supplements) of 4000 IU will ensure that 90% of older adults will have serum 25-hydroxy vitamin D levels of 30 ng/mL.
- Daily supplementation with 4000 IU of vitamin D is safe and nontoxic.
- It is important to receive adequate calcium with vitamin D [53].

The AACE recommends using a range from 30 to 50 ng/mL for serum 25(OH)D levels for most patients as an optimal and safe range [35].

Based on a review of the data on vitamin D needs, a committee of the Institute of Medicine concluded that:

- Persons are at risk of vitamin D deficiency at serum 25(OH)D concentrations <30 nmol/L (<12 ng/mL).
- There is a potential risk for inadequacy at levels ranging from 30 to 50 nmol/L (12–20 ng/mL).
- Practically all people are sufficient at levels ≥50 nmol/L (≥20 ng/mL).
- 50 nmol/L is the serum 25(OH)D level that covers the needs of 97.5% of the population.
- Serum concentrations >125 nmol/L (>50 ng/mL) are associated with potential adverse effects [54].

When evaluating 25-OH levels, be sure to note which measurement unit is being used. Serum concentrations of 25(OH)D and recommended levels are reported in both nanomoles per liter (nmol/L) and nanograms per milliliter (ng/mL). 1 nmol/L = 0.4 ng/mL.

Research on vitamin D continues to evolve and more understanding of how vitamin D affects bone and overall health is expected in the future.

Phosphorus

Phosphorus is an essential building block for bone and generally is easily obtained in Western diets. Some significant sources of phosphorus in the typical Western diet are whole grains, meat, poultry, and dairy foods. The issue with phosphorus is that when an individual consumes significantly more phosphorus than calcium, an excess of phosphorus can result in reduced calcium absorption.

Animal studies indicate that high phosphorus intakes are detrimental to bone. Human studies have also shown that a high phosphate diet has negative effects on bone, especially when combined with low calcium intakes. Phosphorus intake is high in Western countries, often two to three times the recommended intake [55]. The intake of phosphorus in Western diets is increasing due to the widespread use of phosphorus-containing food additives. Phosphorus from food additives is more bioavailable than from foods with naturally occurring phosphorus, which may make it more harmful [56].

An NIH study found that phosphorus-containing additives significantly increased the amount of phosphorus in chicken products and that available nutrient databases did not reflect the higher phosphorus content. The study concluded that variation between similar products makes it impossible for patients and dietitians to accurately estimate phosphorus content [57]. Educate patients that the actual phosphorus level of processed foods may not be known. Advise patients to look for phosphorus-containing additives on ingredient labels. Phosphorus-containing additives include sodium phosphate, sodium aluminum phosphate, sodium acid pyrophosphate, monocalcium phosphate, sodium tripolyphosphate, dicalcium phosphate, hexametaphosphate, phosphoric acid, pyrophosphate, and tricalcium phosphate.

More human research, focused on the effects of high phosphorus and low Ca:P ratios on bone health and fractures, is needed before definite conclusions can be made. Since there are already numerous reasons to discourage the consumption of processed foods, dietary advice related to bone and overall health should include limiting or eliminating the use of additive-containing processed foods.

Magnesium

Magnesium contributes to the structural development of bone and is key in over 300 enzyme systems in the body. Studies have found a positive association between magnesium intake and BMD in both men and women [58]. Some research indicates that magnesium deficiency may be a risk factor for osteoporosis [59]. One study found that women with osteoporosis have lower serum magnesium levels than women with osteopenia and women without osteoporosis or osteopenia [60]. The "What We Eat in America" report found that one-half of all people in the United States do not get adequate magnesium from food and water and that the problem is worse in some gender age groups. More than two-thirds of adults 71 years and older had inadequate intake [61]. Because serum levels have little correlation with total body magnesium levels or concentrations in specific tissues, no single method is considered satisfactory for assessing magnesium status [62].

Good food sources of magnesium include almonds, cashews, peanuts, leafy green vegetables, legumes, seeds, dark chocolate, and whole grains. Magnesium content is lowered substantially when grains are refined by methods that remove the nutrient-rich germ and bran. A bone-healthy and varied diet that is high in vegetables, seeds, nuts, legumes, and whole grains should meet normal magnesium needs. A dietary pattern dominated by meat, containing few vegetables, and limited in whole grains is unlikely to meet magnesium requirements. Magnesium supplements should be considered and tailored to the patient's individual needs if it is not possible to meet magnesium needs with food alone. Magnesium supplements can have a laxative effect, which is a positive for individuals with constipation, but as the dose increases can be a negative for others.

Vitamin K2

There are two forms of vitamin K, K1, and K2. The functions and food sources for the two are different. K2 deficiency is prevalent but K1 deficiency is rare. K2 is key to the body's process of drawing calcium into the bones and incorporating it into the bone matrix. K1 plays a major role in blood clotting.

A Japanese study indicated the regular consumption of natto, a fermented soy food high in vitamin K2, is associated with a lower risk of hip fractures in women compared to women in areas of Japan where natto is not frequently eaten [63]. Vitamin K2 is also key in triggering the body's process responsible for removing excess calcium that can accumulate in arteries and veins. One 10-year study found lower vitamin K2 intakes in individuals diagnosed with significant aortic calcification than individuals with mild or moderate aortic calcification [64]. There are concerns about taking calcium supplements in the presence of K2 deficiency. Patients need to understand that it is important to include good sources of K2 in their diets to be sure calcium is properly utilized in the body. More studies are needed before supplementation is recommended and it is possible that, like other key nutrients, it will be determined that getting K2 from food, not supplements, is best.

K1 is found in leafy greens. K2 is found in animal products such as chicken, beef, egg yolks, and hard whole milk cheeses, all of which are high-acid foods. Patients should understand they can eat these foods in moderate amounts just being sure to balance them out with lots of fruits and vegetables. Meat and dairy from grass-fed animals are higher in vitamin K2 than their grain-fed counterparts because animals can synthesize vitamin K2 from K1, which they obtain from grass. A strain of bacteria used in the fermentation process of natto makes natto the only vegetarian food source of K2. In Japan natto is typically mixed with rice and served for breakfast. Natto has a strong smell and flavor with a sticky consistency so for most people it is an acquired taste. If you want to encourage patients to try natto provide them with some sources and recipes or suggest they google natto to find recipes.

Vitamin B12

Vitamin B12 is necessary for proper blood cell formation, healthy neurological function, and is required to build bones. One osteoporosis study found that men and women with low B12 levels had lower than average BMD [65]. In its natural form, B12 in foods such as meat, fish, poultry, eggs, and dairy products is bound to proteins in the food. Hydrochloric acid and an enzyme in the stomach that breaks down proteins, release the B12 from food so the body can use the B12. Unfortunately, some older adults lack adequate stomach acid for this process to occur. Additionally, the widespread use of PPIs increases the risk of B12 malabsorption. A *Journal of the American Medical Association* study found that individuals taking PPIs for more than 2 years were 65% more likely to be deficient in B12. The study also found that histamine 2 receptor agonists, such as Tagamet®, Pepcid®, and Zantac®, also interfered with B12 absorption with the risk for B12 deficiency in users being 25% higher [66].

Foods fortified with vitamin B12 and B12 supplements use the synthetic form of vitamin B12, which is already in a free form and does not require stomach acids for absorption. Plant foods do not contain vitamin B12. Some nutritional yeast contains B12.

Individuals over 50 years of age as well as those taking acid-blocking medications need to consume foods fortified with purified vitamin B12 or take a B12 supplement to meet their B12 needs. Some experts believe daily intakes should be higher, between 6 and 10 mcg, to better ensure acceptable B12 concentrations in people with adequate vitamin B12 status and absorption [67,68]. Individuals on medications such as metformin, PPIs, and H2 receptor agonists may require more vitamin B12. The body's ability to absorb vitamin B12 from dietary supplements is limited. Only about 10 mcg of a 500 mcg oral supplement is actually absorbed in healthy people. A clinical trial published in the 2003 *British Journal of Clinical Pharmacology* found that B-12 is absorbed just as well from a tablet as from a sublingual form [69]. People with Leber's disease, a hereditary eye condition, should not take B12 supplements because of a risk of harm to the optic nerve possibly leading to blindness [70]. Most B-12 supplements are made with cyanocobalamin, which concerns some people. The rationale for this concern is debatable. If the patient or health care provider is concerned about this, they may use a B-12 supplement made with methylcobalamin, which generally costs a little more, but avoids cyanocobalamin.

Vitamin A

The 2002 Harvard Nurses' Health Study found that postmenopausal women consuming at least 6600 IU of preformed vitamin A per day from food and supplements had nearly double the risk of hip fracture [71]. Additional studies since the 2002 study have produced mixed results with some showing no link between vitamin A and fractures and others reporting a link between osteoporosis and vitamin A.

Vitamin A is available in two forms—as preformed, from animal products, dietary supplements, and fortified foods and as beta carotene (and some other carotenoids) from fruits and vegetables. Vitamin A is essential to good bone health; however, high intakes can stimulate cells involved with bone breakdown and suppress cells involved with bone formation. Some lab research has also determined that high vitamin A intakes could interfere with vitamin D, another important bone nutrient. The bone health concerns and studies relate only to preformed vitamin A, not to beta carotene.

To get the vitamin A needed for healthy bones, and to avoid the worry of too much preformed vitamin A, recommend obtaining vitamin A as beta carotene from fruits and vegetables. Suggest eating lots of colorful carotenoid-rich foods such as leafy greens, broccoli, carrots, cantaloupe, sweet potatoes, and apricots.

Potassium

Many Americans get less than half the potassium they need in their diets. Adequate potassium is thought to help lower blood pressure and protect against heart disease, muscle wasting, osteoporosis, and kidney stones. Potassium is thought to be important to bone health because of its role in neutralizing bone-depleting acids in the body and helping to conserve calcium in the body. It has been suggested that eating foods high in potassium may play a role in osteoporosis prevention. The ideal way to get potassium is to eat lots of fruits and vegetables, which have additional bone benefits beyond the potassium.

Alcohol

Alcohol can impair balance and is a risk factor for falling, which can result in fractures. The results of studies on the effects of moderate alcohol consumption (one drink per day for women and two drinks per day for men) on bones have been mixed. Some research has found that alcohol consumption, especially if long-term and heavy, increases the risk of fractures [72,73]. This is a significant concern since, according to the National Institute on Alcohol Abuse and Alcoholism, a significant number of people engage in heavy and binge drinking [74]. Some researchers believe moderate alcohol intake is not harmful to bone but that chronic alcohol abuse is detrimental to bone health, with one of the mechanisms being a direct toxic effect on bone-forming cells. Since moderate alcohol consumption may reduce the risk of heart disease but increase the risk of some cancers, whether to drink alcohol is already a challenging decision that needs to be made on an individual basis and should always include a recommendation for moderation.

Sodium

A few studies have investigated the effect of sodium on bone density. The results have been mixed with some indicating a high-salt diet reduces bone density and some finding no effect on bone density. The research seems to point toward excessively high sodium intakes as being of the most concern even when bone density is normal. There is still considerable debate as to how effectively the body can adapt calcium absorption in response to high sodium intakes but the higher the sodium intake the more reason for concern.

Sodium in the form of salt, or sodium chloride, increases urinary calcium excretion but the effect on calcium metabolism and balance, as well as on bone, is not fully understood. Calciuria can be the result of numerous metabolic scenarios. Some research suggests that high sodium chloride intakes may be more detrimental to bone when overall calcium intake is low rather than high [75]. Potassium intakes within the recommended ranges may reduce or prevent salt-induced calciuria [76].

The possible relationship between sodium chloride intake and mild metabolic acidosis is also of interest. A small prospective study in young healthy subjects demonstrated that dietary NaCl increases low-grade chronic metabolic acidosis in a dose-dependent effect and is associated with significant dose-dependent increases in urinary calcium excretion and bone resorption markers [77]. It has also been shown that salt-sensitive humans had significantly lower blood pH and plasma bicarbonate levels on high-salt diets compared to salt-resistant humans [78]. Another study found "evidence that, in healthy humans, the diet loads of NaCl and net acid independently predict systemic acid–base status, with increasing degrees of low-grade hyperchloremic metabolic acidosis as the loads increase." The authors stated, "we argue for the biological plausibility of the diet load of sodium chloride as causal of the acidosis-producing effect and discuss the evidence suggesting participation of dietary sodium chloride in increasing the risk of osteoporosis and kidney stones in people eating a net acid-producing diet" [79].

The main source of salt in the American diet is processed food and restaurant food. Everyone should avoid extremely high intakes of salt, which can easily result from eating lots of processed and restaurant food. At this time, it seems wise for sodium recommendations for osteoporosis to be in line with the Dietary Guidelines for Americans recommendation to limit sodium to less than 2300 milligrams per day or 1500 milligrams if 51 years or older, if black or have high blood pressure, diabetes, or chronic kidney disease. In addition, because of the synergies with salt, it is imperative that nutritional advice regarding bone health and sodium intake also include ensuring calcium and potassium intakes are optimal.

Caffeine

High intakes of coffee and caffeine have been associated with an increased risk of fractures in some studies of women yet other studies have failed to find an increased risk. It is hypothesized that caffeine might contribute to bone loss by increasing the excretion of calcium in urine and decreasing the intestinal absorption of calcium.

A 2013 Swedish study published in the *American Journal of Epidemiology* found there was no association between increasing coffee consumption and rate of any type fracture. Compared with an intake level of less than one cup per day, consumption of eight or more cups per day was not associated with a higher rate of any type fracture. A high level of coffee consumption was associated with modestly lower BMD; however, this did not translate into a higher fracture rate [80]. An earlier Swiss study (2006) concluded that a daily intake of 330 mg of caffeine, equivalent to four cups (600 mL) of coffee, or more may be associated with a modestly increased risk of osteoporotic fractures, and may be more of an issue in women with a low calcium intake [81].

At this time, based on the research and the fact that coffee and tea may have other health benefits there does not seem to be good justification for discouraging moderate caffeine intake because of osteoporosis or a concern that caffeine will result in a higher risk of bone fractures in people consuming adequate calcium and other nutrients essential to healthy bones.

Sodas

Studies on the effect of drinking sodas and bone health have conflicting findings with some results, indicating problems, others finding no negative effects and others yielding uncertain results. One Tufts University study only saw a problem with cola drinks in women and not with noncola drinks like Sprite® and Mountain Dew® [82]. Cola drinks generally contain the additive phosphoric acid and Sprite and Mountain Dew do not.

It is possible that people who drink a lot of soda have overall less healthy diets and consume less calcium and less fruits and vegetables, but this has not been proven. Some recent research has found an association between sugar-sweetened sodas and accelerated cellular aging of tissues [83]. Since the use of sodas should be discouraged for a number of nutritional and health reasons, it is best to recommend avoidance of sodas and to offer recommendations for bone-healthy alternative beverages such as mineral water, fruit and vegetable–infused waters, ginger tea, and herbal teas.

Prunes

A 2011 study published in the *British Journal of Nutrition* found that postmenopausal women consuming dried plums (100 g of dried plums—about 10 prunes—each day) had significantly higher BMD in the ulna and spine, compared to postmenopausal women consuming dried apples (100 g). The study was funded by the U.S. Department of Agriculture and the California Dried Plum Board provided the dried plums for the study, as well as some funding to measure markers of oxidative stress [84]. We need more studies to further understand and confirm the effect of prunes on bone health and fracture risk and if less than 10 prunes per day or prune juice has the same effect on bones. Meanwhile, adding some prunes to the diet when possible is a good idea.

Prunes are known to have a laxative effect and not everyone may be able to tolerate, or desire to eat, 100 g of prunes per day, or to afford the 240 calories 100 g of prunes contains. Clinicians can suggest patients gradually incorporate a few prunes into their diets to see how they tolerate them. If they have issues with constipation adding prunes to their diet will have added benefits. It should be emphasized that it is important to not eat prunes at the expense of other fruits and vegetables.

Whole Grains

A 2008 *Journal of Medicinal Food* study found that BMD increased with increasing phytate consumption. The authors concluded that phytate consumption had a protective effect against osteoporosis and suggested that low phytate consumption should be considered an osteoporosis risk factor. This study adds weight to the already prevalent recommendation to regularly include whole grains instead of refined grains in the diet [85].

Fluid Intake

Dehydration is a risk factor for falling. Education to prevent dehydration should be offered with an emphasis on assuring adequate fluid intake when exercising and in warm weather. Patients should understand the need for additional fluid if they are running a fever or experiencing diarrhea or vomiting. There are many good resources available for educating patients about fluid intake. The CDC website "Water: Meeting Your Daily Fluid Needs" at http://www.cdc.gov/nutrition/everyone/basics/water.html offers a good start with multiple links to additional information on meeting fluid requirements.

EXERCISE

The forces of muscle contraction and weight-bearing are the two most important factors needed to strengthen bone [86]. Therefore, appropriate weight-bearing and/or resistance training to optimize whole bone strength is an imperative adjunct to a bone-healthy diet. While one of the primary goals of exercise is to build bone mass and strength, equally important is avoiding muscle loss. Muscle loss leads to frailty and poor balance, which increases the risk of falls. Hip fractures are often the result of falls.

Individuals with osteoporosis should work with physical therapists or follow exercise plans designed by physical therapists or exercise professionals who understand the special needs and precautions to follow with osteoporosis. Not all exercise is acceptable for persons with osteoporosis. Some exercises could be harmful for individuals at risk for vertebral fractures. Forward-bending movements can increase the risk of fractures and contribute to negative postural changes in people with fragile bones. As it is inadequate to limit nutritional advice for osteoporosis patients to "drink lots of milk and take calcium," it is also inappropriate to tell osteoporosis patients to simply exercise, without educating them on appropriate, safe, and effective exercise. Each person's physical condition and degree of bone loss will determine what exercises can most benefit them and what exercises they should avoid. A physical therapist trained to work with osteoporosis patients can teach patients how to do site-specific, weight-bearing exercise designed to target areas of the body where strengthening and flexibility are critical to preventing fractures and pain.

Identify physical therapy partners in your community and share their contact information with your clients. Advise clients of online resources as well. See the resources section for information on professionals specifically focused and trained on the needs of osteoporosis patients.

IDENTIFYING OBSTACLES TO SUCCESS

Practical issues that might prevent the patient from accomplishing the nutritional and exercise goals need to be identified early so that resources or solutions can be developed. Financial, mental, or physical limitations, such as the inability to cook, chew certain foods, and drive or get to a grocery store, can interfere with successful implementation and adherence to the dietary principles. Fracture liaison service (FLS) programs can offer care coordination and transition management and should always include the involvement of a dietitian and physical therapist.

FOLLOW-UP, EVALUATION, AND MEASURING SUCCESS

A good program includes a process for measuring the success and impact of the interventions and education on patient's lives and well-being. Including a tool for evaluating patient's understanding of educational goals will help ensure the educational process has resulted in the knowledge needed to maximize the benefits of food and nutrition. There should be a mechanism for determining if patients successfully avoid fractures and pain and if there are signs of BMD improvement. When patients do succumb to fractures or experience pain, a root cause analysis to determine if there are lessons to be learned and/or improvements to be made in future care plans can facilitate improvement of overall future patient care.

CONCLUSION

The ideal scenario is for patients to work with a registered dietitian nutritionist that can educate them on the best ways to obtain all the nutrients needed for strong bones. An additional option for patients is to use an online eating plan specifically designed for osteoporosis treatment and prevention to help with meal planning. An online program provides an economical alternative and adjunct to working directly with a dietitian nutritionist. An online program facilitates an awareness of evolving nutrition research and changing recommendations as more is learned about the role of nutrition in osteoporosis prevention and treatment. (Disclosure: The author is the owner of food4osteoporosis.com, an online eating plan for osteoporosis.)

As with most medical conditions, the science behind osteoporosis nutrition will continue to evolve and new discoveries and conclusions will further modify what health care professionals recommend to patients. It is critical that anyone giving nutritional advice to individuals with or wanting to prevent osteoporosis and osteoporotic bone fractures offer up-to-date recommendations based on good research. Successfully meeting and overcoming the challenges of osteoporosis and osteopenia will result in a better quality of life for patients, more cost-effective use of limited health care dollars, and an overall improved utilization of health care resources.

RESOURCES

www.food4osteoporosis.com. Reference for patients and health care providers. Food 4 Osteoporosis website offers bone-healthy dietary guidance, including how to meet calcium needs with food, how to incorporate lots of fruits and vegetables into the diet, and how to balance out acid foods with alkaline foods. Includes a subscription online eating plan with dietitian-designed menus that meet osteoporosis nutrient needs and provides recipes and grocery lists for every day of the year. Blog addresses current issues and developments in osteoporosis nutrition research. (Disclosure—author owns this business and website.)

http://nof.org/connect/group. National Osteoporosis Foundation website support group directory to locate osteoporosis support groups in the United States.

www.Consumerlab.com. ConsumerLab.com® for information on supplements, including those that pass their quality tests and are most cost effective (this is a subscription service).

http://www.sarameekspt.com. Website by physical therapist, Sara Meeks PT, MS, GCS, specializing in osteoporosis and low bone mass. The website offers useful information for patients and health care professionals, including how to contact Sara for personal consultations and how to order patient education videos and her book *WALK TALL! An Exercise Program for the Prevention and Treatment of Back Pain, Osteoporosis and the Postural Changes of Aging*. Sara offers training seminars for health professionals in the United States and internationally. Watch her website for a new book Sara is working on.

http://www.melioguide.com/home. Website by physical therapist Margaret Martin, specifically focused on osteoporosis and low bone mass. The website offers useful information for patients and health care professionals, including exercise information, informative blog posts, how to contact for personal consultations, and an online osteoporosis exercise program. Margaret has two excellent books *Strengthen Your Core* and *Yoga for Better Bones*. Margaret's company Melioguide™ also offers continuing education online courses, workshops, and inservices for health and fitness professionals.

http://www.buildingbonevitality.com/page3/page3.html. References to the 1200 studies that form the basis of the book *Building Bone Vitality*.

http://www.capture-the-fracture.org. International Osteoporosis Foundation program, Capture the Fracture®, promotes secondary fracture prevention on a global level by facilitating the implementation of Fracture Liaison Services (FLS), a coordinator-based, post fracture model of care. This website contains information and programs to guide health care systems worldwide to improve the management of secondary fractures through standards, change, and awareness.

http://nof.org/hcp. BoneSource®, a National Osteoporosis Foundation professional program, that promotes excellence in clinical care for all health care professionals involved in the prevention, diagnosis, and treatment of osteoporosis. BoneSource offers a variety of programs, tools, and resources to meet the unique needs of health care professionals who provide bone health care.

BOOKS

Building Bone Vitality by Amy Joy Lanou, PhD, and Michael Castleman
Food 4 Osteoporosis Four Week Eating Plan by Nancy Robinson, RDN, LD
Strengthen Your Core by Margaret Martin, PT
Walk Tall by Sara Meeks, PT, MS, GCS
Yoga for Your Bones by Margaret Martin, PT

REFERENCES

1. Johnell, O., Kanis, J.A. 2006. An estimate of the worldwide prevalence and disability associated with osteoporotic fractures. *Osteoporos Int.* 17:1726.
2. Melton, L.J, Atkinson, E.J., O'Connor, M.K. et al. 1998. Bone density and fracture risk in men. *J Bone Miner Res.* 13:1915.
3. Melton, L.J., Chrischilles, E.A., Cooper, C. et al. 1992. Perspective. How many women have osteoporosis? *J Bone Miner Res.* 7:1005.
4. Kanis, J.A., Johnell, O., Oden, A. et al. 2000. Long-term risk of osteoporotic fracture in Malmo. *Osteoporos Int.* 11:669.
5. Gullberg, B., Johnell, O., Kanis, J.A. 1997. World-wide projections for hip fracture. *Osteoporos Int.* 7:407.
6. International Osteoporosis Foundation. 2000. How fragile is her future?
7. Singer, A., Exuzides, A., Spangler, L. et al. Jan 2015. Burden of illness for osteoporotic fractures compared with other serious diseases among postmenopausal women in the United States. *Mayo Clin Proc.* 90(1):53–62.
8. Lippuner, K., Grifone, S., Schwenkglenks, M. et al. 2012. Comparative trends in hospitalization for osteoporotic fractures and other frequent diseases between 2000 and 2008. *Osteoporos Int.* 23:829–839.
9. American Academy of Orthopaedic Surgeons American Association of Orthopaedic Surgeons Position Statement 1144. 2008. Hip Fracture in Seniors: A Call for Health System Reform. http://www.aaos.org/about/papers/position/1144.asp
10. Ebeling, P. 2014. Osteoporosis in men: Why change needs to happen. International Osteoporosis Foundation. http://share.iofbonehealth.org/WOD/2014/thematic-report/WOD14-Report.pdf (accessed December 22, 2014).
11. WHO Scientific Group Technical Report. 2007. Assessment of Osteoporosis at the Primary Health Care Level. Section 1.1. http://www.iofbonehealth.org/sites/default/files/WHO_Technical_Report-2007.pdf
12. Owusu, W., Willett, W.C., Feskanich, D., Ascherio, A., Spiegelman, D., Colditz, G.A. 1997. Calcium intake and the incidence of forearm and hip fractures among men. *J Nutr.* 127:1782–1787.
13. Bischoff-Ferrari, H.A., Dawson-Hughes, B., Baron, J.A. et al. 2007. Calcium intake and hip fracture risk in men and women: A meta-analysis of prospective cohort studies and randomized controlled trials. *Am J Clin Nutr.* 86:1780–1790.
14. Feskanich, D., Willett, W.C., Stampfer, M.J., Colditz, G.A. 1997. Milk, dietary calcium, and bone fractures in women: A 12-year prospective study. *Am J Public Health.* 87:992–997.
15. Feskanich, D., Bischoff-Ferrari, H.A., Frazier, A.L., Willett, W.C. 2014. Milk consumption during teenage years and risk of hip fractures in older adults. *JAMA Pediatr.* 168(1):54–60.
16. Michaëlsson, K., Wolk, A., Langenskiöld, S. et al. October 2014. Milk intake and risk of mortality and fractures in women and men: Cohort studies. *BMJ.* 28;349:g6015.

17. Newberry, S., Chung, M., Shekelle, P. et al. September 2014. Evidence Report/Technology Assessment Number 217 Vitamin D and calcium: A systematic review of health outcomes (Update) Prepared for: Agency for Healthcare Research and Quality U.S. Department of Health and Human Services 540 Gaither Road. Rockville, MD 20850 www.ahrq.gov Prepared by: Southern California Evidence-based Practice Center Santa Monica, CA AHRQ Publication No. 14-E004-EF. http://www.ncbi.nlm.nih.gov/books/NBK253540/toc/
18. Cosman, F., de Beur, S.J., LeBoff, M.S. 2014. Position paper clinician's guide to prevention and treatment of osteoporosis. *Osteoporos Int.* 25:2359–2381.
19. Moseley, K., Weaver, C., Appel, L., Sebastian, A., Sellmeyer, D. March 2013. Potassium citrate supplementation results in sustained improvement in calcium balance in older men and women. *J Bone Miner Res.* 28:497–504.
20. Meunier, P., Jenvrin, C., Munoz, F., de la Gueronnire, V., Garnero, P., Menz, M. 2005. Consumption of a high calcium mineral water lowers biochemical indices of bone remodeling in postmenopausal women with low calcium intake. *Osteoporos Int.* 16:1203–1209.
21. Burckhardt, P., Waldvogel, S., Aeschlimann, J., Arnaud, M. 2002. Bicarbonate in mineral water inhibits bone resorption. (EMINOS-1). *J Bone Miner Res.* 17(suppl):M360–S476.
22. Wynn, E., Krieg, M.A., Aeschlimann, J.M., Burckhardt, P. 2009. Alkaline mineral water lowers bone resorption even in calcium sufficiency (EMINOS-2). *Bone.* 44:120–124.
23. Burckhardt, P. 2010. Bicarbonate-rich waters with a relatively low calcium content may have no measurable effect on bone metabolism. In *Nutritional Influences on Bone Health*, eds. P. Burckhardt, B. Dawson-Hughes, and C. Weaver, 181–185. Springer, Dordrecht, Heidelberg, London, New York.
24. Fenton, T.R., Eliasziw, M., Tough, S.C., Lyon, A.W., Brown, J.P, Hanley, D.A. 2010. Low urine pH and acid excretion do not predict bone fractures or the loss of bone mineral density: A prospective cohort study. *BMC Musculoskelet Disord.* 11:88.
25. Lanham-New, S.A. 2006. Fruit and vegetables: The unexpected natural answer to the question of osteoporosis prevention? *Am J Clin Nutr.* 83(6):1254–1255 (editorial).
26. Lanham-New, S.A. In *Nutritional Influences on Bone Health*, eds. P. Burckhardt, B. Dawson-Hughes, and C. Weaver, 170. Springer, Dordrecht, Heidelberg, London, New York.
27. Lanou, A.J., Castleman, M. 2009. *Building Bone Vitality.* McGraw-Hill, USA.
28. Paddon-Jones, D., Rasmussen, B.B. January 2009. Dietary protein recommendations and the prevention of sarcopenia: Protein, amino acid metabolism and therapy. *Curr Opin Clin Nutr Metab Care.* 12(1): 86–90.
29. Lucas, M., Heiss, C.J. April 2005. Protein needs of older adults engaged in resistance training: A review. *J Aging Phys Act.* 13(2):223–236.
30. Kobayashi, S., Asakura, K, Suga, H., Sasaki, S. December 2013. High protein intake is associated with low prevalence of frailty among old Japanese women: A multicenter cross-sectional study. *Nutr J.* 12:164.
31. Genaro, P.D., Pinheiro, M.D., Szejnfeld, V.L., Martini, L.A. April 2015. Dietary protein intake in elderly women: Association with muscle and bone mass. *Nutr Clin Pract.* 30(2):283–289. pii: 0884533614545404. [Epub ahead of print].
32. Clark, N. 2014. *Nancy Clark's Sports Nutrition Guidebook,* Fifth edition. Human Kinetics, USA.
33. Vitamin and mineral requirements in human nutrition. 1998. Report of the Joint FAO/WHO Expert Consultation. Geneva, World Health Organization, 59–84 (accessed December 2014).
34. Campbell, T.C., Campbell, T.M. 2004. *The China Study.* Benbella Books, Dallas, TX.
35. American Association of Clinical Endocrinologists AACE Recommendations. Article 106. https://www.aace.com/article/106 (accessed January 2015).
36. Gallagher, J.C., Smith, L.M., Yalamanchili, V. November 2014. Incidence of hypercalciuria and hypercalcemia during vitamin D and calcium supplementation in older women. *Menopause.* 21:1173–1180.
37. Pfeifer, M., Begerow, B., Minne, H.W. et al. 2000. Effects of a short-term vitamin D and calcium supplementation on body sway and secondary hyperparathyroidism in elderly women. *J Bone Miner Res.* 15:1113–1118.
38. Bischoff-Ferrari, H.A., Dietrich, T., Orav, E.J. 2004. Higher 25-OH vitamin D concentrations are associated with better lower-extremity function in both active and inactive persons aged >60 years. *Am J Clin Nutr.* 80:752–758.
39. Flicker, L., Mead, K., MacInnis, R.J. et al. 2003. Serum vitamin D and falls in older women in residential care in Australia. *J Am Geriatr Soc.* 51:1533–1538.
40. Faulkner, K.A., Cauley, J.A., Zmuda, J.M. et al. 2006. Higher 1,25-dihydroxyvitamin D3 concentrations associated with lower fall rates in older community-dwelling women. *Osteoporos Int.* 17:1318–1328.

41. Holick, M.F. 2006. Resurrection of vitamin D deficiency and rickets. *J Clin Invest.* 116:2062–2072.
42. Bischoff-Ferrari, H.A., Giovannucci, E., Willett, W.C. et al. 2006. Estimation of optimal serum concentrations of 25-hydroxyvitamin D for multiple health outcomes. *Am J Clin Nutr.* 84:18–28.
43. Bischoff, H.A., Stähelin, H.B., Dick, W. et al. 2003. Effects of vitamin D and calcium supplementation on falls: A randomized controlled trial. *J Bone Miner Res.* 18:343–351.
44. Bischoff-Ferrari, H.A., Willett, W.C., Wong, J.B., Giovannucci, E., Dietrich, T., Dawson-Hughes, B. 2005. Fracture prevention with vitamin D supplementation: A meta-analysis of randomized controlled trials. *JAMA.* 293:2257–2264.
45. Boonen, S., Lips, P., Bouillon, R., Bischoff-Ferrari, H.A., Vanderschueren, D., Haentjens, P. 2007. Need for additional calcium to reduce the risk of hip fracture with vitamin D supplementation: Evidence from a comparative meta-analysis of randomized controlled trials. *J Clin Endocrinol Metab.* 92:1415–1423.
46. Bischoff-Ferrari, H.A., Dawson-Hughes, B., Willett, W.C. et al. 2004. Effect of vitamin D on falls: A meta-analysis. *JAMA.* 291:1999–2006.
47. Cauley, J. September 13, 2014. American Society for Bone and Mineral Research 2014 Annual Meeting; Houston, Texas. Abstract 1076.
48. Bleicher, K., Cumming, R.G., Naganathan, V. et al. September 2014. U-shaped association between serum 25-hydroxyvitamin D and fracture risk in older men: Results from the prospective population-based CHAMP study. *J Bone Miner Res.* 29(9):2024–2031.
49. ConsumerLab.com.® Vitamin D supplements review. https://www.consumerlab.com/reviews/vitamin_D_supplements_review/Vitamin_D/ (accessed December 2014).
50. Holick, M.F., Binkley N.C., Heike, A. et al. June 2011. Evaluation, treatment, and prevention of vitamin D deficiency: An Endocrine Society Clinical Practice Guideline. *JCEM* 96 (7) http://press.endocrine.org/doi/full/10.1210/jc.2011–0385
51. Dawson-Hughes, B. December 2014. Breaking bad, What you can do to protect your bones. Nutrition Action Newsletter. Center for Science in the Public Interest.
52. American Society for Bone and Mineral Research (ASBMR) 2011 Annual Meeting. November 10, 2011. Experts debate appropriate target levels of serum vitamin d for preventing fracture. *Ann Longterm Care.* 19(11) http://www.annalsoflongtermcare.com/article/american-society-bone-and-mineral-research-asbmr-2011-annual-meeting#sthash.FV0BUckM.kfP9lVpP.dpuf
53. American Geriatrics Society Workgroup on Vitamin D Supplementation for Older Adults. Jan 2014. Recommendations abstracted from the American geriatrics society consensus statement on Vitamin D for prevention of falls and their consequences. *Journal of the American Geriatrics Society* 62(1):147–152. http://onlinelibrary.wiley.com/doi/10.1111/jgs.12631/full
54. National Institutes of Health Office of Dietary Supplements. 2014. Vitamin D fact sheet for health professionals. http://ods.od.nih.gov/factsheets/VitaminD-HealthProfessional
55. Lamberg-Allardt, C., Karp, H., Kemi, V. 2010. Phosphorus and bone. In *Nutritional Influences on Bone Health*, eds. P. Burckhardt, B. Dawson-Hughes, and C. Weaver, 87–89. Springer, Dordrecht Heidelberg London New York.
56. Bell, R.R., Draper, H.H., Tzeng, D.Y.M., Shin, H.K., Schmidt, G.R. 1977. Physiological responses of human adults to foods containing phosphate additives. *J Nutr.* 107:42–50.
57. Sullivan, C.M., Leon, J.B., Sehgal, A.R. September 2007. Phosphorus containing food additives and the accuracy of nutrient databases: Implications for renal patients. *J Ren Nutr.* 17(5):350–354.
58. Tucker, K.L. 2009. Osteoporosis prevention and nutrition. *Curr Osteoporos Rep.* 7:111–117.
59. Rude, R.K., Singer, F.R, Gruber, H.E. 2009. Skeletal and hormonal effects of magnesium deficiency. *J Am Coll Nutr.* 28:131–41.
60. Mutlu, M., Argun, M., Kilic, E., Saraymen, R., Yazar, S. 2007. Magnesium, zinc and copper status in osteoporotic, osteopenic and normal post-menopausal women. *J Int Med Res.* 35:692–695.
61. U.S. Department of Agriculture, Agricultural Research Service. 2012. Nutrient intakes from food: Mean amounts consumed per individual, by gender and age, *What We Eat in America*, NHANES 2009–2010. Available: www.ars.usda.gov/ba/bhnrc/fsrg
62. National Institutes of Health: Office of Dietary Supplements: Magnesium fact sheet for health professionals. 2013. http://ods.od.nih.gov/factsheets/Magnesium-HealthProfessional/ (accessed December 12, 2014).
63. Vermeer, C., Shearer, M.J, Zittermann, A. et al. 2004. Beyond deficiency: Potential benefits of increased intakes of vitamin K for bone and vascular health. *Eur J Nutr.* 43(6):325–335.
64. Geleijnse, J.M., Vermeer, C., Grobbee, D.E. et al. 2004. Dietary intake of menaquinone is associated with a reduced risk of coronary heart disease: The Rotterdam Study. *J Nutr.* 134(11):3100–3105.

65. Tucker, K.L., Hannan, M.T., Qiao, N. et al. January 2005. Low plasma vitamin B_{12} is associated with lower BMD: The Framingham osteoporosis study. *J Bone Miner Res.* 20(1):152–158.
66. Lam, J.R., Schneider, J.L., Zhao, W., Corley, D.A. December 1, 2013. Proton pump inhibitor and histamine 2 receptor antagonist use and vitamin B12 deficiency. *JAMA.* 310(22):2435–2442.
67. Bor, M.V., von Castel-Roberts, K.M., Kauwell, G.P. et al. 2010. Daily intake of 4–7 microg dietary vitamin B-12 is associated with steady concentrations of vitamin B-12-related biomarkers in a healthy young population. *Am J Clin Nutr.* 91(3):571–577.
68. Vogiatzoglou, A., Smith, A.D., Nurk, E. et al. 2009. Dietary sources of vitamin B-12 and their association with plasma vitamin B-12 concentrations in the general population: The Hordaland Homocysteine Study. *Am J Clin Nutr.* 89(4):1078–1087.
69. Sharabi, A., Cohen, E., Sulkes, J., Garty, M. December 2003. Replacement therapy for vitamin B12 deficiency: Comparison between the sublingual and oral route. *Br J Clin Pharmacol.* 56(6):635–638.
70. US National Library of Medicine National Institutes of Health. July 2014. MedLine Plus Vitamin B12. http://www.nlm.nih.gov/medlineplus/druginfo/natural/926.html NIH Medline plus
71. Feskanich, D., Singh, V., Willett, W.C., Colditz, G.A. January 2002. Vitamin A intake and hip fractures among postmenopausal women. *JAMA.* 287(1):47–54.
72. Felson, D.T., Kiel, D.P., Anderson, J.J., Kannel, W.B. 1988. Alcohol consumption and hip fractures: The Framingham Study. *Am J Epidemiol.* 128:1102.
73. Kanis, J.A., Johansson, H., Johnell, O. July 2005. Alcohol intake as a risk factor for fracture. *Osteoporos Int.* 16(7):737–742.
74. National Institute on Alcohol Abuse and Alcoholism. July 2014. Alcohol facts and statistics. http://www.niaaa.nih.gov/alcohol-health/overview-alcohol-consumption/alcohol-facts-and-statistics
75. Bedford, J.L., Barr, S.I. November 2011. Higher urinary sodium, a proxy for intake, is associated with increased calcium excretion and lower hip bone density in healthy young women with lower calcium intakes. *Nutrients.* 3(11):951–961.
76. Heaney, R.P. June 2006. Role of dietary sodium in osteoporosis. *J Am Coll Nutr.* 25(3 Suppl):271S–276S.
77. Frings-Meuthen, P., Baecker, N., Heer, M. 2008. Low-grade metabolic acidosis may be the cause of sodium chloride-induced exaggerated bone resorption. *J Bone Miner Res.* 23(4):517–524.
78. Sharma, A.M., Kribben, A., Schattenfroh, S., Cetto, C., Distler, A. 1990. Salt sensitivity in humans is associated with abnormal acid base regulation. *Hypertension.* 16(4):407–413.
79. Frassetto, L.A., Morris, R.C., Sebastian, A. August 2007. Dietary sodium chloride intake independently predicts the degree of hyperchloremic metabolic acidosis in healthy humans consuming a net acid-producing diet. *Am J Physiol Renal Physiol.* 293(2):F521–F525.
80. Hallström, H., Byberg, L., Glynn, A., Warensjö Lemming, E., Wolk, A., Michaëlsson, K. September 2013. Long-term coffee consumption in relation to fracture risk and bone mineral density in women. *Am J Epidemiol.* 178(6):898–909.
81. Hallström, H., Wolk, A., Glynn, A., Michaëlsson, K. 2006. Coffee, tea and caffeine consumption in relation to osteoporotic fracture risk in a cohort of Swedish women. *Osteoporosis Int.* 17(7):1055–1064.
82. Tucker, K.L., Morita, K., Qiao, N., Hannan, M.T., Cupples, L.A., Kiel, D.P. October 2006. Colas, but not other carbonated beverages, are associated with low bone mineral density in older women: The Framingham Osteoporosis Study. *Am J Clin Nutr.* 84(4):936–942.
83. Leung, C.W., Laraia, B.A., Needham, B.L. December 2014. Soda and cell aging: Associations between sugar-sweetened beverage consumption and leukocyte telomere length in healthy adults from the National Health and Nutrition Examination Surveys. *Am J Public Health.* 104(12):2425–2431.
84. Hooshmand, S., Chai, S.C., Saadat, R.L., Payton, M.E., Brummel-Smith, K., Arjmandi, B.H. September 2011. Comparative effects of dried plum and dried apple on bone in postmenopausal women. *Br J Nutr.* 106(6):923–930.
85. López-González, A.A., Grases, F., Roca, P., Mari, B., Vicente-Herrero, M.T., Costa-Bauzá, A. December 2008. Phytate (myo-inositol hexaphosphate) and risk factors for osteoporosis. A. *Med F.* 11(4):747–752.
86. Jiang, Y., Zhao, J., Rosen, C., Geusens, P., Genant, H.K. 1999. Perspectives on bone mechanical properties and adaptive response to mechanical challenge. *J Clin Densitom.* 2(4):423–433.

Section II

Home Nutrition Support

8 Home Enteral Nutrition

Michelle Romano, RDN, LD/N, CNSC, Elizabeth Bobo, MS, RDN, LDN, CNSC, and Angela Matthewson, MPH, RDN

CONTENTS

INTRODUCTION/OVERVIEW

Enteral nutrition (EN) is defined as "nutrition provided through the gastrointestinal tract via a tube, catheter or stoma that delivers nutrients distal to the oral cavity" [1]. This therapy is used in individuals who are malnourished or at risk for malnutrition because they are unable to consume adequate nutrients by mouth. An early report using representative sampling and the Centers for Medicare and Medicaid Services (CMS) data estimated the home enteral nutrition (HEN) population to be increasing yearly, and was approximately 148,000 in 1991 [2]. More recent estimates place the HEN population at 344,000 people of all ages in the United States [3]. The American Society for Parenteral and Enteral Nutrition (A.S.P.E.N.) has developed Home and Alternate Site Care Standards for clinicians caring for patients requiring home nutrition support stating "a multi-disciplinary team with expertise in nutrition support should be involved in the planning, education, implementation, and monitoring of HEN patients" [4]. Recent studies reporting on the team approach have noted reduced hospitalization rates [5,6]. Successful HEN therapy requires the expertise of multiple clinicians in order to achieve the best possible outcome. This chapter outlines the steps that are needed to achieve clinical and patient goals.

ASSESSMENT

There are several criteria that make up an adult HEN candidate. Ultimately, this individual is one who cannot meet their nutrient requirements orally, who has sufficient bowel length for absorption of nutrients, and who is able to conduct therapy at home [7]. Reduced oral intake can be a result of impaired swallowing, motility disorder, or obstruction. Small bowel length greater than 100 cm is needed for adequate absorption of nutrients. Table 8.1 outlines common diagnoses for patients on HEN. Frequently, HEN is initiated in patients with swallow dysfunction related to stroke or neoplasm of the head and neck, or dysmotility or obstruction of the upper gastrointestinal (GI) tract. Contraindications for EN include patients with obstruction, refractory nausea and vomiting, high output fistulas, and severe malabsorption.

Once the patient undergoes a full nutrition assessment, a plan of care will be developed taking into account the patient's therapy goals. See Table 8.2 for components of a full nutrition care plan.

Assessment of the patient should also include past medical history, available laboratory data, swallowing ability, and bowel habits. The patient may have additional medical conditions that will impact the decision of enteral formula and enteral feeding route choices. For example, a patient that also has heart failure would need a fluid restriction, and a concentrated formula might be used with reduced water flushes. A nutrition-focused physical examination should be undertaken to determine muscle or fat wasting, dehydration, or evident vitamin or mineral deficiency. Medications should

TABLE 8.1
Common Diagnoses for Home Enteral Nutrition

Neoplasm
Crohn's disease (adult and pediatric)
Neurologic swallow dysfunction
Motility disorder (gastroparesis)
Chronic obstruction
Congenital bowel dysfunction (chronic pseudo-obstruction)
Prematurity
Cystic fibrosis
Inborn errors of metabolism
Eosinophilic esophagitis

TABLE 8.2
Home Enteral Nutrition Care Plan

Nutrition goals; short term and long term, anticipated duration of therapy
Patient/caregiver education
Feeding route
Nutrition prescription
Infusion schedule
Drug–nutrient interactions
Care of access device
Infusion equipment
Monitoring frequency
Planned reevaluation of care plan at least every 3 months or as needed based on patient status

be reviewed with special consideration of medication that can or should be crushed, food–nutrient interaction, and dosing schedule (i.e., insulin, medications that need to be taken with or without food). See Table 8.3 for potential enteral nutrition–drug interactions [8].

The patient and/or caregiver, and the home environment need to be considered during the planning of HEN. The patient/caregiver should be assessed for the ability to conduct safe home therapy,

TABLE 8.3
Specific Drug–Enteral Nutrition Interactions

Phenytoin
- Absorption may be reduced due to binding to enteral nutrition components or enteral tubing
- Generally recommended to hold enteral nutrition for 1 hour pre- and postdose

Carbamazepine
- Enteral nutrition can reduce bioavailability, more so for postpyloric feeding than gastric feeding, as it is acid stable
- Adequate dilution of the suspension (or slurry from crushed tablet) at least 1:1 with water prior to administration via feeding tube may help reduce drug loss

Fluoroquinolones
- Bioavailability appears reduced by enteral nutrition formulas
- Although data are limited, it is currently recommended to hold enteral feedings for 1 hour pre- and 2 hours postdose

Warfarin
- Two proposed mechanisms of reduced warfarin absorption are binding with an enteral nutrition component (likely protein) or to polyurethane tubing; however, the interactions have not been clearly delineated
- Potential methods of reducing the warfarin–enteral nutrition interaction include
  - Using concentrated drug administered rapidly to minimize contact with the feeding tube
  - Separating warfarin administration from enteral nutrition administration
  - Increasing the warfarin dose until a therapeutic PT/INR is achieved
  - Changing to an alternate anticoagulation therapy that does not interact with enteral nutrition
  - Holding enteral nutrition for at least 1 hour before and after dose
  - Routine monitoring of PT/INR, especially with changes to enteral nutrition regimen

Source: Rollins, C.J. 2012. Drug–nutrient interactions. In: Mueller C (ed.) *The ASPEN Adult Nutrition Support Core Curriculum*, 2nd Edition. The American Society for Parenteral and Enteral Nutrition, Silver Spring, MD, pp. 298–312.

including willingness, cognitive ability, and physical ability. The home should have adequate water supply, electricity, telephone, and adequate storage area for formula and enteral equipment.

PEDIATRIC INDICATIONS

As practiced in adult care, EN is the preferred route of nutrition support for pediatric patients as it has fewer deleterious effects than parenteral support, and is more physiologic. The primary indications for HEN of a pediatric patient are insufficient oral intake to promote growth and development, oral motor dysfunction, GI abnormality that prohibits sufficient oral nutrient intake, and as primary therapy [9,10].

Insufficient Oral Intake

Insufficient oral intake to meet nutrient needs is a common indicator for HEN in the pediatric population. It may manifest as either a reduction in appetite, such as seen in children undergoing oncologic treatment, or as an inability to meet nutrient needs when needs are elevated above that seen in the general population. For example, children with cystic fibrosis and children with cerebral palsy hypertonicity have increased energy requirements and are often unable to meet their needs via an oral diet alone [11]. Children with congenital heart defects also commonly require home nutrition support [11]. Insufficient oral intake may also present secondary to a developed food aversion, such as seen in some infants with severe gastroesophageal reflux disease, or in children with sensory integration problems or autism. HEN provides the child with additional nutrition so that their needs in relation to their metabolic demands are met.

Oral Motor Dysfunction

Oral motor dysfunction is a common issue in infants born prematurely because the suck, swallow, breathe reflex is not developed until 34 weeks gestation. In addition, after birth, these infants are often intubated for ventilatory support, which inhibits the development of feeding skills and leads to oral motor dysfunction. Thus, it is not uncommon for a premature infant to be discharged with HEN. Children with neurological impairment often require HEN. Issues noted with these children that can lead to HEN include swallowing disorders, esophageal disorders (e.g., gastroesophageal reflux, esophageal dysmotility), and behavioral disorders (aversive feeding behaviors, sensory-based feeding disorders) [12].

Gastrointestinal Abnormality

GI abnormalities that can lead to dependency on HEN are those that inhibit the structure and/or function of the GI tract. For example, congenital malformations (e.g., tracheo-esophageal fistula), short bowel syndrome, tumors of the GI tract, and caustic ingestion). In these instances, HEN may be short term or long term depending on the degree of impact of the abnormality. Also, HEN may be the primary source of nutrition or delivered as an adjunct to parenteral nutrition.

Primary Therapy

HEN is used as primary therapy for the management of pediatric Crohn's disease. Research indicates that a liquid-only diet for 8–12 weeks is as advantageous in inducing remission in Crohn's disease as corticosteroid therapy [13–15]. Because of the difficulty of consuming only liquids to meet nutrient requirements for 2–3 months, many children opt to deliver all or part of the nutrition via a feeding tube. After remission has been achieved, HEN is commonly used as part of the maintenance regimen.

HEN is also used to manage inborn errors of metabolism and eosinophilic esophagitis when the child is not able or willing to follow the required diet via oral intake alone [16]. For example, a child with phenylketonuria may refuse the metabolic formula orally and instead choose to receive it via a feeding tube. HEN may also be used to manage the child with uncontrollable seizures who is following a ketogenic diet given the highly restrictive nature of the ketogenic protocol and its limited palatability.

ENTERAL ACCESS

The type and location of the enteral access device depend on the length of need, and the GI anatomy and function. Adult and pediatric patients with adequate gastric function would be best served with a tube terminating in the stomach, whereas those with gastric dysfunction would best tolerate small bowel feedings. Pediatric access is addressed later in this section. For adults, short-term needs (less than 4 weeks) can be met with nasogastric (NG), nasoduodenal (ND), and nasojejunal (NJ) tubes. The position of the tube should be confirmed radiographically prior to use [17]. When patients are transitioning from hospital to home, it is important to obtain information on the tube tip location, as there are several different manufacturers of tubes, and tube length and position can vary. Use of the ausculatory method or pH testing of aspirate is unreliable in determining feeding tip location [17]. The external tube length should be measured or marked from the nose to monitor for displacement. On occasion, small bowel tubes can migrate upward into the stomach. Changes in tolerance to feedings or increased nausea, or vomiting of tube feedings should prompt radiographic testing of the tube location. Nasal tubes can be used for enteral feeding supplementation while the patient is transitioning to an enteral diet, or to determine enteral feeding tolerance prior to placement of a long-term access, or in patients where long-term access is contraindicated or not desired. Prior to long-term enteral access placement, Bankhead et al. suggests a multidisciplinary review to consider benefits versus risks of placement, in cases of end of life and where oral feeding is improving [17]. In patients with adequate gastric function who will need long-term access, a gastrostomy tube (GT) should be placed. These tubes are larger in diameter and can accommodate different administration methods and medication administration. In cases of inadequate gastric function, a gastrojejunostomy (GJT) or jejunostomy (JT) tube could be placed. Enteral tubes are typically placed endoscopically and radiographically, and less commonly by surgical method. Regardless of access, position should be confirmed [17]. All efforts should be made to avoid tubing not typically used for enteral feedings (e.g., drain tubes or catheters) as there is no internal or external anchoring device and connections with enteral feeding sets may not be compatible. Table 8.4 highlights indications for gastric or small bowel feedings [18]. In patients with gastric dysmotility, a GJT has been useful to vent or decompress the stomach via the gastric port while feeding into the small bowel via the jejunostomy port. For patients who are concerned about the external appearance of a tube, who are active, or who are prone-sleepers, a low-profile device or skin-level device may be an option. These devices have an internal bumper and an external port or ports for gastric or jejunal feedings. Manual dexterity is needed for attaching the extension tubing to the low-profile tube in order to use enteral feeding sets or syringes for tube flush.

Maintenance of the Enteral Access

Efforts should be made to avoid skin irritation at the enteral access site. It is recommended to use mild soap and water to clean the site and avoid occlusive dressings or placement of gauze or cut drain sponges under the external bumper [18]. Topical silver nitrate or steroid can be applied if granulation tissue develops.

Tube clogs can occur due to accumulation of formula sediment and/or improper administration of medications. Flushing the tube with 30 mL of water every 4 hours before and after feedings and medications may prevent or reduce clogging [17].

TABLE 8.4
Indications/Contraindications for Gastric and Small Bowel Access

Gastric indications
Normal gastric and small bowel motility
Adequate anatomy to place access
Small bowel indications
Gastric outlet obstruction
Duodenal obstruction
Gastric or duodenal fistula
Severe gastroesophageal reflux disease
Contraindications
Mechanical obstruction
Active peritonitis
Bowel ischemia
Relative contraindications
Ascites
Recent GI bleeding

PEDIATRIC ENTERAL ACCESS CONSIDERATIONS

Orogastric

Orogastric tubes are generally not used in the outpatient setting. Rarely, they may be seen in the home patient who has a facial dimorphism that prohibits the use of a NG tube. Even so, these tubes are generally replaced with a permanent tube for long-term nutrition support.

Nasogastric

NG tubes are used for children requiring short-term enteral access (i.e., less than 12 weeks) [19], for example, infants/children with failure to thrive who are expected to become independent of nutrition support or children with altered appetite due to oncologic treatment. NG tubes can be used long term for children who are placing a tube nightly for enteral access as part of their treatment method for Crohn's disease. NG tubes are appropriate for children with little or no gastroesophageal reflux, normal gastric function, and a low risk for aspiration [9]. Ideally, NG tube placement should be verified using abdominal x-ray [17,20]. However, repeat exposure to radiation is a concern in the pediatric cohort. In addition, obtaining an x-ray to consistently verify tube placement is not feasible in the home setting. Thus the best approach in the home setting to assure proper tube placement is to monitor tube insertion length and to measure the pH of aspirated gastric secretions. Gastric secretions have a pH of 1–4. The literature supports using a pH of <4 to verify correct tube placement [20]. The auscultation method should not be used. NG tubes generally can remain in place for 4 weeks before being changed. Placement of an NG tube is not a contraindication to initiating or continuing an oral diet provided that the child is medically safe to ingest oral nutrition [19].

Nasojejunal

NJ tubes are indicated for short-term enteral access and are appropriate for the child with gastroesophageal reflux, gastroparesis, aspiration risk, or acute pancreatitis. Tube placement should be verified using x-ray. Because these tubes are located in the small intestine, they are not appropriate for bolus feedings. Generally, these tubes may remain in place for 4 weeks before being replaced.

Gastrostomy/Gastrojejunostomy

GTs are indicted for children who require EN support long term (suggested for 12 weeks or more) and have a functioning GI tract [19]. Conversely, GJTs are indicated for children with severe gastroesophageal reflux who are not appropriate candidates for a Nissen fundoplication or for children who have a GT in place, but are temporarily not tolerating feeds. In this case, the jejunal port should be used for pump-assisted feedings and the gastric port should be used for venting to improve feeding tolerance.

Jejunostomy

Jejunostomy tubes (JTs) are indicated for children with significant gastroesophageal disease and/or gastroparesis. They are also indicated for children with a high aspiration risk. Typically, these tubes are considered if enteral access is going to be needed for 6 months or longer [19]. Like GJTs, these tubes are only appropriate for pump-assisted feedings. They also require routine flushing to prevent clogging.

ENTERAL FORMULA SELECTION

Planning the HEN regimen should take into consideration the patient's medical history, GI capabilities, enteral access, administration method, short-term and long-term nutrition goals, and the patient/caregiver wishes.

There are enteral formulas that are manufactured for specific disease states; however, a standard polymeric formula will meet the nutritional needs of most home patients. The nutrient concentration of a polymeric formula can range from 1–2 calories/mL, and meet the Recommended Daily Allowance (RDA) for vitamins and minerals within 1.5 L per day. For a pediatric patient, the volume needed to meet the RDA is dependent on the age of the child and the type of formula being used. For example, a standard 1 calorie/mL formula is designed to meet the needs of a child 1–8 years of age in 1 L, but for a child 9–13 years of age, 1.5 L is required. It is important to consider the medical status of the child when choosing a formula. For example, a child that is neurologically impaired and hypotonic may do best with a calorie-reduced formula that will still provide ample protein, vitamins and minerals for age. Fiber-containing formula may help to regulate frequency or consistency of stool. Table 8.5 describes the categories and characteristics of the various enteral formulas available. Occasionally, the patient may require a higher amount of macronutrient, such as protein or fiber. Modular products are available that can be given in separate doses to meet the patient's requirements. Protein modulars are available in liquid and powder forms. Fiber supplements are available as soluble fiber, and when mixed with water will dissolve and reduce risk of tube clogging.

Since the patient or caregiver will be responsible for the feedings, collaboration should take place to determine a feeding schedule. Several goals can be accomplished: the patient will begin feedings and advance as tolerated to the goal volume to meet his/her nutritional requirements, the feeding schedule and advancement will minimize complications and intolerance, and the tube feeding schedule itself is adaptable to his/her lifestyle. For adults with gastric access, formula can be administered intermittently (bolus, gravity drip) or by pump-assisted (cycle or continuous) method. One benefit of bolus or gravity drip is that it can mimic a meal time schedule, and may allow flexibility in daily activities. In some cases, where oral intake has been diminished for a period of time or the patient is undergoing radiation or chemotherapy, the gravity drip method may be better tolerated, as this allows for slower infusion. Initiation of enteral feedings for pediatric patients will be addressed later in this section.

For adults with jejunal access, feedings are best tolerated using a pump-assisted method. Consideration should be given to a cycle infusion to allow the patient freedom from feeding

TABLE 8.5
Characteristics of Enteral Formulas and Recommendations for Use

Formula Type	Characteristics	Recommendations for Use
Polymeric	• Contain macronutrients as nonhydrolyzed protein, fat, and carbohydrate • Range in concentration from 1 to 2 kcal/mL • 1–1.5 L usually meets RDA for vitamins and minerals • May be disease specific and/or contain pre- and probiotics	Patients with normal or near-normal GI absorptive capacity
Fiber-containing	Fiber content intended to improve the health of the GI tract, regulating frequency and/or consistency of stool by maintaining healthy GI flora Fiber content is typically below total daily fiber recommendations May contain prebiotics in the form of fructooligosaccharides, oligofructose, or inulin May also contain probiotics	Recommended for use among patients with diarrhea and/or to promote/maintain gut microbiota
Commercial blenderized	Contains whole food ingredients in carton or ready-to-feed packaging. Available for adults and pediatrics	Patients with normal or near-normal GI absorptive capacity
Homemade whole food/ blenderized	Blenderized whole foods designed to allow patients to receive qualities of food not found in standard enteral formulas, such as phytochemicals	Due to infection/food-borne illness risk, use in medically stable patients with healed enteral access site Best suited for patients with safe food practices and tube maintenance techniques Should be provided as bolus/gravity drip administration to maintain safe food practices (hang time <2 hours) RDN should be involved in the development of feeding composition to ensure adequate nutrient delivery
Diabetes/ glucose intolerance	Intended to reduce hyperglycemia with macronutrient composition of 34%–36% carbohydrate, 40%–44% fat, and 20% protein Fat and soluble fiber content may slow gastric emptying and prevent elevated blood glucose	Use of DM-specific enteral formulas is not currently supported by strong research; instead efforts should be made to prevent overfeeding
Renal	Fluid restricted	Research does not strongly support renal formulas over standard polymeric formulas with renal insufficiency
	Contains lower amounts of electrolytes, specifically potassium and phosphorus, to prevent excessive delivery to patients with renal insufficiency Protein content varies	If significant electrolyte abnormalities exist or develop, a renal formula should be considered until electrolytes stabilize Patients receiving maintenance hemodialysis (MHD) may benefit from a renal formula with regard to electrolyte balance In some cases, a standard formula may be used in MHD patients along with monitoring electrolytes
Elemental/ semielemental	Macronutrients are hydrolyzed to maximize absorption	Intended for patients with malabsorptive disorders

Source: Adapted from Brown B, Roehl K, Betz M. *Nutr Clin Prac* 2015;30(1):72–85.

TABLE 8.6
Enteral Access, Administration Method, and Initiation of Enteral Feedings

Access	Administration Method	Initiation
Gastric	Bolus (5–10 minutes) Gravity drip/intermittent (20–60 minutes)	3–8 times per day, starting with 60–120 mL formula and increase by 60–120 mL each feeding or each day until goal is reached
Gastric or small bowel	Pump-assisted cycle (<24 hours/day, commonly 8–14 hours/day) Pump-assisted continuous (24 hours/day)	Start at 10–40 mL/hour For cycle schedule, increase by increments of 10–20 mL/hour every 12–24 hours depending on the length of the infusion cycle For continuous infusion, advance by 10–20 mL/hour every 8–12 hours until goal is reached

equipment. The hours of infusion should be discussed with the patient/caregiver, and the tube feedings advanced accordingly. For patients with some oral intake, a nighttime cycle schedule may be ideal to supplement daytime intake. Table 8.6 provides recommendations on initiation and advancement.

PEDIATRIC INITIATION

Initiation of enteral feedings for a younger pediatric patient is generally done in the hospital over the course of several days to test for tolerance and advance the feeding volume [17]. However, feeds may also be initiated in the homecare setting provided that proper tube placement has been verified and caregiver support is adequate. When providing HEN to a pediatric patient, it is important to implement measures that ensure safe and proper delivery of the nutrition. For example, locking the settings on the enteral pump is beneficial so that the child will not change them when touching the buttons. It is also sometimes beneficial to use clamps to secure the extension tubing to prevent separation when tugged on. For infants, running the tubing out of the bottom of a sleeper outfit for nighttime feeds prevents the infant from grabbing the tubing and disconnecting it. Applying facial tape to secure NG/NJ tubes is essential to reduce the incidence of tube dislodgment in infants. Using access covering equipment (i.e., tube protective belts) can be helpful with toddlers and small children as a deterrent from playing with or pulling the access device, such as a GT. One must also consider the most appropriate regimen that will nourish the child, but also support age-appropriate development. For example, assuring that the child has a small backpack to hold the pump/formula so that they can be mobile during the day while receiving feeds. In addition, providing oral stimulation in the form of nonnutritive sucking or oral feedings, if medically safe to do so, is important to foster the development of feeding skills in children [21–23]. Speech therapy services may also be needed to assist with the development of oral/motor skills.

Bolus and Gravity Feedings

When initiating bolus/gravity feedings, it is suggested that the regimen be initiated at 25% of the feeding goal, divided by the number of desired feedings. For example, if the desired volume is 400 mL/day over the course of 4 feedings, start at 100 mL/day and give 25 mL per feeding. Increase the volume by 25% of the feeding goal each day as tolerated [17]. It is prudent to not administer the feeding over a period of time that is less than one would expect the child to consume the formula orally as this practice may lead to intolerance of the feeding. One should also be cognizant of the child with a Nissen fundoplication. If a Nissen is intact, then venting of the feeding tube after feeds may be necessary to lessen discomfort by allowing gas to escape.

Pump-Assisted Feedings

Guidelines suggest initiating the regimen for a child at 1–2 mL/kg/hour and advancing by 0.5–1 mL/kg/hour every 6–24 hours as tolerated until goal feedings are achieved [17]. Feedings may need to be started at a slower rate for children who are malnourished to avoid refeeding syndrome. It is best to use a nondiluted isotonic formula to reduce the risk of bacterial contamination [17]. Sterile formula in an open system can hang for up to 12 hours, unless it is being provided to a neonate in which case it should only hang for 4 hours [24]. Similarly, human breast milk and nonsterile powder formulas should only hang for 4 hours [17]. Pump accuracy is of utmost importance as small volumes are often administered to pediatric patients. The calibration of the pump should be verified. An accuracy of 5% of the set volume is acceptable in pediatrics [17].

MONITORING

The next step in nutrition care is monitoring the therapy to be sure that the goals are achieved. Monitoring enteral therapy should take place at regular intervals as determined by the healthcare providers. Table 8.7 describes recommended monitoring parameters.

The enteral access should be monitored for leakage or peristomal infection. Peristomal infections are the most common complication and in most cases are mild and can be treated with antibiotics and local wound care. Stoma leakage can be caused by infection, tension on the external portion of the tube, or cleansing with irritating solutions. Patients with excessive tension between the external and internal bumpers, poor wound healing, or significant weight gain are at risk for buried bumper syndrome. The external bumper should be monitored and loosened to at least 1 cm [18].

PATIENT/CAREGIVER EDUCATION

The goals of education are to provide the skills needed to provide safe and effective HEN, and to reduce potential complications. Ideally, hospitalized patients transitioning to home would receive

TABLE 8.7
Home Enteral Nutrition Monitoring

Observations for signs and symptoms of intolerance to therapy
Evaluation of weight changes and/or growth rates as appropriate
Evaluation of hydration status
Review of systems and/or physical examination
Periodic review of biochemical, vitamin, mineral, or other pertinent laboratory data
Assessment for clinical signs of nutrient deficiencies or excesses
Assessment of other disease states or conditions that may affect the nutrition therapy
Review for evidence of an interaction between the nutrition therapy and medications or other disease states
Evaluation of functional status and performance
Psychosocial status
Evaluation of access device and site
Patient/caregiver compliance with techniques and procedures
Assessment of the need for continued therapy
Monitoring intake (fluid, nutrient, oral) and output (urine, stool, GI losses)
Review the appropriateness of the feeding route

Source: Durfee SM et al. *JPEN J Parenter Enteral Nutr* 2014;29(4):542–555. Copyright © 2014 by American Society for Parenteral and Enteral Nutrition. Reprinted by permission of SAGE Publications.

TABLE 8.8
Patient/Caregiver Education for HEN Administration

Name and phone numbers of resources available 24 hours per day to troubleshoot and answer questions
The name, composition, intended use, and expected outcome from the formulation
Medication information and administration, including dosage, route, frequency, and the potential for adverse effects and drug interactions
Timing, method of administration, and feeding schedule
Route of administration and duration of nutrition therapy
Care of the enteral access device and site
Product hang time and stability at room temperature
Inspection of enteral products for contents and expiration date
Clean technique for preparation of HEN, administration, and reuse of supplies and equipment
Techniques for self-monitoring of therapy and identification of potential complications
Proper storage of ready-to-use products and HEN formulas that require mixing
Use and storage of enteral feeding equipment, supplies, and pump
Proper disposal of used containers, tubing and unused or expired feeding formulations, and/or medications
Action to be taken in the event of late or missed administration of HEN
Process to order additional feeding formulation and supplies
Infection prevention and control
Basic home safety (fire, electrical, environment, mobility, bathroom)
Information on emergency preparedness to assist patients and caregivers if an emergency should interrupt service
Patients and caregivers shall be educated based on the teach-back method
Patients and caregivers shall display competency in the understanding and performance of techniques

Source: Durfee SM et al. *JPEN J Parenter Enteral Nutr* 2014;29(4):542–555. Copyright © 2014 by American Society for Parenteral and Enteral Nutrition. Reprinted by permission of SAGE Publications.

some basic education prior to discharge, and then follow-up education would occur in the home. Trends have been noted with increasing home nutrition support population, decreased hospital length of stay, and decreased time for patient training in the hospital [25]. Table 8.8 describes specific education and training in order to provide safe and effective therapy. Training should be aimed at the home regimen versus the hospital schedule. For example, the home schedule could be adjusted so that patients/caregivers are not waking in the middle of the night for water flushes, adding formula, or feeding set changes.

All formula and equipment should be available in the home for comprehensive training. The patient/caregiver should be educated one-on-one in a quiet environment. Limitations of physical pain, dexterity, vision, hearing, or immobility may be taken into account, as well as anxiety or stress in learning a new task. The healthcare provider should provide an initial demonstration, and then allow the patient/caregiver to "teach back," verbalizing the task and return demonstrate [26]. Reassurance and encouragement should be provided with each task accomplishment.

Patient education materials used for training should have several components. The content should be accurate and based on current practice standards. The literacy level should be at a fifth- to sixth-grade level, with definitions provided for unfamiliar words or terms [27]. Graphics or visual presentation of information will help understanding and recall of health information. The layout of the material should be uncluttered, and type of at least 12-point font should be used. The material should be individualized to the patient/caregiver, and a chart can be used as a reminder of the schedule. Involving them in the process will help to foster learning and recall [27]. Cultural relevance is helpful in the patient/caregiver's identification with the material, so the target audience needs to be considered. Lastly, feasibility of the material refers to access to the information and materials provided in the patient's/caregiver's spoken language. There are some online videos and materials that may be helpful [28–30].

NEW INNOVATIONS IN EN

Home Blenderized Tube Feedings

There is a revitalized interest in alternatives to the primary commercial tube feeding formulas. Commercial formulas have been in the ascendant for the last 40 years. The main rationales have been lower risk of microbial contamination, predictable nutrition content, and better compatibility with tubing. However, no randomized controlled trials exist to unequivocally support any clinical benefit of commercial formulas compared to homemade recipes [5]. Early studies of home-prepared formulas report a contamination rate up to 80% [17]. Commercial formulas remain the professional standard as per the 2014 A.S.P.E.N. Standards for Nutrition Support: Home and Alternate Site Care [4]. If BTF are used, A.S.P.E.N. recommends regular sanitization of home preparation equipment [4].

Some of the ingredients that contribute to shelf stability and calorie density have become increasingly unpopular with patients/caregivers over the last several years. In particular, some patients/caregivers are opposed to certain ingredients or preservatives used in the formulas. Others may require specialized oral nutrition and therefore EN such as low fermentable oligo-, di-, and monosaccharides, and polyols (FODMAP) intake [31]. Currently, options are quite limited for prepackaged completely organic formulas. Achieving reimbursement for these formulas may be difficult. While supply is lacking, demand is not. Eighty-one percent of American families report buying organic foods at least some times, and growth in organic agriculture was 240% compared to 3% in nonorganic [32,33]. Given the growth in demand for organics, development in supply is likely to follow.

Until affordable, ready-to-use formulas are more widely available, some patients will choose to make their own mixtures to put down their feeding tubes. Consultation with registered dietitian/nutritionist (RDN) should be strongly encouraged for evaluation of the nutrient adequacy of the home BTF, education on food safety practices, and avoidance of tube clogging. There are no "hang time" practice guidelines for BTF formulas; however, Bankhead et al. suggests less than 4 hours for prepared formulas [17]. Because of the potential viscosity of the formula, a tube size of at least 14 French may be needed. Blended formulas would be best used via GT access versus JT due to the short infusion time and diameter of the tube. Patients with malabsorption will likely not benefit from these formulas.

The Oley Foundation provides several references for BTF recipes. Oley also provides purchasing information for high-speed blenders that are more capable of producing formula that will not clog a feeding tube [30]. It is imperative that practitioners maintain open communication with patients and caregivers, even if their strong preferences conflict with general practice.

Pediatric Considerations in Home Blenderized Feedings

Home BTF are becoming more commonplace in the pediatric cohort for a variety of reasons. Some caregivers believe that BTF are better tolerated than commercial formulas in that they help to regulate bowel function and reduce gagging and vomiting. Further, with a BTF, unprocessed ingredients can be used, which is appealing to some caregivers as a means of providing their child with what they perceive as optimal nutrition. A BTF also offers a nurturing aspect to the nutrition care of a child that formula feeding does not. With a BTF, caregivers may feel as if they are more involved in feeding their child and directing the nutrition that the child receives.

As with adults, there are a variety of issues that should be considered when initiating BTF. For example, the size of the feeding tube, feeding schedule, overall feeding volume, food allergies and/or intolerances, and immunosuppression should all be considered. The feeding volume and feeding schedule can be particularly problematic in pediatrics. Owing to the viscosity of the blend and because it is not sterile, feeds should be given via bolus, not continuously. This mode of feeding can be problematic for some children from a tolerance standpoint. The total volume of the feeds is also an issue as most children will require a minimum of 30 oz. of BTF a day to meet nutrient requirements due to blend compositions [34–36]. One should also be cognizant that a BTF for a pediatric patient is not stagnant. As the child ages, nutrient needs change and the blend will require adjusting. Thus, it is imperative that a child on a BTF receive regular medical nutrition therapy from an RDN. The RDN should analyze multiple days of the blend using a nutrition software program to assess the overall nutritional appropriateness of the blend since nutrients change depending on which ingredients are used. For example, changes in fruits and vegetables will alter the nutrient profile of the blend. The RDN should also monitor the child's anthropometrics and nutrition-related laboratory values as a means of determining the appropriateness of the blend [37].

Enteral Access Design

In 2006, the Joint Commission issued a sentinel event alert regarding enteral tubing misconnections [38]. This alert stemmed from more than 100 incidences of enteral tubing misconnections, some with fatal outcomes, whereby small-bore connectors commonly used with medical devices were connected inappropriately with enteral tubing (e.g., enteral feedings connected with venous access). The sentinel alert called for a design change in enteral feeding connector than would make inappropriate connections impossible. A redesign process was implemented by the International Organization of Standardization (ISO) in 2008 to develop a new connector that would only be compatible with enteral access. These new products, called ENFit connectors, have been developed, which include the connector for the enteral set, syringes, and enteral feeding access [39]. As of this writing, the anticipated roll-out of these products in the United States should take place by the beginning of 2016. For more information, visit www.stayconnected.org.

Technology-Based HEN Care

Recent changes in healthcare legislation will have a direct impact on the evolution of care of patients receiving HEN. The Health Information and Technology for Economic and Clinical Health (HITECH) Act, enacted in 2009, requires the use of electronic health records (EHR) to improve healthcare quality, safety, and efficiency [40]. The Patient Protection and Affordable Care Act (PPACA), enacted in 2010, includes the promotion and funding for a patient-centered medical home. "The patient-centered medical home delivery model is designed to improve quality of care through team-based coordination of care, treating the many needs of the patient at once, increasing access to care, and empowering the patient to be a partner in their own care" [41]. Strategies for clinicians to use technology to monitor HEN therapy is evolving. In 2010, Boisseau et al. used an automated telephone call system whereby patients could answer questions by phone and the results would be available by website to the healthcare providers [42]. Now, patient portals have been developed in order for home patients to communicate with their healthcare providers and access their medical information. There will likely be further innovations. A study currently in progress is evaluating the use of mobile technology in the care of home parenteral patients [43]. Use of the EHR and other technology will hopefully aid in timely care of HEN patients and provide insight into ways to avoid or improve clinical complications.

SPECIAL CONSIDERATIONS IN LONG-TERM EN PATIENTS

Population Characteristics

Particularly in the United States, patients on tube feeding at home represent a large and growing population. From 1989 to 1992, the population grew from 34,000 to 73,000 [44]. More recent numbers are not available for the overall U.S. population. Comparisons of U.S. population to European population are also difficult due to scarcity of data. Heburterne's survey in the late 1990s indicated roughly 3 times higher prevalence per million in the United States versus the European median [45], while Klek estimated HEN prevalence in the United States at 4–10 times higher than Western Europe [46]. Klek et al. also reports much higher per patient costs in the United States. In the year 2000, each U.S. HEN patient incurred an annual cost of 9000–25,000 USD, compared to annual per patient European costs of 9048–10,140 USD [46].

Current utilization data for the United States is difficult to obtain. Specific data are last available from a 1987–1991 survey. At that time, the major indication for HEN in the United States was primary cancer, causing poor oral intake, followed by swallowing disorders related to stroke or neuromuscular disease [47]. In Hebuterne's survey of European HEN use, the main indication was dysphagia, largely related to neurologic impairment or head and neck cancers [45]. There was significant country-to-country variation. A major difference between United States and Europe is higher usage among older patients. For example, a survey in the early 1990s showed much more frequent usage in the United States compared to Great Britain [47]. The United States also has a large population of tube-fed patients in nursing homes. A 2006 survey of administrative data from the CMS showed 70,000 patients in nursing homes receiving feedings via enteric tube [48].

Management guidelines are nonspecific for monitoring patients on long-term HEN at home [47]. A.S.P.E.N. recommends that practitioners develop protocols that allow them to ensure that the nutrition care plan is being carried out as intended and the patient is able to meet his/her nutritional goals [4]. Prior to tube feeding initiation, a case manager, RDN, or other providers should review financial considerations with the patient/caregiver. Reimbursement levels vary based on insurance plans and diagnoses. Providers should also ensure that the patient and caregivers have adequate understanding of HEN procedures and that the home environment is appropriate for infusion [4]. Transition from HEN to an oral diet should be gradual and monitored to ensure adequacy [4]. Discontinuation of HEN should take place when oral intake is adequate or when the care plan dictates it, for example, if a patient's advance directive indicates that nutrition support is no longer appropriate [4].

For the pediatric patient, long-term HEN requires close monitoring as the macro- and micronutrient needs change as the child ages. For instance, the calorie, protein, vitamin, and mineral needs change as an infant progresses to a toddler and then to a young child. With the evolution in needs come alterations in the type of formula provided and feeding schedule. One should be mindful to provide a formula that is designed for the age of the child so as to most appropriately meet his/her nutrient needs. Adult formulas should not be given to children younger than 10–13 years of age. The child's growth (weight, length/height, and head circumference for children <3 years of age), hydration status, laboratory markers, clinical status, and overall physical development should be monitored to assure that the nutrition regimen is appropriate [21]. It is suggested that weight be monitored weekly, monthly, or at clinic visits and length/height be measured monthly or at clinic visits [7,22]. It is also recommended that nutrient intake (calories, protein, fluid, vitamins and minerals) be evaluated monthly [7]. The access device needs to be assessed prior to each feeding [22]. The device may need to be replaced periodically to accommodate periods of growth. Overall, the monitoring schedule should be developed based on the child's overall nutrition status at the time of initiation of nutrition support the child's medical condition(s), the child's age and the tolerance to nutrition support regimen [22].

Complications

Pulmonary aspiration can be a major complication; however, caregivers can significantly reduce the risk by following guidelines to avoid. Checking gastric residual volumes has not been proven effective [17]. In fact, checking of gastric residuals is rarely recommended in the HEN patient. Instead, patient positioning is of utmost importance. Risk of aspiration is much higher among

patients receiving their feedings in a supine position, versus those in a semirecumbent position [17]. Although a few studies question the value of elevated head of bed, it is still the accepted standard of care [17].

Tube clogging is another complaint common among long-term tube-fed patients. While most studies show clogs requiring replacement are more common in patients with jejunostomies versus gastrostomies, some reports have shown the opposite. Theoretically, jejunostomy clogs would be related to the smaller tube diameter. Owing to greater peristaltic forces in their distal location, jejunostomies are also prone to more frequent dislodgement. Clogging tends to increase with improper medication administration, inadequate water flushes, and too frequent checking of gastric residuals [17]. When clogs do occur, water is the recommended fluid to declog them. Although studies support water as the most effective solution, some patients do still choose to use carbonated drinks and cranberry juice [17]. Preventing clogging is the primary goal, and frequent water flushes are recommended [17].

Other tube complaints include discharge from the tube site, tender stoma, granulation tissue, clogs, breakage of the tube, and dislodgement [49]. In a single-center study, 10% of children that received GT had complications within the first year, which included cellulitis, granulation tissue, tube malpositioning, or dislodging [50]. Although supporting studies are small and have limitations, there appears to be a strong need for close, long-term follow-up of patients with feeding tubes.

GI complaints (i.e., nausea, vomiting, diarrhea, constipation, abdominal bloating) are the most frequently reported in the HEN population. Changes in bowel habits may occur after initiating enteral feedings. One multicenter observational study, reported 63% of patients experienced one or more GI complication [51]. Both diarrhea and constipation can occur with HEN, but studies looking at causes and treatment options in the home population are sparse. An early study by Shankardass et al. reported the addition of fiber to enteral formula significantly improved incidence of constipation in long-term enterally fed patients [52]. Current recommendations support this use of a fiber-blended formula (soluble and insoluble) to promote bowel function in long-term patients [14]. Table 8.9 outlines treatment options for common complications.

Factors Contributing to Diarrhea

Diarrhea is a commonly reported complication of tube feedings, both in and out of hospitals and other institutions [53]. Reported incidence of diarrhea can vary as widely as 2% to 95%, in part due to inconsistencies in definition [54]. Diarrhea can contribute to fluid and electrolyte abnormalities [53]. Where fecal incontinence is also present, it can lead to skin breakdown with concurrent or separate wound infections [53]. In addition, diarrhea may result in orders to hold tube feeding altogether, thereby contributing to worsening malnutrition [54]. Aside from the feedings themselves, medications (especially antibiotics) and infections increase the risk of diarrhea [53]. Other risk factors include age, disease state, and altered GI anatomy [54]. Although contamination of feedings has been shown to increase the risk of diarrhea, the link is not uniformly reported [55]. Bacterial contamination can be either endogenous (retrograde growth from the patient) or exogenous (relating to poor hand and equipment hygiene) [17]. Control protocols, such as handwashing, have decreased diarrhea incidence [54]. Aspects related to tube feedings have been postulated to have connections to diarrhea, including delivery method (either bolus or continuous administration) and formula composition [53]. Continuous administration (especially at very low rate) may not induce adequate response in the gut. On the other hand, the bolus method may be more than the GI tract, especially the small bowel, can handle. There are no randomized controlled trials to support either causation [53].

Fiber content in formula may reduce diarrhea, although the exact type of fiber that is most beneficial remains unproven [53]. There have been no studies conducted in the HEN population; however, a meta-analysis by Elia et al. reported a reduction in diarrhea in the non-ICU hospitalized population [56]. In general, soluble fiber is the major beneficial actor. Bacteria in the colon ferment soluble fiber to short-chain fatty acids (SCFAs), which are preferred fuel for colonocytes. The colonocytes

TABLE 8.9
Enteral Feeding Complications and Prevention/Treatment Suggestions

Complication	Cause	Prevention/Treatment
Diarrhea	Formula temperature	Infuse formula at or near room temperature
	Formula infusion rate	Reduce infusion rate and increase hours
	Medications	Consult with pharmacist regarding medications that may cause diarrhea
	Bacterial contamination	Ensure good hand hygiene and clean preparation surfaces
		Do not use out-of-date formula. Rinse containers prior to opening
		Store partial cans, covered, in the refrigerator for no more than 24 hours
		Ensure safe water source
		Equipment: Discard infusion bags after 24 hours. When using syringes for feedings, wash with soap and water after each use
Constipation	Inadequate fluid	Increase fluid intake
	Inadequate or absent fiber	Consider fiber-containing formula
	Relative or total inactivity	As able and tolerated, recommend increased physical activity
	Underlying disease	Multidisciplinary interaction regarding any potential medication changes
Bloating	Formula infusion rate	Decrease infusion rate and increase hours
	Air in tubing	Remove air by "priming" the tubing of feeding set
	FODMAP content	
Clogged tube	Formula clinging in tube lumen	Fill syringe halfway with very warm water (that is still comfortable to the touch). Rapidly flush small amounts at a time into the tube
	Medication clinging to tube lumen	If unable to flush, try clearing the tube first. Use an empty syringe and draw back the plunger repeat until fluid flows freely
		If unable to clear clog, contact your healthcare provider
		Use liquid medications whenever able. Ensure that any tablet can be crushed
		Crush tablets to fine powder and mix in warm water
		Flush with water before and after each medication
		Do not mix medications

Source: Mayo Foundation for Medical Education and Research. Patient education: Tube feeding at home. Rochester, MN: Barbara Woodward Lips Patient Education Center. 2011. Used with permission.

are then able to increase their uptake of water [54]. However, the exact type of soluble fiber is still in question. For example, partially hydrolyzed guar gum can reduce diarrhea, whereas inulins and fructooligosaccharides (FOS) can increase it (Blumenstein).

There is emerging interest in FODMAPs and in the high FODMAP content of enteral formulas relating to the incidence of diarrhea [53]. The FODMAP content of enteral formulas can vary between 10.6 and 36.5 g/day [31] (measurements based on volume required to provide needs for typical patient). Enteral formula composition may change at any time and vary in content between the country from which they are produced and therefore must be reevaluated often. In a single-center study of 160 hospitalized patients, the lowest FODMAP formula was protective against diarrhea, showing a fivefold reduction in diarrhea incidence [31]. People with irritable bowel syndrome (IBS) respond proportionally to reductions in FODMAPs, and recognized maximum levels are <0.5 g per sitting or <3 g per day [53]. Certainly, all tube-fed patients do not have IBS. However, their symptoms are remarkably similar [53]. This is an area of further study for the HEN population and something for the clinician to consider especially in the IBS population.

Changes in colonic microflora may also contribute to diarrhea during enteral feeding. In a small study of 10 patients, samples demonstrated significant decreases in fecal bacteria and total SCFA, as well as increases in fecal pH. The reduction in SCFA may decrease the ability of colonocytes to absorb water [55]. Many practitioners look to manipulation of the gut microbiome as a potential solution to EN-associated diarrhea. The most promising strains are *Lactobacillus acidophilus*, *Lactobacillus bulgaricus*, and *Saccharomyces boulardii* [55]. In the realm of prebiotics, FOS and inulin fibers have the most research. In healthy patients, the consumption of both has been shown to increase fecal bacteria and SCFA counts [55]. Research is lacking in the HEN population.

Ethical Concerns

Nutrition support at end of life remains controversial. Patients and caregivers should be aware of the supportive role of nutrition, that tube feeding is not capable of improving outcome in terminal situations. [57]. Tube feeding does not prevent aspiration completely, as it is still possible to aspirate oral secretions or have GI reflux [57].

Placement of feeding tubes is common in patients in nursing homes. Up to 34% of patients with severe cognitive impairment, living in nursing homes, receive a feeding tube. However, placement is not without risks. In fact, a 2006 survey indicated cognitive impairment increased risk of emergency department visits and hospitalizations, and that risk increased with the degree of impairment. Not only do hospital visits incur added healthcare expenses, but they also represent significant setback to most patients, and there is the potential for iatrogenic complications, as well as simple burden to the patient [48].

Some of the most common complaints regarding long-term HEN relate more to psychosocial aspects rather than physical issues. In a series of semistructured interviews with 15 adult patients and 19 caregivers, they reported sleep disturbance, restricted activity, limited clothing options, finding places to do feeding while out, missing the act of eating, awkwardness in social situations, negative attitudes of others toward tube feedings, and being a burden to the family [58].

Considerations of quality of life (QOL) are important, particularly in light of the high mortality rates for many patients getting G-tubes [59]. Loeser's study of 211 patients confirmed a role for HEN in improving QOL as well as nutrition status [59]. In fact, their results even questioned the previous research indicating that mentally incompetent patients cannot benefit from tube feeding, as half their patients improved their competency during follow-up [59]. However, several studies do suggest worse outcomes and decreased QOL with HEN [46].

Use of HEN in pediatrics is often viewed by caregivers as a means to help their children and also improve the family dynamics [60]. For example, HEN reduces the amount of time spent on feeding, which allows for more time to dedicate to other family activities. Caregivers also report feeling that their children are more appropriately nourished with HEN. However, it is important to monitor the overall well-being of the primary caregiver, who frequently is the mother, as there have been reports in the literature of increased risk for psychological distress in this population, which can affect the family dynamics [61,62]. Satisfaction with HEN appears to be directly related to the length of time on HEN and the age at which it was started. Caregivers are more satisfied as the time on tube feedings increases and at an earlier age of initiation [60].

Food has tremendous emotional importance in all societies. Patients and their families tend to understand nutrition therapy better than other aspects of medical care [57]. Families and patients may choose HEN out of fear of starvation [57]. However, physiologic adaptations at end of life mean that patients do not suffer feelings of hunger. Families also need reassurance that typically the underlying disease causes death, very rarely starvation [57].

It is important for healthcare providers to present benefits and risks openly. HEN practitioners can take the lead in helping patients best cope with their nutritional changes. Thompson presents a small qualitative study of HEN patients who identified themselves as "coping well." These patients found that healthcare providers helped them cope by providing adequate initial education, adjusting their HEN prescriptions to best fit their needs, and providing good continuum of care after starting HEN [63]. HEN practitioners should also share all available resources with patients. Another qualitative study reported increased QOL with membership in the Oley Foundation, which is a national support group for home enteral and parenteral nutrition support patients [64]. Only 46% of those surveyed found out about this organization through their healthcare provider and all reported a wish that they had known about the group sooner [64].

REIMBURSEMENT

Once the patient has been assessed for HEN and therapy is planned, insurance reimbursement should be explored for home therapy. Patients are typically insured by Medicare, Medicaid, or commercial/private insurance. However, the criteria under which formula and supplies are covered can vary, and clinicians can aid the process by obtaining necessary documentation of medical necessity.

Medicare

The CMS oversee the Medicare program. HEN (formula and supplies) are covered under Medicare Part B as a durable medical equipment (DME) prosthetic device. HEN is covered at 80% of the allowed amount set by Medicare. To qualify for reimbursement, the beneficiary should meet the following criteria: (a) permanent nonfunction or disease of the structures that normally permit food to reach the small bowel or (b) disease of the small bowel that impairs digestion and absorption of an oral diet, either of which requires tube feedings to provide sufficient nutrients to maintain weight and strength commensurate with the beneficiary's overall health status [65]. "Permanence" under Medicare criteria is defined as greater than 3 months [65]. Coverage is not provided for psychological disorders or end-stage disease with anorexia or nausea, or home-blended formula. Additional documentation may be required for pump feedings, specialized formulas, malabsorption, or feedings providing <750 or >2000 calories per day [65].

Patients may also have Medicare secondary or supplemental insurance, which may or may not cover any co-pays or the remaining 20% not covered by Medicare Part B. Medicare Advantage (also known as Medicare Part C) provides coverage by private insurers approved by Medicare and will typically follow Medicare criteria.

Private or commercial insurance coverage will vary depending on the policy contract. The insurance company will need to be contacted directly to determine the individual patient's coverage. In some cases, enteral feeding supplies will be covered, but not the formula.

Medicaid is a state-run program; therefore, coverage will vary from state to state. In 2005, the Government Accountability Office (GAO) surveyed state Medicaid reimbursement, compared to criteria of Medicare coverage. The survey questioned whether each state's Medicaid matched Medicare in five categories. The results show a patchwork of coverage with little discernable pattern. A few states do follow Medicare guidelines exactly—Alaska, Iowa, Maine, North Dakota, South Carolina, Texas, and Vermont. Several others follow all guidelines but do not require the condition be permanent (3 months per Medicare). Many states cover some parts for children but not for adults. West Virginia is unique in providing no coverage at all [66]. Clinicians should contact the Medicaid office to determine coverage because the GAO report is now several years old (www.medicaid.gov).

Commercial/Private Insurance

Commercial insurance coverage for HEN will vary depending on the patient's individual policy. The coverage can encompass full coverage for formula and supplies, partial coverage, or no coverage at all.

Financial Assistance

Enteral formula companies and other medical supply providers may have programs to provide financial assistance to those uninsured or underinsured who need HEN formula and supplies. The

TABLE 8.10
Home Enteral Equipment Providers[a]

Type	Length of Need	Ongoing Clinical Monitoring	HEN Supplies/Equipment
DME provider	Any	Sometimes	Equipment for gravity/syringe/ pump feeding method Supplies for site care: Gauze Enteral formulas; large selection Enteral pumps: Portable/stationary IV pole
Home infusion company	Any	Yes, while clinically necessary. Can continue to provide DME once patient does not need nursing care	Equipment for gravity/syringe/ pump feeding method Supplies for site care: Gauze Enteral formulas; large selection Enteral pumps: Portable/stationary IV pole
Hospital-based home-care agencies	Any	Yes, but may only be able to provide supplies while receiving nursing care	May or may not provide all the above supplies

Source: Pattinson A, Epp L. *Pocket Guide to Enteral Nutrition*, Charney P and Malone A (eds.), pp. 198–229. Academy of Nutrition and Dietetics, © 2013. Reprinted with permission.

[a] All types of providers listed here offer 24-hour support and often provide delivery and/or ship directly to patients. They may qualify for third-party coverage if they meet the coverage criteria and may provide direct billing to the insurance company.

Oley Foundation (www.oley.org) is a national support organization for HEN and parenteral nutrition patients that may have donated formula and supplies.

HEN PROVIDERS

Depending on insurance coverage, the patient may have options in who will be providing skilled nursing and home enteral formula equipment. In keeping the A.S.P.E.N. home care standards, home care equipment providers should encompass a multidisciplinary approach to the patient receiving HEN therapy. In addition, the home care provider should be able to meet the needs of those requiring more intensive nursing and nutrition monitoring. HEN providers should be knowledgeable about enteral formula equipment, enteral access, and care, and provide 24-hour on-call services. Table 8.10 outlines various home care/home equipment providers.

SUMMARY

The HEN population continues to increase yearly. The needs of these patients require a multidisciplinary approach to meet treatment goals and to keep the patient at home. Clinician expertise in the areas of assessment, intervention, and monitoring will aid in the success of HEN therapy.

RESOURCES

Association of Gastrointestinal Motility Disorders, Inc (AGMD). http://www.agmd-gimotility.org

Brantley SL, Mills ME. Overview of enteral nutrition. And Cresci G, Lefton J, Esper DE. Enteral formulations. In: Mueller CM (ed.) *The ASPEN Adult Nutrition Support Core Curriculum*, 2nd Edition, Silver Spring, MD, 2012, pp. 170–184.

Centers for Medicare and Medicaid Services (CMS) 1984. National coverage determination for enteral and parenteral nutrition therapy. http://www.cms.gov/medicare-coverage-database/details/ncd-details

Pattinson A, Epp L. Home enteral nutrition. In: Charney P and Malone A (eds.) *Pocket Guide to Enteral Nutrition*, 2nd Edition, pp. 198–229. Academy of Nutrition and Dietetics. 2013.

Oley Foundation. www.oley.org

The A.S.P.E.N. Nutrition Support Patient Education Manual. Contains pertinent patient education material in English and Spanish. www.nutritioncare.org

Tube Feeding Awareness Foundation. http://www.feedingtubeawareness.com

REFERENCES

1. Teitelbaum D, Guenter P, Howell WH et al. Definition of terms, style and conventions used in ASPEN guidelines and standards. *Nutr Clin Pract* 2005;20:281.
2. Oley Foundation. 1993. *North American Home Parenteral and Enteral Nutrition Patient Registry Annual Report—1985–1991*. Oley Foundation, Albany, NY.
3. Ireton-Jones C. 2007. Home enteral nutrition support in adults. In: Delegge M, Ireton-Jones C (eds.) *Handbook of Home Nutrition Support*. Jones & Bartlett Publishers, Sadbury, MA, pp. 83–102.
4. Durfee SM, Adams SC, Arthur E et al. ASPEN standards for nutrition support: Home and alternate site care. *JPEN J Parenter Enteral Nutr* 2014;29(4):542–555.
5. Klek S, Szybinski P, Sierzega M et al. Commercial enteral formulas and nutrition support teams improve the outcome of home enteral tube feedings. *J Parenter Enteral Nutr* 2011;35(3):380–385.
6. Hall BT, Englehart MS, Blaseg K et al. Implementation of a dietitian-led enteral nutrition support clinic results in quality improvement, reduced readmissions and cost savings. *Nutr Clin Prac* 2014;29(5);649–655.
7. A.S.P.E.N. Board of Directors and the Clinical Guidelines Task Force. Guidelines for the use of enteral and parenteral nutrition in adult and pediatric patients. *JPEN J Parenter Enteral Nutr* 2002;26: 1SA–138SA.
8. Rollins CJ. 2012. Drug–nutrient interactions. In: Mueller C (ed.) *The ASPEN Adult Nutrition Support Core Curriculum*, 2nd Edition. The American Society for Parenteral and Enteral Nutrition Silver Spring, MD, pp. 298–312.
9. Baker SS, Baker RD, Davis AM. 2007. *Pediatric Nutrition Support*. Jones & Bartlett Publishers, Sudbury, MA.
10. Schwenk WF, Olson D. 2001. Pediatrics. In: Gottschlich M (ed.) *The Science and Practice of Nutrition Support A Case-Based Core Curriculum*. Dubuque, IA, pp. 347–372.
11. Hannah E, John RM. Everything the nurse practitioner should know about pediatric feeding tubes. *J Am Assoc Nurse Pract* 2013;25:567–577.
12. Schwartz S. Feeding disorders in children with developmental disabilities. *Infants Young Children* 2003;16:317–330.
13. Critch J, Day A, Otley A et al. Use of enteral nutrition for the control of intestinal inflammation in pediatric Crohn disease. *JPEN J Parent Enteral Nutr* 2012;54:298–305.
14. Lochs H, Dejong C, Hammarqvist F et al. ESPEN (European Society for Parenteral and Enteral Nutrition). ESPEN guidelines on enteral nutrition, gastroenterology. *Clin Nutr* 2006;25:260–274.
15. Canani RB, Terrin G, Borrelli O et al. Short- and long-term therapeutic efficacy of nutritional therapy and corticosteroids in pediatric Crohn's disease. *Dig Liver Dis* 2006;38:381–387.
16. Monzka J. 2015. Enteral nutrition support: Determining the best way to feed. In: Corkins MR (ed.) *The A.S.P.E.N. Pediatric Nutrition Support Core Curriculum*, 2nd Edition, Silver Spring, MD, pp. 583–592.
17. Bankhead R, Boullata J, Brantley S et al. Enteral nutrition practice recommendations. *JPEN J Parenter Enteral Nutr* 2009;33(2):122–167.
18. Itkin M, DeLegge MH, Fang JC et al. Multidisciplinary practical guidelines for gastrointestinal access for enteral nutrition and decompression from the Society of Interventional Radiology and American Gastroenterological Association (AGA) Institute, with endorsement by Canadian Interventional Radiological Association (CRIA) and Cardiovascular and Interventional Radiological Society of Europe (CIRSE). *Gastroenterology* 2011;141:742–765.
19. Lyman B, Shah R. 2015. Nutrition access. In: Corkins MR (ed.) *The A.S.P.E.N. Pediatric Nutrition Support Core Curriculum*, 2nd Edition, Silver Spring, MD, pp. 567–582.
20. Irving S, Lyman B, Northington L, Bartlett J, Kemper C, NOVEL project work group. Nasogastric tube placement and verification in children: Review of the current literature. *Nutr Clin Pract* 2014;29:267–276.

21. Corkins MR, Griggs KC, Groh-Wargo S et al. Standards for nutrition support: Pediatric hospitalized patients. *Nutr Clin Pract* 2013;28(2); 263–276.
22. Szeszycki E, Cruse W, Beitzel M. 2015. Evaluation and monitoring of pediatric patients receiving specialized nutrition support. In: Corkins MR (ed.) *The A.S.P.E.N. Pediatric Nutrition Support Core Curriculum*, 2nd Edition, Silver Spring, MD, pp. 615–639.
23. Edwards S, Davis A, Bruce A, Mousa H, Lyman B, Cocjin J, Dean K, Ernst L, Almadhoun O, Hyman P. Caring for Tube-Fed children: A review of management, tube weaning, and emotional considerations. *JPEN* 2015 (Epub ahead of print).
24. Lyman B, Gebhards S, Hensley C et al. Safety of decanted enteral formula hung for 12 hours in a pediatric setting. *Nutr Clin Pract* 2011;26:451–456.
25. Metzer LC. Education materials for home nutrition support patients. *Nutr Clin Prac* 2010;25(5):451–470.
26. Kornburger C, Gibson C, Sadowski S et al. Using "teach-back" to promote a safe transition from hospital to home: An evidence-based approach to improving the discharge process. *J Pediatr Nurs* 2013;28:282–291.
27. Clayton LH. Strategies for selecting effective patient nutrition education materials. *Nutr Clin Prac* 2010;25(5):436–442.
28. Mayo Clinic. 2014. Home enteral nutrition feeding tube overview. https://www.youtube.com/watch?v=pqxzRyfUq6k. 2/14/14, Accessed 5/30/15.
29. AGMD Association of Gastrointestinal Motility Disorders, Inc. Enteral and parenteral nutrition access and complications. https://vimeo.com/channels/gimotility. Published 2013, Accessed 5/30/15.
30. Oley Foundation. 2006. Tools for living better on home IV & tube feedings. Making your own food for tube feeding. http://oley.org/lifeline/TubetalkSO07.html. Accessed 1/19/2015.
31. Halmos EP, Muir JG, Barrett JS et al. Diarrhoea during enteral nutrition is predicted by the poorly absorbed short-chain carbohydrate (FODMAP) content of the formula. *Aliment Pharmacol Ther* 2010;32:925–933.
32. Daniels S. US organic food market to grow 14% from 2013–2018. http://www.foodnavigator-usa.com/Markets/US-organic-food-market-to-grow-14-from-2013–2018. Accessed 10/6/2014.
33. Dixon S. Nutrition in complementary and alternative medicine. *Seminars Oncol Nurs* 2012;28(1):75–84.
34. Mortensen M. Blenderized tube feeding clinical perspectives on homemade tube feeding. *PNPG Post* 2006;17:1–4.
35. Novak P, Wilson K, Ausderau K. Cullinane D. The use of blenderized tube feedings. *ICAN* 2009;1:21–23.
36. Klein MD, Morris SE. *Homemade Blended Formula Handbook*. Mealtime Notions, LLC, Tucson, Arizona, 2007.
37. Malone A. Enteral formula selection: A review of selected product categories. *Pract Gastroenterol* 2005;28:44.
38. The Joint Commission Sentinel Event Alert. Tubing misconnections—A persistent and potentially deadly occurrence. 2006; http://www.jointcommission.org/sentinel_event_alert_issue_36_tubing_misconnections%E2%80%94a_persistent_and_potentially_deadly_occurrence/. Accessed 3/2/15.
39. Global Enteral Device Supply Association (GEDSA). Stay Connected 2015. http://www.stayconnected.org/index.html. Accessed 3/2/2015.
40. Office of the National Coordinator for Health Information Technology (ONC) 2014. Health IT legislation and regulations. http://www.healthit.gov/policy-researchers-implementers/health-it-legislation-and-regulations. Last update 9/25/14. Accessed 3/19/15.
41. Health and Human Services. 2014. The Affordable Care Act supports patient centered medical homes in health centers. http://www.hhs.gov/news/press/2014pres/08/20140826a.html. Accessed 3/19/15.
42. Boisseau N, Burde A, Bachmann P et al. A telephone-linked computer system for home enteral nutrition. *J Telemed Telecare* 2010;16(7):363–367.
43. Smith CE. 2014. Home parenteral nutrition families' mobile distance to care research. https://clinicaltrials.gov/ct2/show/NCT01900288.
44. Majka AJ, Wang Z, Schmitz KR et al. Care coordination to enhance management of tong-term enteral tube feeding: A systematic review. *JPEN J Parenter Enteral Nutr* 2014;38(1):40–52.
45. Hebuterne X, Bozzetti F, Moreno Villares JM et al. Home enteral nutrition in adults: A European multicentre survey. *Clin Nutr* 2003;22(3):261–266.
46. Klek S, Hermanowicz A, Dziwiszek G et al. Home enteral nutrition reduces complications, length of stay and health care costs: Results from a multicenter study. *Am J Clin Nutr* 2014;100:609–615.
47. DeLegge M. Home enteral nutrition. *JPEN J Parenter Enteral Nutr* 2002;26(5):S4–S7.
48. Stephens CE, Sackett N, Govindarajan P et al. Emergency department visits and hospitalizations by tube-fed nursing home residents with varying degrees of cognitive impairment: A national study. *BMC Geriatr* 2014;14:35–42.

49. Crosby J and Duerksen DR. A prospective study of tube- and feeding-related complications in patients receiving long-term home enteral nutrition. *JPEN J Parenter Enteral Nutr* 2007;31(4):274–277.
50. McSweeney ME, Jaing H, Deutsch AJ et al. Long-term outcomes of infants and children undergoing percutaneous endoscopy gastrostomy tube placement. *J Pediatr Gastroenterol Nutr* 2013;57(5):663–667.
51. Blumenstein I, Shastri YM and Stein J. Gastroenteric tube feeding: Techniques, problems and solutions. *World J Gastroenterol* 2014;20(26):8505–8524.
52. Shankardass K, Chuchmach S, Chelswich et al. Bowel function of long-term tube fed patients consuming formulae with and without dietary fiber. *JPEN J Parenter Enteral Nutr* 1990;14(5):508–512.
53. Halmos EP. Role of FODMAP content in enteral nutrition-associated diarrhea. *J Gastroenterol Hepatol* 2013;29(suppl 4):25–28.
54. Chang SJ and Huang HH. Diarrhea in enterally fed patients: Blame the diet? *Curr Opin Clin Nutr Metab Care* 2013;16:588–594.
55. Whalen K. Enteral tube feeding diarrhea: Manipulating the colonic microbiota with probiotics and prebiotics. *Proc Nutr Soc* 2007;66:299–306.
56. Elia M, Engler MB, Green CJ, Silk DB. Systematic review and meta-analysis; The clinical and physiological effects of fibre-containing enteral formulae. *Aliment Pharmacol Ther* 2008;27(2):120–145.
57. McMahon MM, Hurley DL, Kamath PS et al. Medical and ethical aspects of long-term enteral tube feeding. *Mayo Clin Proc* 2005;80(11):1461–1476.
58. Brotherton A, Abbott J, Aggett P. The impact of percutaneous endoscopic gastrostomy feeding upon daily life in adults. *J Hum Nutr Diet* 2006;19(5):355–367.
59. Martinez-Costa C, Calderon C, Gomez-Lopez L et al. Satisfaction with gastrostomy feeding in caregivers of children with home enteral nutrition, application of the SAGA-8 questionnaire and analysis of involved factors. *Nutr Hosp* 2013;28(4):1121–1128.
60. Boebel V, Musil CM, Carl JC. Families with children who are technology-dependent: Normalization and family functioning. *Wes J Nurs Res* 2012;34(1):52–71.
61. Calderon C, Gomez-Lopez L, Martinez-Costa et al. Feeling of burdon, psychological distress, and anxiety among primary caregivers of children with home enteral nutrition. *J Pediatr Psychol* 2010;36(2):188–195.
62. Thompson C. Fostering coping skills and resilience in home enteral nutrition (HEN) patients. *Nutr Clin Pract* 2006;21:557–565.
63. Chopy K, Winkler M, Schwartz-Barcott D et al. A qualitative study of perceived value of membership in the Oley Foundation by home parenteral and enteral nutrition patients. *JPEN J Parenter Enteral Nutr* 2015;39(4):426–433.
64. Centers for Medicare and Medicaid Services (CMS) Local Coverage Determination (LCD) 2013. Enteral nutrition. http://www.medicarenhic.com/viewdoc.aspx?id=1635. Accessed 3/20/15.
65. Parver AK, Mutinsky SE. Enteral nutrition reimbursement—The rationale for the policy: The US perspective. *Nestlé Nutr Inst Workshop Ser Clin Perform Program* 2009;12:53–70.
66. Brown B, Roehl K, Betz M. Enteral nutrition formula selection: Current evidence and implications for use. *Nutr Clin Prac* 2015;30(1):72–85.

9 Home Parenteral Nutrition

Kristen Roberts, PhD, RDN, LD

CONTENTS

INDICATIONS FOR USE

Intestinal failure (IF) is defined as a condition resulting in an inability to maintain hydration and electrolyte and nutritional status without intravenous support. For many patients with IF, home parenteral nutrition (HPN) is a life-saving modality when IF extends beyond the hospital stay. In the 1970s, HPN became more readily available to patients with infusion pharmacy and homecare services becoming involved in the treatment of these patients. Over the last several decades, HPN providers have reported the main causes of IF, leading to the initiation of HPN [1]. Commonly reported conditions are listed below [1–3]:

- Inflammatory bowel disease (IBD)
- Bowel ischemia
- Short bowel syndrome (SBS)
- Radiation enteritis
- Motility disorder
- Gastrointestinal (GI) fistulae
- Bowel obstruction

Not all patients with IF are appropriate for HPN due to the complexity of the therapy. Determining appropriateness requires a team of nutrition professionals, preferably a nutrition support team (NST), to evaluate nutritional status, GI function, and disease severity of each patient leading to the need for HPN. Specifically, these nutrition professionals include a physician, registered dietitian (RD), registered nurse (RN), pharmacist, social worker, and case manager [4]. This chapter deals primarily with adults requiring HPN. Pediatric HPN is discussed in Chapter 3 with additional references.

The physician oversees the full HPN evaluation process and puts extensive emphasis on conducting a thorough evaluation of the GI tract. Briefly, the RD works with the patient to establish a nutrition prescription to achieve one or several nutrition-related goals. Typical goals include losing, maintaining, or gaining weight and/or to correct or prevent micronutrient deficiencies and dehydration. The RD along with the RN contributes to educating the patient on documenting daily weights, temperatures, and intake and output records. In addition to educating the patient on HPN procedures, the

RN assists the patient in selecting a vascular access device (VAD). This is an essential component of the HPN process as the RN ensures that the patient understands the risks and benefits to each VAD prior to making a selection (see Chapter 10). Once the VAD is selected, education on care ensues to allow the patient to be autonomous with the VAD at discharge. The pharmacist inspects the PN solution for stability and compatibility and provides recommendations for medication management in the HPN solution. Cognitive and psychosocial concerns are evaluated by the team social worker with the goal of assessing patient safety with a VAD and intravenous therapies [5,6]. Also, the social worker evaluates the home environment to ascertain if electricity, running water, and telephone access are suitable [7]. Lastly, owing to the extraneous costs of HPN, the case manager will confirm the indication for HPN with the insurance company and verify insurance benefits.

A proficient case manager is critical to preparing the patient for discharge on HPN to ameliorate costs associated with the therapy. Accurately documenting a patient as having permanent IF (>90 days) requiring HPN is critical for financial reimbursement [8]. Knowledge of this documentation is critical for determining insurance benefits (see Chapter 11). Many patients utilize Medicare or Medicaid for HPN coverage, but the majority rely on private insurance to supplement their primary insurance coverage [8]. Determining insurance coverage early on in the discharge process and appropriately documenting the indications for HPN in the medical record is key. Documentation of IF and concurrent insurance approval permits the NST to complete the education sessions and stabilize the PN formula for discharge.

INITIATING HPN

Initiation of HPN can occur in the hospital or home; however, hospital initiation is favored to minimize risk in certain cases. The American Society of Parenteral and Enteral Nutrition (A.S.P.E.N.) recommends hospital initiation for patients with severe medical conditions and/or electrolyte disorders [9]. This chapter will primarily address initiation of PN in the hospital. Initiation of PN in the hospital (or home) should only be started once all significant electrolyte abnormalities are corrected and the patient is metabolically stable. Once electrolyte status is stable, initiating a low-dextrose PN solution on the first day of therapy is warranted to prevent adverse events (i.e., severe hyperglycemia, cardiac dysfunction). In cases of extreme malnutrition or organ dysfunction, reaching the caloric goal may take several days to achieve and daily monitoring of laboratory parameters and weights is necessary to safely advance the PN solution. When the low-dextrose PN is tolerated (i.e., no significant electrolyte or blood sugar abnormalities), the caloric content of the solution can slowly be increased to goal calories. Once a patient is identified as appropriate for HPN, a nutrition-related goal for the PN prescription should be established, as well as other steps in the discharge process (see Figure 9.1). Patients who have an appropriate indication for PN in the home, are clinically stable, have proper access for HPN, and are capable of being educated in the safe administration of HPN, may be initiated in the home setting [9].

PN Prescription

Macronutrient, fluid, and micronutrient components of the PN prescription are established based on the nutrition assessment completed by the RD and the nutrition-related goals of each patient. These nutrient components are established prior to initiation and can then be adjusted in response to therapy as needed [7,10]. Total energy needs are established based on the patients' long-term goal to gain, maintain, or reduce total body weight. Calculating energy needs can be determined by multiple predictive equations or by indirect calorimetry. For most patients, 20–30 kcal/kg of body weight is sufficient for weight maintenance [4,10–12]. Yet, patients requiring weight gain may require up to 42 kcal/kg [13]. Of these calories, lipid should be provided to patients unable to consume adequate dietary fat to prevent essential fatty acid deficiency (EFAD). Prevention of EFAD requires a minimum of 3%–4% total calories delivered from an intravenous fat emulsion (IVFE) unless dietary

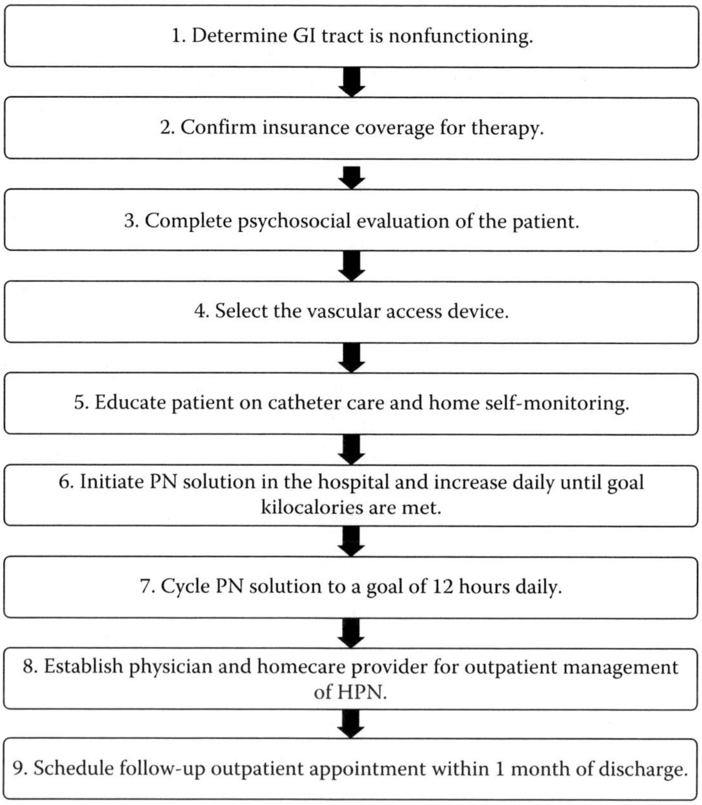

FIGURE 9.1 Steps for discharging a patient on home parenteral nutrition.

fat absorption is adequate as EFAD can develop within 1–2 weeks on lipid-free PN prescriptions [10,14,15]. Although A.S.P.E.N. recommends that the lipid content not exceed 2.5 g/kg/day, most clinicians utilize a maximum of 1.0 g/kg/day for long-term HPN therapy [10,16–18]. The current US IVFE is soybean oil based; however, newer alternative lipid sources may allow for a more diverse lipid type and therefore administration tolerance [16]. Protein (i.e., amino acids) and carbohydrate (i.e., dextrose monohydrate) requirements fluctuate based on patient tolerance, medical condition, and the response to therapy and therefore, must be adjusted accordingly [10]. Typically, protein should provide 1.2–2.0 g/kg/day depending on body mass and disease severity and delivered as a concentrated amino acid solution ranging from 3% to 20% [10,12]. Carbohydrate needs are met by infusion of a dextrose monohydrate solution ranging from 5% to 70% with each gram supplying approximately 3.4 kcal. Fluid needs can be estimated by providing 30–40 mL/kg of dry weight [10]. Ultimately, fluid delivery should cover GI and insensible losses while allowing for a minimum of 1000 mL of urine daily for the adult patient [2,4,19]. Electrolyte, vitamin, and mineral additives should be added to the PN bag daily and adjusted based on individual needs. Estimated micronutrient requirements for parenteral nutrition solutions have been reviewed and guidelines are available for dosing [10].

With ongoing drug shortages affecting the HPN prescription of many patients with IF, tactics for preventing micronutrient deficiencies have been suggested [20]. Specifically, these guidelines recommend that multivitamin (MVI) and multiple trace element (MTE) solutions should be given orally in those HPN patients with adequate functionality of the GI tract to tolerate and absorb oral doses. In patients without adequate functionality of the GI tract, intravenous MVI and MTE solutions should be reduced from daily to 3× per week [20].

Once the nutritional goals are established, the clinician formulates the PN solution as a 3-in-1 (carbohydrate, lipid, and protein delivered in the same bag) or 2-in-1 (carbohydrate and protein

TABLE 9.1
Stability Guidelines for 3-in-1 Admixtures

Nutrient	Parameters
Macronutrient	≥4% Amino acid
	≥10% Dextrose
	≥2% Lipid
Divalent cations	Between 16 and 20 mEq/L
Iron	Omit iron dextran from PN solution

Source: Adapted from Mirtallo JT et al. *JPEN J Parenter Enteral Nutr* 2004; 28 (6):S39–70; Boullata, JI et al. *JPEN J Parenter Enteral Nutr* 2014; 38 (3):334–77; Driscoll DF. *Nutr Clin Pract* 2006; 21 (4):381–6.

delivered in the same bag and lipids given separately). Several factors determine how the PN solution is formulated, such as fluid requirements, stability parameters, presence of organ failure (i.e., hepatic, renal, and/or pulmonary diseases), and energy needs [10,21]. It is not uncommon for a patient to receive 2-in-1 solutions 6/days per week and a 3-in-1 solution for the remaining day to meet lipid and/or caloric requirements. Guidelines for maintaining stability and compatibility in 3-in-1 admixtures are listed in Table 9.1.

Infusion Parameters

Infusion parameters such as the infusion time, infusion rate, and tapering of the solution are established based on the patients tolerance of fluid and macronutrient infusion. Typically, HPN solutions are infused over 8–12 hours when feasible due to the psychological and hepatic benefits [23,24]. The process of cycling a PN prescription over a shorter infusion time (<24 hours) can take several days during hospitalization. Although cycling in a long-term care facility or in the home can be done, data on the frequency and adverse events associated with this is unknown. Each adjustment to the infusion cycle requires calculation of a new infusion rate. The infusion rate is determined by calculating the total fluid volume needed in the PN bag divided by the number of hours the patient will be infusing the solution at home (hours in the cycle). Most patients will require the PN solution to be tapered up and down one-hour to prevent blood sugar abnormalities [25]. A metabolically stable patient will likely be able to tolerate a 12-hour PN cycle that tapers off over the last hour (see example below for a patient requiring 2 L of fluid daily over 12 hours).

Main rate: 2000 mL ÷ (12 hours – 1/2 hour) = ~174 mL/hour × 11 hours
Taper down rate: 174 mL/hour ÷ 2 = ~87 mL/hour × 1 hour
Infusion instructions: Start PN solution at 174 mL/hour × 11 hours and then decrease the infusion rate to 87 mL/hour for the last hour

On the other hand, a metabolically unstable patient may require longer infusion times to gain stability (see example below for a patient requiring 4 L of fluid daily over 18 hours).

Main rate: 4000 mL ÷ (18 hours – 1 hour) = ~235 mL/hour × 16 hours
Taper up rate: 235 mL/hour ÷ 2 = ~118 mL/hour × 1 hour
Taper down rate: 235 mL/hour ÷ 2 = ~118 mL/hour × 1 hour
Infusion instructions: Start PN solution at 118 mL/hour × 1 hour, then increase the infusion rate to 235 mL/hour × 16 and then decrease the infusion rate to 118 mL/hour for the last hour

MONITORING

All patients on HPN must be monitored for complications due to the complexity of the therapy and the reported complications associated with this therapy. Monitoring should include tactics for preventing short- and long-term complications associated with HPN. Short-term complications include metabolic abnormalities such as fluid and electrolyte imbalances, blood glucose abnormalities, and VAD problems (i.e., occlusions, breakage, and infection) [10]. Long-term complications include metabolic bone disease (MBD) and liver disease. Fortunately, guidelines have been proposed for monitoring HPN patients to prevent both short- and long-term complications (see Table 9.2) [7,10]. A monitoring plan should be established with the patient prior to discharge and should include laboratory parameters, intake and output record keeping, body weight, and temperature logs [26].

Laboratory Measurements

Laboratory parameters are assessed at baseline prior to discharge home and are tailored to each individual from that point forward. Most patients on HPN will have laboratory parameters monitored weekly after discharge with the frequency being decreased over time to monthly or fewer blood draws (see Table 9.2). This allows clinicians to identify laboratory trends that may require adjustment within the HPN prescription. It is important to remember that with HPN patients, HPN solutions are delivered a few times each month depending on the homecare pharmacy. Therefore, adjustments to the HPN prescription should be subtle to avoid metabolic abnormalities in-between HPN deliveries and blood draws.

TABLE 9.2
Guidelines for Monitoring Patients on HPN

Parameter	Baseline	Daily	Weekly	Monthly	Yearly
Laboratory parameters					
Blood glucose assessment	Yes	Yes, until stable	–	–	–
Electrolytes, blood urea nitrogen (BUN), and creatinine	Yes	Yes, until stable	Yes	Yes	–
Liver enzymes and bilirubin	Yes	Yes, until stable	Yes	Yes	–
Albumin or prealbumin	Yes	Yes, until stable	Yes, until stable	Yes	–
Trace elements	Yes	–	–	Every 6 months as needed	–
Vitamins	Yes, depending on disease state	–	–	Every 6 months as needed	–
Anthropometric and other measurements					
Intake and output records	Yes	Yes	–	–	–
Body weight	Yes	Yes	–	–	–
Body temperature	Yes	Yes	–	–	–
Dual-energy x-ray absorptiometry	Yes	–	–	–	Yes, as needed

Source: Adapted from Shatnawei A et al. *Arch Surg* 2010; 145 (6):521–7; Rhoda KM, Suryadevara S, Steiger E. *Surg Clin North Am* 2011; (4):913–32; Ireton-Jones C et al. *Nutr Clin Pract* 2003; 18 (4):310–7.

Anthropometric and Other Measurements

Self-monitoring includes daily recording of dietary and intravenous intake, GI losses, and body weight and temperature measurements. Prior to discharge home, patients should be educated on the importance of self-monitoring to prevent metabolic imbalances from occurring. Each component of home self-monitoring can alert the HPN prescriber that adjustments in the HPN prescription may be warranted (see Table 9.3). Significant fluctuations in dietary intake and GI output can quickly alter

TABLE 9.3
Acute Changes during HPN Therapy and Prescriber Considerations

Reported Change	Common Differential Diagnoses	Considerations for PN Prescription
Vomiting	Exogenous toxins Mechanical obstruction Infection (viral or bacterial)	Additional IVFs and/or oral rehydration solution Adjust electrolyte and/or energy components of PN prescription
Diarrhea	Increased oral intake Medication change (type, dose) Infection (viral or bacterial) Obstruction SIBO	Additional IVFs and/or oral rehydration solution Adjust electrolyte and/or energy components of PN prescription Initiate antidiarrheal therapy as needed
Reduced stool output	Decreased oral intake Inadequate fiber or fluid intake Improved GI absorption Medication change (type, dose) Obstruction	Adjust electrolyte and/or energy components of PN prescription Adjust antidiarrheal therapy as needed
Decrease urine output	Decreased fluid intake (oral and/or IV) Dehydration	Additional IVFs and/or oral rehydration solution
Increased urine output	Increased fluid intake (oral and/or IV) Overhydration	Reduce PN fluid volume and/or infusion days per week Hold PN infusion
Decreased oral/EN intake	Worsening GI function	Adjust electrolyte and/or energy components of PN prescription Assess need for initiating IVFE
Increased oral/EN intake	Improved GI absorption	Reduce IVFE needs Adjust electrolyte and/or energy components of PN prescription Consider reducing PN infusion days
Increase in body weight	Improved GI absorption Fluid overload	Adjust electrolyte and/or energy components of PN prescription Consider reducing PN infusion days Reduce PN fluid volume and/or hold PN infusion if weight gain ≥1lb for 2 consecutive days
Decrease in body weight	Malnutrition Decreased oral/IV intake Dehydration	Adjust electrolyte and/or energy components of PN prescription Consider increasing PN infusion days Additional IVFs and/or oral rehydration solution
Elevated body temperature	Infection (viral and/or bacterial)	Hold PN infusion until source of infection is determined

Source: Adapted from Kumpf VJ, Tillman E. *Nutr Clin Pract* 2012; 27 (6):749–57; Barco, KT et al. In: *The Health Professional's Guide to Gastrointestinal Nutrition*. Eds: LE Matarese, GE Mullin, and JL Raymond, Academy of Nutrition and Dietetics. 2014.

Note: IVF: intravenous fluids, SIBO: small intestine bacterial overgrowth, EN: enteral nutrition, IVFE: intravenous fat emulsion; IV: intravenous, CRBSI: catheter-related bloodstream infection, GI: gastrointestinal, PN: parenteral nutrition.

fluid and electrolyte balance, requiring an adjustment of the HPN prescription and/or GI-related medications (i.e., antidiarrheals, motility medications). Acute changes in fluid balance can easily be ascertained from daily body weights especially when blood draws are infrequent. Weight fluctuations of ≥1 pound for two consecutive days can identify significant fluid shifts associated with dehydration or overhydration [26]. Elevated body temperature with or without tremors and chills during the HPN infusion can quickly identify any infectious complications associated with the VAD [26]. These tactics for home self-monitoring can prevent significant adverse events from occurring [26].

Metabolic Bone Disease

HPN monitoring schedules include a baseline assessment of bone mineral status to determine the presence of MBD. MBD is a condition of reduced bone mass such as osteomalacia and osteoporosis that is prevalent in as many as 67% of patients on HPN [28]. Nutrient deficiencies and toxicities may play a role in the pathogenesis of MBD, but a definitive cause is yet unknown [29]. Historically, PN ingredients, particularly amino acid solutions, were highly contaminated with aluminum, which was associated with MBD. Since this time, aluminum contamination has been minimized in HPN solutions in accordance with the FDA mandate that all manufacturers list the aluminum concentration on drug packaging. This allows NSTs to accurately calculate the contribution of aluminum in the HPN bag and ensure that patients are receiving less than 5 mcg/kg/day [30]. Management of MBD should start with a baseline dual-energy x-ray absorptiometry (DEXA) measurement. HPN prescriptions should maximize the intravenous delivery of calcium and phosphorus, supplementation of vitamin D should be given as needed and patients should be encouraged to participate in routine exercise [29]. DEXA scans should be assessed at baseline and then every 6–12 months until discontinuation of HPN with abnormal readings being monitored by endocrinology [4].

Hepatobiliary Disease

HPN monitoring schedules include an assessment of the liver to prevent and/or identify hepatobiliary diseases such as cholestasis, steatosis, steatonecrosis, and cirrhosis associated with HPN. Etiology of liver disease in HPN patients is multifactorial and has been associated with SBS, overfeeding, or intolerance of enteral nutrition [17,31,32]. Prevalence rates are largely unknown; yet monitoring schedules of HPN patients must include assessment of liver function [8,17,33]. Liver-associated enzymes (LAEs), such as bilirubin, alkaline phosphatase, and aspartate transaminase (AST), as well as routine radiographic imaging of the liver and spleen can be used to assess for liver injury while on HPN [4,7]. Liver biopsy, although invasive, may be the most effective tool for determining the presence of liver damage since laboratory parameters may not indicate disease until the final stages when liver transplantation is necessary [33]. Early identification of hepatobiliary diseases in HPN patients is more common when followed by an NST for HPN management. Gupte and colleagues reported in a retrospective analysis of children referred for intestinal transplantation that 58% of children managed by an NST had fewer incidence of liver disease compared to management by a physician alone [34]. The multidisciplinary approach used by an NST includes the prevention of hepatobiliary disease by preventing infectious complications associated with the VAD, providing EN when feasible, preventing overfeeding, and ensuring adequate micronutrient supplementation [17].

CONCLUSION

Selecting patients appropriate for HPN is imperative to successful outcomes. Once patients are identified as appropriate for receiving HPN, careful initiation and monitoring for potential complications reduce adverse events from occurring. The management of HPN is best by an NST, whether in the hospital or at home, and by including the patient in the establishment of the long-term goals of therapy.

REFERENCES

1. Pironi L, Goulet O, Buchman A et al. Home Artificial Nutrition and Espen Chronic Intestinal Failure Working Group. Outcome on home parenteral nutrition for benign intestinal failure: A review of the literature and benchmarking with the European prospective survey of ESPEN. *Clin Nutr* 2012; 31 (6):831–45.
2. Shatnawei A, Parekh NR, Rhoda KM et al. Intestinal failure management at the Cleveland Clinic. *Arch Surg* 2010; 145 (6):521–7.
3. Howard L, Heaphey L, Fleming CR et al. Four years of North American registry home parenteral nutrition outcome data and their implications for patient management. *JPEN J Parenter Enteral Nutr* 1991; 15 (4):384–93.
4. Rhoda KM, Suryadevara S, Steiger E. Home parenteral nutrition support for intestinal failure. *Surg Clin North Am* 2011; (4):913–32.
5. Winkler MF, Smith CE. Clinical, social, and economic impacts of home parenteral nutrition dependence in short bowel syndrome. *JPEN J Parenter Enteral Nutr* 2014; 38 (1 Suppl):32S–37S.
6. Srp FE, Steiger E, Gulledge AD et al. Psychosocial issues of nutritional support. A multidisciplinary interpretation. *Nurs Clin North Am* 1989; (2):447–59.
7. Ireton-Jones C, DeLegge M, Epperson L et al. Management of the home parenteral nutrition patient. *Nutr Clin Pract* 2003; 18 (4):310–7.
8. Hendrickson E, Corrigan M. Navigating reimbursement for home parenteral nutrition. *Nutr Clin Pract* 2013; 28 (5):566–71.
9. Durfee SM, Adams SC, Arthur E et al. A.S.P.E.N. Standards for nutrition support: Home and alternate site care. *Nutr Clin Pract* 2014; 29 (4):542–55.
10. Mirtallo JT, Canada T, Johnson D et al. Safe practices for parenteral nutrition. *JPEN J Parenter Enteral Nutr* 2004; 28 (6):S39–70.
11. De DeBiasse MA, Wilmore SW. What is optimal nutritional support? *New Horiz* 1994; 2 (2):122–30.
12. McClave SA, Martindale RG, Vanek V et al. Guidelines for the provision and assessment of nutrition support therapy in the adult critically ill patient: Society of Critical Care Medicine (SCCM) and American Society for Parenteral and Enteral Nutrition (A.S.P.E.N.). *JPEN J Parenter Enteral Nutr* 2009; 33 (3):277–316.
13. Matarese LE., Steiger E, Seidner DL et al. Body composition changes in cachectic patients receiving home parenteral nutrition. *JPEN J Parenter Enteral Nutr* 2002; 26 (6):366–71.
14. Jeppesen PB, Hoy CE, Mortensen PB. Differences in essential fatty acid requirements by enteral and parenteral routes of administration in patients with fat malabsorption. *Am J Clin Nutr* 1999; 70 (1):78–84.
15. Ling PR, Ollero M, Khaodhiar L et al. Disturbances in essential fatty acid metabolism in patients receiving long-term home parenteral nutrition. *Dig Dis Sci* 2002; 47 (8):1679–85.
16. Vanek VW, Seidner D, Allen P et al. ASPEN position paper: Clinical role for alternative fat emulsions. *Nutr Clin Prac* 2012; 27 (2):150–92.
17. Jeejeebhoy KN. Management of PN-induced cholestasis. 2005 In *Practical Gastroenterology*, 62–8. www.practicalgastro.com/pdf/February05/Feb05Jeejeebhoy.pdf.
18. Buchman A. Total parenteral nutrition-associated liver disease. *JPEN J Parenter Enteral Nutr* 2002; 26 (5 Suppl):S43–8.
19. Burnes JU, O'Keefe SJ, Fleming CR et al. Home parenteral nutrition—A 3-year analysis of clinical and laboratory monitoring. *JPEN J Parenter Enteral Nutr* 1992; 16 (4):327–32.
20. Hassig TB, McKinzie BP, Fortier CR et al. Clinical management strategies and implications for parenteral nutrition drug shortages in adult patients. *Pharmacotherapy* 2014; 34 (1):72–84. doi: 10.1002/phar.1350.
21. Boullata, JI, Gilbert K, Sacks G et al. A.S.P.E.N. clinical guidelines: Parenteral nutrition ordering, order review, compounding, labeling, and dispensing. *JPEN J Parenter Enteral Nutr* 2014; 38 (3):334–77.
22. Driscoll DF. Lipid injectable emulsions: 2006. *Nutr Clin Pract* 2006; 21 (4):381–6.
23. Suryadevara S, Celestin J, DeChicco R et al. Type and prevalence of adverse events during the parenteral nutrition cycling process in patients being prepared for discharge. *Nutr Clin Pract* 2012; 27 (2):268–73.
24. Jensen AR, Goldin AB, Koopmeiners JS et al. The association of cyclic parenteral nutrition and decreased incidence of cholestatic liver disease in patients with gastroschisis. *J Pediatr Surg* 2009; 44 (1):183–9. doi: 10.1016/j.jpedsurg.2008.10.033.
25. Bendorf K, Friesen CA, Roberts CC. Glucose response to discontinuation of parenteral nutrition in patients less than 3 years of age. *JPEN J Parenter Enteral Nutr* 1996; 20 (2):120–2.

26. Kumpf VJ, Tillman E. Home parenteral nutrition: Safe transition from hospital to home. *Nutr Clin Pract* 2012; 27 (6):749–57.
27. Barco, KT, Alberino, MJ, Roberts, KM, Wolff, J, Parekh, NR. In: *The Health Professional's Guide to Gastrointestinal Nutrition*. Eds: LE Matarese, GE Mullin, and JL Raymond, Academy of Nutrition and Dietetics, Chicago, Illinois. 2014.
28. Cohen-Solal M, Baudoin C, Joly F et al. Osteoporosis in patients on long-term home parenteral nutrition: A longitudinal study. *J Bone Miner Res* 2003; 18 (11):1989–94.
29. Buchman AL, Moukarzel A. Metabolic bone disease associated with total parenteral nutrition. *Clin Nutr* 2000; 19 (4):217–31.
30. Aluminum in large and small volume parenterals used in total parenteral nutrition—FDA. Proposed rule. 1998; *Fed Regist No.* 63 (2):176–85.
31. Teitelbaum DH, Tracy T. Parenteral nutrition-associated cholestasis. *Semin Pediatr Surg* 2001; 10 (2):72–80.
32. Javid PJ, Collier S, Richardson D et al. The role of enteral nutrition in the reversal of parenteral nutrition-associated liver dysfunction in infants. *J Pediatr Surg* 2005; 40 (6):1015–8.
33. Salvino R, Ghanta R, Seidner DL et al. Liver failure is uncommon in adults receiving long-term parenteral nutrition. *JPEN J Parenter Enteral Nutr* 2006; 30 (3):202–8.
34. Gupte GL, Beath SV, Protheroe S et al. Improved outcome of referrals for intestinal transplantation in the UK. *Arch Dis Child* 2007; 92 (2):147–52.

10 Parenteral Nutrition Access

Marianne Opilla, RN, BSN, CNSC

CONTENTS

INTRODUCTION

Vascular access for parenteral nutrition support at home is a challenging and complex facet of the overall therapy. Diligent maintenance and care of the access site and device by the patient or home caregiver is vital in reducing catheter complications, extending device life, reducing hospitalizations, and improving quality of life.

VASCULAR ACCESS

Home parenteral nutrition (HPN) formulations are usually hypertonic in order to provide the nutrients and electrolytes the patient needs. The large vessels of the central venous system have the rapid blood flow necessary to dilute the HPN solution and prevent venous damage [1]. Central venous access refers to a device whose distal tip terminates at the junction of the superior vena cava (SVC) and the right atrium or the inferior vena cava above the level of the diaphragm [2].

Figure 10.1 shows the sites used for central venous catheter (CVC) placement. The most common insertion sites are the subclavian and internal jugular into the SVC. Other sites that may be cannulated in patients with limited venous access are the femoral vein or translumbar vessels leading into the inferior vena cava. Central venous access can also be achieved by venipuncture of the basilic and cephalic peripheral veins in the arm and the CVC is advanced to the junction of the SVC and the right atrium.

CVCs appropriate for HPN infusion include the peripherally inserted central catheter (PICC), tunneled catheter, and implanted port. Each device has specific characteristics and benefits tailored to meet the patient's individual needs. Pediatric patients use the same types of devices as adults. It

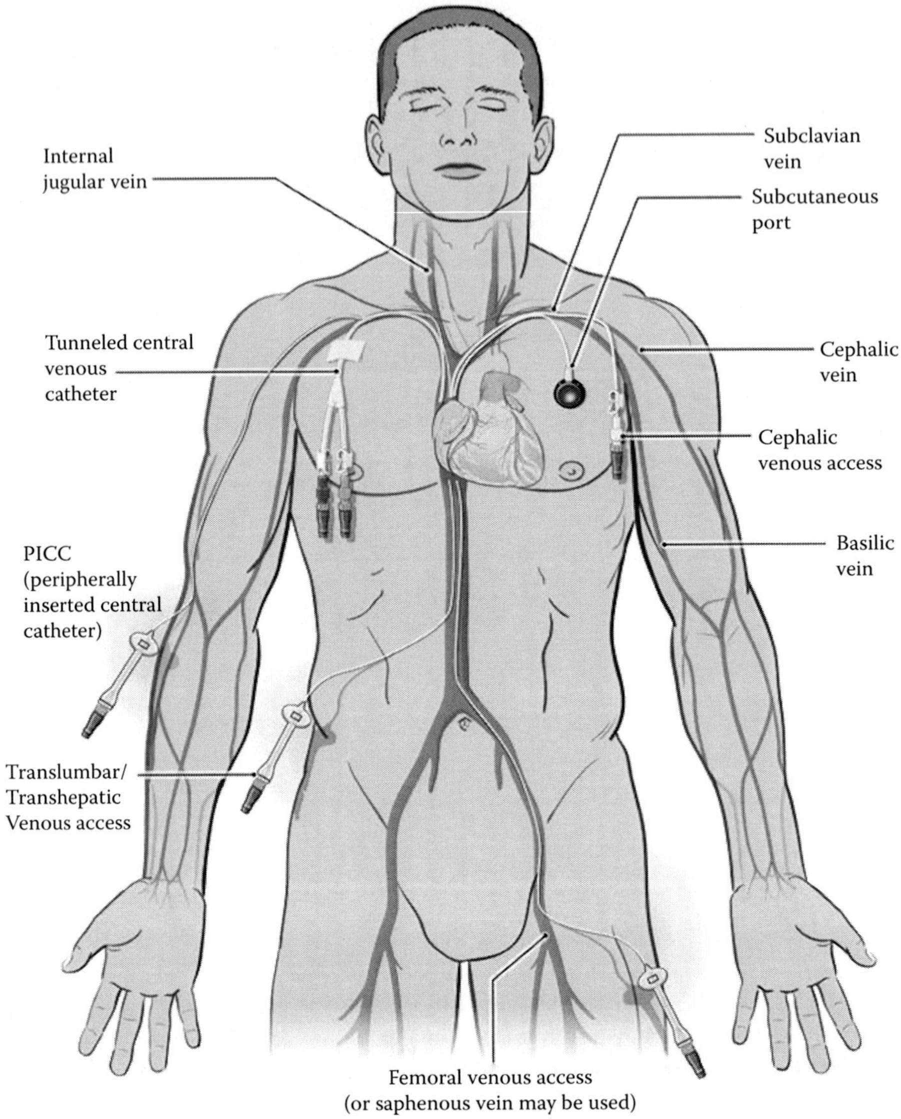

FIGURE 10.1 Femoral venous access. (Reproduced with permission of the Cleveland Clinic Center for Continuing Education. Kirby DF, Corrigan ML. Principles of Nutrition Support. Disease Management Project (http://www.clevelandclinicmeded.com/medicalpubs/diseasemanagement/gastroenterology/principles-of-nutrition-support/). Copyright 2000–2014. The Cleveland Clinic Foundation. All rights reserved.)

is recommended that placement be reconfirmed for pediatric CVCs on a yearly basis due to growth that could change the position of the catheter tip [3].

Prior to CVC insertion, careful patient assessment by the clinical insertion team helps to ensure successful placement. In addition, discussion with the patient and caregiver should include age, ability to care for self, body image, length of therapy, lifestyle characteristics, and caregiver availability. Dialogue between the patient, caregivers, and clinicians will ensure the patient receives the device most suited to their lifestyle.

CVC insertion may be performed at the bedside, in the radiology department, or in the operating room. Local anesthetic with intravenous sedation or general anesthesia may be given depending upon the individual patient needs. CVCs are inserted by a variety of clinicians with expertise in the field. These include specially trained registered nurses, nurse practitioners, physician's assistants, and physicians.

DEVICE FEATURES

Designs

Tunneled catheters and PICCs and are available as single, double, or triple lumen. Implanted ports are single or double lumen. Multiple lumens provide access for more than one infusion, but may have a higher incidence of infection due to increased manipulations at the hub. A single lumen catheter is the preferred option for patients infusing HPN only [4]. Catheter lumens are either open-ended or valved at the distal tip. An open-ended catheter requires clamping to prevent air embolism and heparin flush to prevent clotting at the tip. Valved catheters have a pressure slit at the distal tip which opens with flush, infusion, or aspiration, but remains closed when not in use. The valve helps to prevent air embolism, blood reflux, and clotting, and it does not require heparin flush.

Materials

The implanted port reservoir is either magnetic resonance imaging (MRI)-compatible plastic or titanium with a silicone septum. Silicone and polyurethane polymers are used for port catheters, PICCs, and tunneled catheters. Both products have superior compatibility with body tissue and fluids. The polyurethane is stiffer to provide easier insertion, but softens once it is within the body. Silicone is a very soft flexible material, which, although may be more challenging to insert, is more comfortable for long-term wear and more compatible with infusates and antiseptics. Polyurethane may crack with exposure to antiseptics and certain medications. Valved catheters are silicone. Although appropriate for use with HPN, polyurethane was primarily developed to administer high-flow-rate power injection therapies and is therefore a highly durable catheter material compared to silicone, which may tear or develop pinholes over time [5].

Measurements

A catheter's French (Fr) size describes the circumference of the outer diameter in millimeters. The internal lumen will vary depending upon catheter design and material. Polyurethane catheters have narrower walls, so a 5 Fr polyurethane catheter has a larger internal volume than a 5 Fr silicone catheter. All types of catheters come in various lengths to accommodate different heights and weights. Silicone catheters may be trimmed to fit the anatomy of the patient, but valved and polyurethane length cannot be adjusted. French size and lumen volume may be imprinted on the hub of PICCs and tunneled catheters. The patient should receive a wallet-sized ID card, which contains important catheter information and is helpful in determining measurements.

Pressure per square inch (PSI) is important to understand in the care of CVCs. Excessive PSI can cause catheter rupture. Silicone catheters are very soft and can only withstand about 25 PSI compared to polyurethane at 300 PSI.

CENTRAL VASCULAR ACCESS DEVICES

Peripherally Inserted Central Catheters

A PICC is inserted into the peripheral cephalic or basilic vein near the antecubital fossa and advanced into the central venous system to the distal SVC. Traditionally, PICCs were indicated for therapies lasting 6 months or less, but have been reported to remain in place for months to years without complications [6]. Figure 10.1 shows placement of a PICC. It is usually anchored in place on the skin at the insertion site using a stabilization device rather than tape or sutures. These devices reduce catheter movement at the site and within the vessel and help to prevent dislodgement [2]. PICC site care is generally provided by weekly home health nursing visits to closely observe the site and maintain the stabilization device.

Tunneled Catheters

The tunneled catheter is inserted into the vessel through a small incision or cut down and threaded into desired distal SVC tip position. Figure 10.1 shows tunneled catheter placement. A subcutaneous tunnel is created with an exit site on the chest, abdomen, or rarely, the thigh. A Dacron cuff is placed above the exit site within the subcutaneous tissue of the tunnel. This cuff provides catheter stability, as well as a barrier against bacteria migrating from the exit site into the central venous system. Additional anchoring is provided with external sutures at the exit site. The subcutaneous tissue adheres to the Dacron cuff in about 10–14 days and then sutures at the exit site can be removed. Many HPN patients and caregivers are taught to perform their own site care and in some cases a dressing is not required at the exit site once it is well healed [4]. The tunnel and cuff feature of these catheters increase patient independence with self-care and reduce catheter malposition and dislodgement.

Implanted Port

The implanted port reservoir is placed in a subcutaneous pocket on the chest, abdomen, or thigh and the tubing is threaded into the central venous system. Figure 10.1 demonstrates implanted port placement in the chest area. It is completely under the skin and must be accessed for infusion with a noncoring 90° needle with extension to connect the HPN infusion. Once the infusion is completed, the needle can be removed or left in place for up to 7 days covered with a sterile dressing. Implanted ports are an appropriate choice for HPN patients desiring a concealed device, when infusion days are less than 5 days per week, or for patients, such as children, who manipulate the external catheter. The port site requires no dressing or routine flushing when HPN is not infusing. Careful consideration should be given before implanted ports are placed, since the needle insertion requires home health nursing, a skilled caregiver, or an individual willing to learn self-accessing.

COMPLICATIONS

Catheter-Related Bloodstream Infection

Catheter-related bloodstream infection (CRBSI) is a serious complication associated with HPN therapy. Reported CRBSI rates in HPN patients range from 0.74 to 3.0 per 1000 catheter days [7]. The most common pathogen is *Staphylococcus* followed by Gram-negative and fungal organisms, as well as polymicrobial infections. The main portal of entry for pathogens into the bloodstream is the catheter hub and skin flora from the entry site of PICCs and implanted ports. The Dacron cuff on the tunneled catheter provides a protective barrier against migration of skin bacteria into the bloodstream.

Suspected CRBSI requires immediate medical intervention. Symptoms include fever and chills, especially at the beginning of the infusion, headache, nausea, vomiting, body aches, and malaise. Peripheral and catheter paired blood cultures should be obtained prior to initiation of antibiotics. CRBSI diagnosis is made when the same organism is growing from the peripheral and catheter cultures [8]. When blood cannot be obtained from the CVC and/or the peripheral site, available cultures and assessment of the patient's medical condition will indicate diagnosis of CRBSI. The preferred route of treatment for HPN patients should be intravenous antibiotics since altered intestinal anatomy and gastrointestinal function may prevent absorption of oral antibiotics. Often, lock therapy is administered in conjunction with the appropriate systemic antibiotic. Locking solutions available in the United States include concentrated antibiotics and medical-grade alcohol [9].

The decision to remove the CVC as part of the treatment plan is dependent upon the patient's condition. In cases of septic shock, persistent positive blood cultures, endocarditis, osteomyelitis, and fungal infections, catheter removal is indicated [8]. In uncomplicated Gram-negative and Gram-positive infections, the CVC may be salvaged [10]. This is important for the HPN patient who needs to maintain a CVC for a lifetime.

Often, the therapy can be completed in the home setting after the HPN patient is symptom free and negative blood cultures are obtained. Teaching of antibiotic administration can be completed by home health nursing or the infusion pharmacy.

Numerous risk factors have been identified as contributing to the incidence of CRBSI. Some of these include multiple therapies increasing manipulations at the hub, frequent blood draws from the catheter, use of narcotics, daily lipid infusions, and multiple lumens [11]. Awareness and identification of risk factors can be helpful in reducing an HPN patient's CRBSI rate.

Hand hygiene is the main strategy for prevention of CRBSI and should be practiced often. Antibacterial soaps or alcohol-based hand rubs are acceptable for CVC procedures [4].

Disinfection is necessary with each access into the CVC port or end adapter. An antiseptic agent such as 70% alcohol, chlorhexidine and alcohol combination solution, and povidone-iodine are all acceptable when applied with a scrubbing friction technique and allowed to dry prior to access [12]. Caps containing an alcohol foam insert are also effective when used to cover the end adapter and they offer a protective barrier against skin bacteria and ostomy and enteric tube contamination at the hub [13].

Locking solutions may be used as a preventative strategy in patients who have frequent incidents of CRBSI [4]. A lock solution is instilled into the catheter and allowed to dwell for a specific time period with the goal of reducing microbial biofilm within the catheter lumen. Concentrated antibiotic solutions with or without heparin, and medical-grade alcohol are available as lock solutions in the United States [9]. They are generally used daily or several times a week for an indefinite period of time.

Reduction of lab draw frequency from the CVC has been shown to reduce infection rates in HPN patients [11]. Fibrin that collects within the catheter lumen and hub when blood is withdrawn provides an environment for bacteria to thrive and grow, eventually causing CRBSI. Peripheral lab draws should be encouraged whenever possible.

Catheter care should be performed with minimal conversation and in a private setting with clean work surface. Sterile gloves and masks are recommended for CVC site care with newly inserted catheters or when immune function is depressed. Well-healed older catheters may not require sterile dressing and site care depending upon the individual patient and physician recommendation [4].

Involvement in HPN support and networking groups has been shown to reduce the incidence of CRBSI [14].

Occlusion

CVC occlusion occurs when there is partial or complete obstruction of the CVC lumen. It presents as resistant or sluggish flushing and infusing, inability to aspirate, also known as withdrawal occlusion, and persistent increasing pump occlusion alarms. Occlusion is a significant complication that delays or interrupts therapy. The cause of occlusion is either nonthrombotic or thrombotic.

The first nonthrombotic occlusion to be ruled out should be assessment for mechanical causes. All components of the CVC and infusion system should be checked for kinks, clogged filters, malfunctioning clamps, and misconnections. The entrance or exit skin sites should be examined closely for constricting sutures, tight securing devices, or crimped tubing.

Implanted ports may be more challenging to troubleshoot due to inability to visualize since they are placed under the skin. Changing or repositioning the noncoring needle may relieve an occlusion, but in most cases, radiological evaluation is indicated in order to assess for a flipped port and kinked or separated tubing [15].

Internal mechanical causes in tunneled CVCs and PICCs may also result in occlusion and will require radiological assessment and intervention. These include kinks within the tunnel or vessel, migration of the CVC out of position, and pinch-off syndrome. Although rare, pinch-off syndrome occurs when the CVC tubing is compressed by the clavicle and the first rib. Symptoms may be intermittent during position change of the arm and shoulder, or there may be actual tearing or fracture of the CVC resulting in migration into the venous system.

Other nonthrombotic occlusions may be caused by drug and mineral precipitate and lipid deposits within the catheter lumen. Precipitates are formed when incompatible drugs are administered without adequate flushing between each drug. Calcium, phosphorus, and magnesium may precipitate in HPN solutions when concentrations are too high. Lipid emulsion residue may also build up in the CVC lumen over time.

Incompatible drug precipitates can be avoided by not mixing drugs together in a syringe or infusion solution. Drugs should be administered individually with a 10 mL sodium chloride flush between each medication.

Pharmacy compounding protocols are established to prevent mineral precipitate in HPN solutions. Review of medications and solutions with the home care pharmacist is indicated if precipitate occlusion is suspected.

Drug and mineral participate may be cleared depending upon the pH of the offender. Sodium bicarbonate, sodium hydroxide, hydrochloric acid, and L-cysteine have all been shown to clear various precipitates [16]. Lipid deposit occlusions are usually suspected if sluggishness or clogging occurs following a lipid infusion. Ethanol lock 70% with a 2-h dwell time may remove lipid residue from the CVC lumen [16].

Thrombotic occlusions occur when fibrin builds up within or around the tip of the CVC lumen or noncoring needle. Thrombotic occlusions can be prevented by maintaining good catheter patency. Proper CVC flushing and use of positive or neutral end adapters prevent blood reflux into the CVC lumen.

A thrombolytic drug called Alteplase can be used to dissolve fibrin clot within the catheter lumen. A 2 mg dose is instilled into the CVC lumen or port and allowed to dwell 30 min to 2 h. It may be repeated if patency is not restored. Alteplase is safe for use in outpatient and home settings for adult and pediatric patients without bleeding disorders and often helps to reduce emergency room and hospital visits [17]. When thrombotic occlusion is not resolved by flushing or Alteplase injection, radiological studies or venogram may be indicated to determine the extent of the thrombus and further treatment plan for CVC salvage.

Thrombosis

Venous thrombosis is the formation of a localized clot within a vein, causing narrowing or obstruction. Extensive thrombosis of the major vessels used for CVC cannulation and subsequent loss of venous access is an indication for small bowel transplant.

Virchow's triad describes three factors contributing to the formation of venous thrombus: vessel wall trauma, blood flow stasis, and hypercoagulability [18]. Other contributing risk factors include age, cancer, diabetes, pregnancy, estrogen therapy, dehydration, immobility, multiple CVC insertions, catheter diameter, and multiple lumens.

Symptoms of CVC-related thrombosis are extremity, face, and neck swelling and vein engorgement, pain during infusion, extremity numbness and discoloration, development of collateral vessels most often visible in the chest and neck area, pump alarms, and incomplete HPN infusions. Often, thrombosis is asymptomatic and only noted when radiological studies are performed.

Prevention of thrombosis includes correct tip location at the junction of the SVC and the right atrium. Proximal tip location in the SVC has been shown to increase thrombosis for each type of

CVC [19]. Use of the smallest-diameter CVC with the least number of lumens, maintaining good hydration and regular exercise have been shown to help reduce thrombosis formation.

Prophylactic anticoagulation has not been shown to reduce CVC-associated thrombosis [17].

Treatment for CVC-related thrombosis includes leaving the CVC in place if tolerated and long term anticoagulation. Increased risk for CRBSI, recurrent thrombosis, and persistent vascular occlusion are associated complications with chronic CVC thrombosis.

Dislodgement

Despite sutures, securing cuffs and devices, or being totally implanted, all CVCs have the risk of becoming dislodged. This can occur with inadvertent pulling of the CVC or strenuous activity. Signs of dislodgement are leaking, cuff exposure on tunneled CVCs, longer tubing, or a moveable implanted port. Other less obvious signs are infusion problems, partial or complete occlusion, inability to aspirate, and burning or pain sensation with flush and infusion.

When dislodgement is suspected, the physician should be notified immediately, infusions held, and usually radiology assessment will be required.

Dislodgement can be prevented by anchoring the CVC with a securing loop or device. Patients should be educated on ways to secure the CVC to reduce pulling, such as a securing loop. Physical activities that involve strenuous arm movement or over the head exercise should be avoided. PICCs should be measured upon insertion and periodically to ensure they are not advancing out of position.

Tip migration out of the junction of the SVC and the right atrium may occur with vigorous coughing or sneezing, reduced blood flow from a disease process, tumor, or large thrombosis. There may be difficulty with infusion, flushing, or aspiration. The patient may complain of swishing sounds when flushing the CVC, headache, pain or swelling in the neck, face, or shoulder [18].

Breakage

Pulling, use of scissors, and excessive force flushing may cause CVC rupture and damage. Small pinholes may develop over time from clamps or pinched tubing. The patient may notice a wet dressing or leakage while infusing or flushing. Internal rupture may occur with pinch off syndrome or forced flushing and is exhibited by swelling or burning within the tunnel during flushing and infusing. Damaged leaking implanted port tubing causes swelling into the soft tissue of the port pocket and surrounding area.

Silicone is the softest CVC material. A silicone tunneled catheter can be safely repaired with a specified kit. Repairs include a spliced section that is glued into place and can last for many years. HPN patients should keep an individualized repair kit in their home supply stock. Polyurethane catheters are very durable and rarely develop breaks. They cannot be repaired and must be replaced if damage occurs. Implanted ports cannot be repaired and must be replaced before resuming HPN.

PATIENT EDUCATION

The HPN patient is the keeper of their lifeline and the best person to monitor and care for the CVC. If home nursing is initiated at the onset of HPN, eventually the patient or family member will become the primary caregiver. Education should include ability to provide self-care for dressing changes, administration of medication and solutions, and troubleshooting the CVC device for all possible complications. It is important to identify a back-up caregiver in case the patient becomes incapacitated. HPN patients should not be discharged from home health until they are able to independently return demonstrate all HPN and CVC care procedures correctly.

REFERENCES

1. Bullock-Corkhill, M. Central venous access devices: Access and insertion. In: Alesander M, Corrigan A, Gorski L, Hankins J, Perucca R (eds.), *Infusion Nursing: An Evidence-Based Approach.* Missouri: Saunders Elsevier, 2010: 480–94.
2. Alexander M, Gorski LA, Corrigan A et al. Technical and clinical application. In: *Core Curriculum for Infusion Nursing.* Philadelphia: Lippincott Williams & Wilkins, 2014: 1–85.
3. Gibbons S, Richardson DS. Central venous catheter care. In: *Clinical Management of Intestinal Failure.* London: CRC Press, 2011: 331–58.
4. O'Grady NP, Alexander M, Burns LA et al. Guidelines for the prevention of intravascular catheter-related infections. *Clin Infect Dis* 2011;52(9): e162–93.
5. Cohen AB, Dagli M, Stravropoulos SW et al. Silicone and polyurethane tunneled infusion catheters: A comparison of durability and breakage rates. *J Vasc Interv Radiol* 2011;22(5): 638–41.
6. Cotogni P, Barbero C, Garrino C et al. Peripherally inserted central catheters in non-hospitalized cancer patients: 5-Year results of a prospective study. *Support Care Cancer* 2015;23(2): 403–9.
7. Elfassy S, Kassam Z, Amin F et al. Epidemiology and risk factors for bloodstream infections in a home parenteral nutrition program. *JPEN* 2015;39(2):147–53.
8. Mermel LA, Allon M, Bouza E et al. Clinical management for the diagnosis and management of intravascular catheter-related infection: 2009 Update by the Infectious Diseases Society of America. *Clin Infect Dis* 2009;49(1): 1–45.
9. John BK, Khan MA, Speerhas R et al. Ethanol lock therapy in reducing catheter-related bloodstream infections in adult home parenteral nutrition patients: Results of a retrospective study. *JPEN* 2012;36(5): 603–10.
10. Dibb MJ, Abraham A, Chadwick PR et al. Central venous catheter salvage in home parenteral nutrition catheter-related bloodstream infections: Long term safety and efficacy data. *JPEN* September 15, 2014. pii: 0148607114549999. [Epub ahead of print] http://www.ncbi.nlm.nih.gov/pubmed/25224728.
11. Buchman AL, Opilla M, Kwasny M et al. Risk factors for the development of catheter-related bloodstream infections in patients receiving home parenteral nutrition. *JPEN* 2014 38(6): 744–9.
12. The Joint Commission. CLABSI prevention strategies, techniques, and technologies. In: *Preventing Central Line-Associated Bloodstream Infections: A Global Challenge, A Global Perspective.* Oak Brook IL: Joint Commission Resources, 2012: 39–70.
13. Merrill K, Sumner S, Linford L et al. Impact of universal disinfectant cap implementation on central line-associated bloodstream infections. *Am J Infect Control* 2014;42(12):1274–7.
14. Smith CE, Curtas S, Werkowitch M et al. Home parenteral nutrition: Does affiliation with a national support and educational organization improve patient outcomes? *JPEN* 2002;26(3): 159–63.
15. Kansagra AP, Yu J-PJ, Naeger DM et al. Risk stratification and radiologic evaluation of central venous port malfunction. *JAVA* 2014;19(2): 77–83.
16. Ast D, Ast TS. Nonthrombotic complications related to central vascular access devices. *J Infus Nurs* 2014;37(5): 349–58.
17. Baskin JL, Pui C-H, Reiss U et al. Management of occlusion and thrombosis associated with long-term indwelling central venous catheters. *Lancet* 2009;11(374): 159–69.
18. Gorski L, Perucca R, Hunter MR. Central venous access devices: Care, maintenance, and potential complications. In: *Infusion Nursing: An Evidence-Based Approach.* Missouri: Saunders Elsevier, 2010: 495–15.
19. DeChicco R, Seidner DL, Brun C et al. Tip position of long-term central venous access devices used for parenteral nutrition. *JPEN* 2007;31(5): 382–7.

11 Parenteral Nutrition Solutions

Kevn McNamara, PharmD, RPh, CNSC, PRS, CVAA(c) and Brenda Gray, PharmD, CNSC, BCNSP, CVAA(c), PRS

CONTENTS

Parenteral nutrition (PN) can be a life-sustaining and life-enhancing therapy but does not come without significant risks. Safe administration of PN requires a solution that is sterile, stable with components that are compatible in solution, in addition to being clinically appropriate. A solution may be proposed that has the carefully determined components to meet the patient's needs but these components must be able to safely form a stable solution to be administered. This chapter focuses on how to determine if a proposed clinically appropriate formulation can be safely compounded and administered.

PN is essentially a combination of electrolytes, macro- and micronutrients, and trace elements mixed into a single solution instead of being administered separately to allow for an effective administration of nutrition support. Medications that are compatible with the solution may also be incorporated into the PN formulation. In many cases, especially in the outpatient or home environment, a patient receiving PN is receiving a custom mixture designed specifically to meet their needs based on the individual's electrolyte levels, nutritional needs, and medical history. Because each solution is unique and customized to the patient, the stability and the compatibility of each component and the entire mixture must be evaluated on an individual basis with each change.

In order to understand this concept, a good working definition of stability, sterility, and compatibility is necessary. Compatibility is best explained as the type and amount of an ingredient that can safely be combined with other components into a PN solution. Many different ingredients can be placed in a PN; however, the "safe" concentration of the ingredient may vary with the agent, the salt form of the ingredient, and the concentration of the other components in the solution. Calcium and phosphate are the best-known examples of concentration-based compatibility. Other factors that affect compatibility are pH, temperature, and order of mixing of the ingredients.

Stability is best defined as how well all the ingredients are able to *remain* compatible. In general, stability is assessed with a product maintaining the desired activity within 10% of original levels. The same factors that impact compatibility also impact the stability of the solution. Additionally, over time, a product may slowly degrade in a solution and result in either insufficient activity of the product or a new opportunity to interact with another product due to molecular changes from degradation. A solution may be compatible in the short term but maintaining that compatibility over a minimum of the storage period plus infusion period is required for a solution to be determined to be stable.

MACRONUTRIENT COMPATIBILITY

Macronutrient compatibility is often of limited concern for the amino acid, dextrose, and water components. Most clinically suitable concentrations are compatible for the commercially available amino acid products. The stability of these products can far exceed the sterility limitations of a compounded product. Commercially compounded products are often stabile for a period of years in clinically suitable ready-to-administer solutions. General compatibility guidelines for PN macronutrients in solution to ensure 9 days refrigerated and 24 h room temperature stability would be as follows:

Dextrose	≥10%
Amino acid	≥4%
Fat emulsion	≥2% final concentration (more than 2 g fat emulsion/100 mL or 20 g/L)

The greatest concern that does arise with macronutrients comes from environmental influences on longer-term stability with both the concentrated bulk solutions and ready-to-use (RTU) formulations. This is not due to compatibility with other macronutrients but in the solution itself maintaining stability in varying environments. Extremes in temperature, exposure to light, and changes in humidity can have significant impact on the macronutrients, resulting in oxidation of lipid products and denaturing of proteins. The denaturing of a protein is extremely dangerous as this breaks the protein into foreign proteins, which may no longer be physiologically acceptable to the human body. These foreign proteins can cause significant systemic reactions. It is important to note that the solution may appear visibly unchanged and therefore monitoring of environmental conditions and education of patients at home regarding proper handling of solutions is critical in preventing this occurrence.

The impact of the environmental factors is more significant for the outpatient than in an inpatient acute care setting. In general, the outpatient environment is less monitored, more difficult to control, and less stable. Individual patients prefer different environmental conditions and this is more customized in the outpatient setting where one home may have a very different climate than another and both considered "room temperature." Additionally, fewer patients monitor their refrigerator temperatures and may use less reliable appliances that create uneven cooling. Patient's lifestyle may impact the temperature extremes to which the solution is exposed. The actual dispensing and delivery of the product is also different as generally multiple units are made at one time and stored by the clinic, patient's home, or long-term care facility outside the monitoring of the pharmacy and the solutions may undergo shipping and handling extremes during transit. All of these factors can cause a greater risk to stability for the same solution for the outpatient versus the inpatient.

Macronutrients

Macronutrient compatibility can vary based on the pH of the base solution as determined by the concentration and components of the solution. Amino acid solutions are the main drivers of the pH of the PN solution. Amino acids have similar pH (5.2–6.5 is the range of the commonly used products). Because of the concentration of bulk amino acids (maximum of 20% vs. the concentration of dextrose 70%), amino acids are commonly the primary macronutrient component of the PN solution. Therefore, the overall pH of the PN solution is generally governed by the amino acid component. While there are no true clinical studies that validate this, one can look at the calcium–phosphate solubility curves published by the amino acid manufacturers and observe that the higher the amino acid and dextrose concentration of the test solution, the more calcium and phosphate that can be safely added to the solution. Thus, there is a relationship between the pH of the PN solution, and the lower the pH, the better the calcium–phosphate solubility.

Inherents—Every amino acid solution has some amount of sodium, potassium, chloride, and acetate. These are commonly referred to as the "inherents" or inherent cations and anions and are electrolytes used to buffer and stabilize the solution. Many prescribers do not address these since they are actually part of the amino acid solution and cannot be changed. Other prescribers will include the inherents in the total amount of electrolytes to be provided to the patient. The exact amount varies between products and can be found in the package insert provided by the manufacturer for each product (Table 11.1). The pharmacist should verify with the prescriber or pharmacy that is making the PN solution if inherents need to be taken into consideration when determining the amount of electrolytes added to each PN solution compounded.

FreAmine® (B Braun, California) is the exception because it includes phosphorous and not potassium as inherents. Like other amino acids, it has inherent sodium, chloride, and acetate. Unlike other amino acids, it also has phosphorus but does not have potassium. In the early days of PN, patients would become hypophosphatemic because the PN solutions did not contain sufficient amounts of phosphorous. In order to combat this issue, B Braun, the original manufacturer of FreAmine, began adding phosphorus to their amino acid formulation. Each liter of FreAmine 10% contains 10 mmol phosphorus.

TABLE 11.1
Inherents in Common Amino Acid Formulations

Amino Acid Formulations	Manufacturer	Sodium (Na) (mEq/L)	Potassium (K) (mEq/L)	Phosphorus (PO_4) (mmol/L)	Chloride (Cl) (mEq/L)	Acetate (OAc) (mEq/L)
Aminosyn II® 10%	Hospira, Inc.	38				72
Travasol® 10%	Baxter				40	88
FreAmine® III 10%	B Braun Medical, Inc.	10	0	10	<3	~89
Aminosyn II® 15%	Hospira, Inc.	62.7				107.6
Clinisol® 15%	Baxter					137
Prosol® 20%	Baxter					140

Specialty Amino Acids

Certain patient populations require more customized amino acid profiles to optimize PN therapy (Table 11.2). While there is some controversy over the value of specialty amino acids, for liver or kidney disease, there is much less controversy over the use of specialty amino acids for premature infants and very young children. The debate here is related to the duration of use. The neonatal specialty amino acids are designed to provide higher concentrations of amino acids needed in early childhood development. They contain cysteine, which is necessary for growth and development and has been found to increase the calcium–phosphate solubility that is very important in the young child population. The manufacturers have published solubility curves; however, the curves cannot be interchanged. If a precipitate forms, the entire solution and tubing should be disposed of immediately.

3-IN-1 SOLUTIONS OR TOTAL NUTRIENT ADMIXTURES

A significant concern arises when a "3-in-1" or "total" nutrient admixture in which an emulsion is formed with dextrose, amino acid, and lipid is being combined in a single solution. This emulsion can be very fragile. The ability to maintain a safe emulsion can be influenced by concentration of bases, the impact of micronutrients, temperature, light exposure, and even the handling of the product by the patient. An early "cracking" of the emulsion (separation of the lipid from the nonlipid component) can be difficult to identify, but once cracked, the solution is no longer considered stabile and not safe to administer. A cracked emulsion should never be agitated with a goal of reemulsification as the solution is already damaged.

The stability of the emulsion is significantly impacted by the activity and concentration of the other components of the solution. The exact conditions that cause emulsion cracking are not well understood and opinions vary greatly as to how to ensure a safe solution. Maintaining an appropriate concentration range and limiting the impact of multivalent ions on the fat cell walls will allow for the highest level of reliable stability. The micelle membrane of the fat molecule has an attraction to other fat molecules and this attraction allows the emulsion to stay evenly distributed and thus maintain a smooth homogenous emulsion. When this attraction undergoes stress from competing attractions, the molecules may pull apart or stick together and crack the emulsion. The higher the valence of the molecule (e.g., trivalent iron molecules), the stronger this attraction becomes and the greater the risk for emulsion instability. Observational literature has demonstrated that the very low

TABLE 11.2
Specialty Amino Acids

Specialty Amino Acid	Content	Indication/Contraindication
Hepatamine®—B Braun Medical, Inc.	High in branched-chain amino acids (36%) leucine, isoleucine, and valine	Specifically for the treatment of hepatic encephalopathy in patients with cirrhosis or hepatitis Contraindicated in patient with anuria, inborn errors of metabolism *Note*: Verify that all documentation is available for reimbursement purposes as Hepatamine is billed using different codes than traditional amino acids
Nephramine®—B Braun Medical, Inc.	Contains only essential amino acids in a 5.4% solution	Indicated in patient with chronic renal failure
Premasol®—Baxter	6% and 10% amino acid solution	For neonatal and pediatric use only
Trophamine®—B Braun Medical, Inc.	6% and 10% amino acid solution	Better calcium and phosphate solubility than Premasol due to differences in the manufacturing process as reflected on the manufacturers' solubility curves

(less than 2%) concentrations of lipids can cause the molecules to be pulled too far apart in solution, causing an uneven distribution or large variance in particle size. Therefore, this guideline is used by most clinicians as an indicator to increase caution when evaluating solution stability closer. There are multiple opinions as other factors with lipid emulsion stability, including particle size and solution components, that require further research.

Micronutrients and Electrolytes

Electrolyte additives may be ordered in many different ways although they can only be added as a salt since an ion cannot exist alone but will always bind to another ion in the environment to be electrically neutral then separate and rebind to other ions in solutions. However, ordering is not always simple. Electrolytes may be ordered as salts, or as ions, as mEq, mmol, mg of elemental Ca, for example, per bag, per day, per L, per 100 mL, or per kg. The person ordering and compounding the PN must ensure they know exactly what the desired outcome is for the formula. Owing to the risks associated with "misunderstanding" the PN order and possible impact on patient safety, the American Society of Parenteral and Enteral Nutrition (A.S.P.E.N.) has created safety guidelines for ordering PN solutions. These guidelines can be found on the A.S.P.E.N. website (www.nutritioncare.org) and should be reviewed often to minimize the risk of patient harm from misreading a PN order.

Monovalent Anions and Cations Balancing

Monovalent anions and cations include sodium, potassium, chloride, and acetate. Additionally, phosphorus presents as phosphate, which is a monovalent compound. All of these must match in quantity to create an electrically neutral solution. In order to balance a solution, one will determine the amount of Na and K ordered. Since phosphorus requires a monovalent anion to form a dissolvable salt, first determine the amount of Na or K that will be used in providing the phosphate. The remaining Na and K will be provided combined with acetate and chloride.

- $NaPO_4$ = 4 mEq Na and 3 mmol PO_4/mL
- KPO_4 = 4.4 mEq K and 3 mmol PO_4/mL

Note: Some prescribers and some facilities include the "inherent" cations and anions that are part of the amino acid solutions. In this case, these will be calculated and subtracted from the order prior to "balancing" the formula. It is important to know if this is included in the order and be consistent in calculations. For the following examples, one will assume the inherents either are not included in the order or have already been subtracted.

A desired ratio should be noted on the order or it is assumed to be balanced as 1:1. Shifting this balance can shift the overall pH of the formula as well as affect the patient's acid–base balance and thus the lab values seen for CO_2 and Cl^-. Once this ratio is determined, the chloride (Cl) and acetate (OAc) salts can be assigned. It is a best practice to reduce the number of ingredients and create the formula with the least number of salts.

Ion Balancing Example K, Na, Cl, and OAc

The PN orders say 40 mEq K^+ and 120 mEq Na^+. Cl^- to OAc^- 1:1

K^+ (40) + Na^+ (120) = 160^+ charges. Need 160^- charges (80 as Cl^- and 80 as OAc^-)
In the PN, the following could be added: KCl 40 mEq, NaCl 40 mEq, and NaOAc 80 mEq.
(There are additional options available for each formula presented based on salts available. This is one example for demonstration purposes.)

The PN orders say 40 mEq K^+ and 120 mEq Na^+. Cl to acetate 3:1.

K^+ (40) + Na^+ (120) = 160^+ charges. Need 160^- charges: (120 Cl^- and 40 OAc^-)
In the PN, KOAc 40 mEq, NaCl 120 mEq could be added

or

In the PN, KCl 40 mEq, NaCl 80 mEq, and NaOAc 40 mEq added depending on compounder choice and availability of salts. The second option is less desirable due to increased number of additives.

Ion Balancing Example K, Na, Cl, OAc, and PO_4

The PN orders say 40 mEq K^+ and 120 mEq Na^+. Cl^- to OAc^- 1:1 and 15 mmol PO_4 (the amino acid is *not* FreAmine)

K^+ (40) + Na^+ (120) = 160^+ charges. Need 160^- charges (15 mmol PO_4^-, 50% remainder as Cl^- and 50% as OAc^-)

The PN could have an additional KCl 40 mEq, $NaPO_4$ 15 mmol (representing 20 Na^+ charges and thus 20 negative charges since every 4 mEq of Na for every 3 mmol of PO_4 as noted above) and NaCl 30 mEq and NaOAc 70 mEq. Thus, the formula has the 40 of K^+, 120 of Na^+ balanced with the 15 mmol of phosphate, 70 mEq of Cl^-, and 70 mEq of OAc^-

ADDITIONAL CONSIDERATIONS BASED ON FORMULATIONS

Sodium: Na

- Avoid exceeding 154 mEq/L. When administering hypertonic solutions, undesired fluid and electrolyte shifts may occur between extracellular and intracellular fluids.

Potassium: K

- The primary limitation is administration rate, which should not exceed 10 mEq/h in the absence of cardiac monitoring.

Chloride and Acetate: Cl and OAc

- Both may influence the pH of the solution, leading to instability. If provided in excess, it may also impact the pH of the patient.
- In cases of low CO_2, sodium bicarbonate should *not* be added to the PN due to stability concerns.

Phosphorus: PO_4

- Generally ordered in mmol of phosphate (1 mmol of phosphate = 31 mg elemental phosphorous).
- When receiving a PN order, *always* verify the units the PO_4 is ordered in. Some institutions may order as mg phosphorus or mEq. This is a significant opportunity for medication error prevention. If unsure, always verify with the prescriber.
- If FreAmine is the amino acid, allow for the inherent PO_4 in FreAmine.
- When compounding, PO_4 is generally added to the PN solution by hand at the very end of the compounding process to ensure maximum volume and solubility of the solution.

Magnesium: Mg (Generally Ordered as $MgSO_4$)

- Divalent cation.
- Verify units used in the ordering of Mg. Some hospitals may order in mg of Mg, mg $MgSO_4$, or mEq $MgSO_4$. This is a potential area for medication errors.

Calcium: Ca (Preferred as Ca Gluconate)

- Divalent cation.
- Verify units used in the ordering of Ca. Some hospitals may order in mg of elemental Ca, mg of the Ca salt, or mEq Ca gluconate. This is a potential area for medication errors.
- In emergency cases of shortages, $CaCl_2$ can be used. If $CaCl_2$ is used, patient safety is a major concern due to changes in the overall solubility of the solution. Of note, if the chloride salt is being used, the sulfate salt for magnesium should be discouraged to avoid the formation of calcium sulfate in the solution which may pass through a traditional PN tubing filter.
- Although this can also occur when magnesium is added to other calcium-containing solutions, the calcium chloride salt is more likely to separate in solution and result in this insoluble compound. The microprecipitates formed are too small to be filtered out using the typical filters and can silently accumulate in the body over time, causing injury.

Other Additives

- Iron
  - Iron has a significant impact on lipids due to being a trivalent cation, and immediately separates from its carbohydrate carrier once in the presence of the active amino acid solution and then the ion affects the fat cell wall.
  - Be aware of its presence in some trace element formulations. At the time of this publication, the only iron product studied with PN is iron dextran.
  - Other iron salts may be administered to patients receiving PN, but should *not* be added to the PN solution or infused via the PN dedicated line.
- Cysteine
  - Not actually a direct impact of cysteine but an indirect impact of the salt formulation from the HCl acid molecule tied to the cysteine (see discussion below).
  - Since nutritional requirements for additional cysteine are limited, the cysteine may get removed at a certain age but then the formulation must be reevaluated. This pH shift creates changes that may affect stability.
- Zinc
  - Solubility is concentration and pH dependent; current literature does not recommend a total of more than 10 mg/L in any PN solution.
  - Individual trace elements should be added at the time of mixing. Current literature should be reviewed prior to adding individual trace elements and additions should be based on patient's needs and disease state.

Limits and Guidelines for Stability and Solubility

The solubility of a solution is a concentration- and pH-dependent interaction. The pH of the solution (as determined by the concentration of the macronutrients and the additives) is the main determinant of the solubility. Additional influence comes from temperature, so a solution that is soluble at room temperature may not be as the formula is heated or cooled. The order in which the products are added into the solution can also impact solubility. The shaking of a solution can break the amino acids and thus impact pH and create instability.

There are very limited guidelines for stability and solubility and many are anecdotal. Additionally, the information that is published in standard reference guides such as Trissel's *Handbook of Injectable Drugs*©, *Extended Stability for Parenteral Drugs*©, or *King Guide*© is from single solutions that are tested. Therefore, the data are specifically related to that formula and the information should be extrapolated to other solutions carefully.

Specific additives and medications can also impact solubility. Certain medications will precipitate in the PN solution or cause amino acids or additives to become insoluble through changes in pH or direct binding. Calcium and phosphorus are one of the most common causes of solution instability and precipitation and the reference solubility curves provided by the manufacturer should be extrapolated carefully.

EXAMPLES OF COMMON CAUSES OF PRECIPITATION OR SOLUTION INSTABILITY

- Using the incorrect amino acid curve or incorrect units (mg/mmol/mEq)
- Adding an additive that impacts the pH
  - Too high of a concentration of acetate
  - Using a traditional amino acid, but the solubility curve from Trophamine or Premasol
- Using a different salt
  - Calcium chloride instead of calcium gluconate
- Dispensing or compounding in a smaller volume such as pooling or using dual-chamber bags
- Adding calcium and phosphorus too close together or in too small of a volume. Examples of this include
  - Adding both calcium and phosphorus to a pool solution instead of adding second to the diluted final volume
  - Dispensing in a dual-chamber bag but calculating solubility based on the final volume
- Not agitating solution between ingredients to ensure distribution in solution
- Improper compounding temperatures (exceeding United States Pharmacopeia [USP] guidelines) or storage conditions. The presence of a light source, such as bili-lamps or prolonged exposure to sunlight, may lead to solution instability

Cysteine is one additive that is known to impact the pH and is often used to increase the solubility of the formulation by creating a significant shift in the pH. It is not cysteine that actually creates this effect but the HCl molecule that is released when the cysteine solution separates in the formulation. This impact on pH creates an increase in solubility for calcium and phosphate while still keeping the formula at a safe pH to administer. This is commonly used in pediatric solutions as this population often has an increased need for calcium and phosphorus and thus benefits from the increased solubility instead of having to increase the overall volume. Specific curves are available. Although generally the curves are based on 40 mg of L-cysteine per gram of protein (based on controlling the pH shift within appropriate boundaries), this should be verified with the data on the curves to ensure applicability of the curve. Of note, at the time of publication, no published study has verified how long this pH shift benefit will last, so use in the outpatient setting can be controversial. All PNs should be observed prior to administration for any signs of instability on precipitation.

MEDICATION COMPATIBILITY

When considering medication compatibility, there are additional variables to consider. In addition to considering the pH, concentration, temperature, and salt form, we must also consider the duration of the infusion. For example, morphine may be compatible with all the components of a PN solution; however, to clinically administer morphine at a continuous rate over 12 h may not be the ideal situation for the patient.

COMMON ADDITIVES TO PN IN THE PHARMACY

Some additives may be added by the pharmacy in the compounding room while others have variable or poor stability and must be added immediately prior to administration. The most common example of a "patient additive" is multivitamins.

- H_2 antagonists
  - Famotidine
  - Ranitidine
- Antiemetics
  - Promethazine
  - Ondansetron
- Iron dextran—This is a very controversial additive and there is only minimal information, which is mostly anecdotal. There are reports of iron dextran in very small amounts being compatible with a nonlipid-containing formulation but the data are weak and difficult to extrapolate. Additionally, the European trace element product has minute doses of iron in it and is undergoing stability studies.
- Carnitine
- Octreotide—Anecdotal gas formation; efficacy varies from independent administration.

COMMON ADDITIVES TO PN IN THE HOME

Owing to very short stability, patients may have to add some medications to the PN solution immediately prior to administration. Home health nurses will teach patient how to prepare the PN bag and the additive for addition to the solution to prevent contamination.

- Multivitamins
- Ascorbic acid
- Folic acid
- Insulin
- Octreotide
- Phytonadione

Coadministration of medications—Can be administered via a "Y-site," non-PN lumen, or a separate infusion site. When administering via the Y-site, all components should have a minimum of 4 h stability based on the closest PN formula referenced in published guidelines.

- Proton pump inhibitors
  - Pantoprazole may become discolored and should not be used if this occurs
- Antibiotics—Varies by medication—check stability charts
- Analgesics—Varies by medication and concentration—check stability charts

Medications Not to Be Administered While PN Infusing

- Albumin
- Ceftriaxone (if calcium is in PN solution)
- Fluorouracil (5-FU)

STERILITY

In order to discuss stability, we must also talk briefly about sterility. As stated previously, safe solution assessment includes the stability as well as the sterility and the "beyond use date" is determined by the more restrictive of the two. Beyond use date is the date placed on the label as the last day the product can be considered safe for administration and is based on guidelines from USP 797 and product-specific variables.

As a review, stability is how long the compounded solution is safe to administer. In other words, for how many days is the solution safe (no chemical degradation or breakdown) and can be analyzed within 10% of the amount of nutrition, medication, and electrolytes as ordered by the prescriber, as well as remain particulate free. In many cases, this may be much longer than the time in which the sterility of the solution can be ensured. Sterility is the absence of microorganisms or contaminants in the solution.

Sterile compounding should only occur in an environment with specific engineering controls that limit the presence of viable and nonviable particles. In addition, sterile supplies and appropriately trained staff should be utilized to further limit the risk of product contamination. Solutions and supplies should remain sealed until the time of use. Nurses and patients should be trained in administration technique that limits the entry of viable and nonviable particles. However, no system outside of a full patient isolation can remove all risk of product contamination.

A properly compounded product should be free of any contaminants. However, since PN is temperature sensitive and contains large molecules for some nutrients, end product sterilization is not an option. Because sterile ingredients and proper controls are used, the solution is generally considered to be safe; however, there are always a small number of particulates present in a clean room, including microorganisms. Every time a product is manipulated, there is a risk of those particulates entering the product and the more the manipulations, the greater the risk. Generally, the body's immune system can respond and eliminate a small number of particles or organisms that may enter a product at compounding or administration.

As a nutrition source, the solution can support the growth of the microorganism. Therefore, if an organism does enter the product and it is not administered immediately, the organism can "feed" on the solution and reproduce rapidly. This growth can result over time with exponential numbers that the body can no longer fight off. This is the principle behind limiting the storage of the product. Whereas the tiny amount of organisms on day 1 may be safe, this multiplied colony is no longer safe.

Many specific nutrient supplementations and medications have very short-term stability and thus must be added to the formulation just prior to administration. In the home, this is generally performed by the patient or the caregiver after learning from the home health nurse. Since these individuals have less training and experience and this is being done in an uncontrolled environment, there are certain risks such as coring the injection port with multiple injections, contamination, and incorrect dose (incorrect measurement if not using a full vial), and thus jeopardizing the integrity of the formula and container.

Custom Formulations versus Premixed Formulations

PN solutions are available as custom solutions compounded by a pharmacy or "premixed" standard solution available from a manufacturer. Although opinions as to the benefits and limitations of the premixed solutions vary greatly, some literature claims as many as 80% of patients can be maintained on premixed solutions at least short term. The premixed solutions may be used as the foundation for custom formulations by some pharmacies.

Premixed solutions are available in several variations:

1. Macronutrient only
2. Macronutrient and electrolyte
3. Full formulations, including lipids: available in triple-chamber bags to allow longer storage life

Premade formulations can often meet short-term needs such as travel, short-term admissions, or emergency situations. Some patients may be able to continue the long-term use of premixed solution; however, many times, the premixed solutions are used as a bridge until the custom formulation is available. Long-term needs and certain medical conditions require custom formulas to be used in order to replace losses and meet specific metabolic needs (such as high protein needs-specific electrolyte losses, etc.).

Premade Solutions

1. All-in-one solutions
   a. Dual-chamber RTU bag
      i Amino acids + dextrose
      ii Amino acids + dextrose + electrolytes
      iii Multiple concentrations
   b. Triple-chamber RTU bags
      i Amino acids + dextrose + lipids
      ii Contain electrolytes
      iii Multiple concentrations
2. Advantges
   a. Prolonged stability
   b. No refrigeration required
   c. Less risk for contamination
   d. Ready to use
3. Disadvantages
   a. Set concentrations, volumes, and amounts of electrolytes
   b. No stability data when adding additional products if needed
   c. Limited flexibility to meet clinical needs of the patient
   d. Must add trace elements and other additive, which can be added to the PN (H_2 blockers, antiemetics, etc.)
   e. Only approved in patients over the age of 2 years

ADDITIONAL PN INNOVATIONS

As with everything in pharmacy, research continues to attempt to develop ideal products and meet the needs of the patient. Innovations can come from many sources, including new understandings of pathophysiology and products activities, new chemical developments, and new clinical discoveries. Developments and research can also be driven by impacts on product availability such as addressing product shortages due to loss of base ingredients or changes in manufacturing processes.

One of the biggest challenges facing pharmacy is to find a better tolerated and more appropriate intravenous fat emulsion (IVFE).

1. Clinolipid—Approved by the U.S. Food and drug Administration (FDA) in October 2013. The product received an expedited review due to shortages of other IVFE.

   a. Contains refined olive oil and refined soybean oil. Although the fatty acids are an important source of energy, the ratio of omega-3 fatty acids to their omega-6 cousins in the new drug "has not been shown to improve clinical outcomes compared to other lipid emulsion products," according to the FDA.
   b. Caloric density is 2 kcal/mL.
   c. Each liter contains 15 mmol phosphorus.
2. Omegaven™—Remains investigational in the United States with many teaching institutions participating in the clinical research.
   a. Fish oil-based fat emulsion designed primarily for pediatric patients or others experiencing liver problems associated with IVFE administration.
   b. Caloric density 1.12 kcal/mL.
   c. Dosing—1–2 mL/kg/day.
   d. Maximum infusion rate—0.5 mL/kg/h.
   e. Because of limited data on formulation stability and long-term use data in the United States, it is only available through compassionate use and research protocols.

SELECTED REFERENCES AND RESOURCES

Aminosyn III®. Prescribing information, Hopsira Inc., 2014.

Bouchand, L., Fonzo-Christe, C., Klingmuller, M., and Bonnabry, P. Compatibility of intravenous medications with parenteral nutrition: *In vitro* evaluation. *Journal of Parenteral and Enteral Nutrition*, May 2013; 37:3:416–424.

Boullata, J. et al. A.S.P.E.N. clinical guidelines: Parenteral nutrition ordering, order review, compounding, labeling, and dispensing. *Journal of Parenteral and Enteral Nutrition*, March–April 2014;38(3):334–377.

Clinimix®. Prescribing information, Baxter Healthcare Corp., 2014.

Derenski, K. Standardized PN using commercial premix. *Pharmacy Purchasing & Products*, February 2012;9(2):1–7.

Driscoll, D.F. Lipid injectable emulsions: Pharmacopeial and safety issues. *Pharmaceutical Research*, 2006;23(9):1959–1969.

Durfee, S. et al. ASPEN standards for nutrition support: Home and alternate site care. *Nutrition in Clinical Practice*, August 2004; 29:4;542–555.

Hazards of Precipitation Associated with PN, FDA letter from 4/18/1994.

http://www.medsafe.govt.nz/profs/datasheet/o/Omegaveninf.pdf

Kabiven®. Prescribing information, Fresenius-Kabi USA LLC, 2014.

King Guide to Parenteral Therapy, Total Parenteral Nutrition, 2003. www.kingguide.com Accessed 2015.

Mirtallo, J. et al. Safe practices for parenteral nutrition. *Journal of Parenteral and Enteral Nutrition*, November, 2004; 28:6:S39–70.

Newton, D. Y-site compatibility of intravenous drugs with parenteral nutrition. *Journal of Parenteral and Enteral Nutrition*, May 2013;37:416–424, first published on October 30, 2012.

Perikabiven®. Prescribing information, Fresenius-Kabi USA LLC, 2014.

Premasol®. Prescribing information, Baxter Healthcare Corp., 2014.

Travasol®, Clinisol®, Prosol®. Prescribing information, Baxter Healthcare Corp., 2014.

Trissel, L. *Handbook on Injectable Drugs*, 17th edn., American Society of Health-System Pharmacists, Bethesda, MD, October 2013.

Trophamine®, Hepatamine®, Nephramine®. Prescribing information, B Braun Medical, Inc., 2015.

USP 797 Guidebook to Pharmaceutical Compounding—Sterile Preparation, Rockville, MD: United States Pharmacopeia Convention, 2012.

Zaloga, G. et al. Safety and stability of lipid emulsions. *Nutrition in Clinical Practice*, June 2007; 22:3:367–369.

12 Home Parenteral Nutrition Reimbursement

Marianne Duda, MS, RDN, LDN, CNSC, Deborah Pfister, MS, RDN, CNSC, and Jody Strain

CONTENTS

While home parenteral nutrition (HPN) is life saving and life sustaining, it is a medical therapy for which reimbursement is also essential for the patient due to the cost. Third-party insurance coverage for HPN includes commercial or private payers (group and individual plans), federal government payers (Medicare), and state-run programs (Medicaid). Coverage under these payer types can include HMOs (Health Maintenance Organizations), PPOs (Preferred Provider Organizations), ACOs (Accountable Care Organizations), medical benefit, pharmacy benefit, government exchanges, and the list goes on. A physician's order is necessary and accompanying documentation is often required to substantiate the need for HPN. The hospital-based team and home nutrition support clinicians are the essential link between the insurer's medical policy and payment for HPN, related supplies, and services. It is important for the clinicians, home infusion provider, and insurance company to work in partnership with the patient to understand options for coverage.

With the passage of the Patient Protection and Affordable Care Act in 2010, lifetime caps on insurance coverage have been lifted, family coverage has been extended to include children up to 26 years old, and preexisting condition clauses have been eliminated.[1] Despite this standardization, qualification and reimbursement for the provision of HPN continues to vary by payer. Commercial insurers offer varying degrees of coverage for HPN and related supplies that are based on individual policy limitations. Government payers include Medicare and Medicaid, whose original legislation established publicly run insurance for the elderly and the poor based on mid-1960s medical practice and life expectancy. Government and commercial payers often reimburse for a limited number of visits by home health nursing, but as of this writing, few insurers provide payment for other clinical services involved in the management and monitoring of PN consumers in the home setting.

Within the hospital setting, PN therapy is usually initiated at the discretion of the medical team and may be provided for a variety of reasons. All clinicians should have a basic understanding of how HPN is covered by commercial and government payers when managing patients who may require home nutrition support. The home infusion provider with expertise in reimbursement should work with the prescriber in collecting appropriate documentation that supports medical necessity and expected length of need for HPN.

In addition to records obtained from the attending and consulting physicians, the progress notes from dietitians, pharmacists, nurses, wound and ostomy specialists, and other members of the health care team can assist in documenting clinical need. The medical record is not limited to hospital documents, but may include records from physician offices, clinics, nursing facilities, home health agencies, other professionals, etc. A.S.P.E.N's 2014 Home and Alternate Site Standards also specify that the medical record include documentation supporting the criteria for HPEN as set by the insurance carriers.[2] Additionally, A.S.P.E.N. standards recommend verification of insurance benefits for HPEN, obtaining insurance authorization prior to the provision of service, an explanation of benefits and cost of service be provided to the patient and caregiver, and a system for payment for out-of-pocket expenses for medically ordered enteral and parenteral formulations, supplies, and services be in place.[2] Records from suppliers or healthcare professionals with a financial interest in the claim outcome are not considered sufficient on their own to determine that HPN is reasonable and necessary.

MEDICARE

HPN therapy is a covered benefit as long as the patient carries Part B coverage and meets the coverage criteria in the Parenteral Nutrition Medical Policy and Local Coverage Documentation (http://www.medicarenhic.com/viewdoc.aspx?id=1661). Part B coverage was enacted in 1965 with the original Medicare program (Part A) and implemented in 1966. Medicare began providing coverage for HPEN (Home Parenteral and Enteral Nutrition) under the Part B, Prosthetic Device Benefit in 1976.[3] The Centers for Medicare and Medicaid Services (CMS), a component of the Department of Health and Human Services, has administrative oversight of Medicare, Medicaid, and other programs.

Enrollment in Part A, which covers hospital care, physician charges, skilled nursing facility care, nursing home care, hospice and home health nursing, is automatic at retirement age or disability and completed through the Social Security Administration. Medicare Part B coverage is optional and may be selected at the required time period when eligible, or at special enrollment. Part B has a monthly premium that can be automatically deducted from the beneficiary's monthly Social Security payment.

Medicare Part B pays 80% of the allowable charge when criteria are met. The remaining 20% of charges are billed to a secondary or supplemental insurance, Medicaid, or to the patient. In the event that the patient's medical condition does not meet criteria as set by Medicare Part B, and when a denial of payment is obtained from Medicare, a "true secondary" insurance policy will often provide benefits for HPN. (Once the denial from Medicare is obtained, the secondary insurance becomes the primary payer.) Supplemental insurances will provide payment for the remaining 20% of allowable charges, but only if approved and paid by Medicare Part B. Medicare Advantage plans, also known as Medicare Part C, are managed by commercial insurance companies, also have a monthly premium and generally follow the Part B guidelines for medical necessity of HPN. These plans can also have coinsurance responsibilities.[4]

Information verifying Medicare Part B coverage criteria have been met *must* be present in the patient's medical record. It is recommended that home infusion providers proactively obtain and review appropriate medical records and maintain a copy in their files. These records are not routinely submitted to Medicare with the initial claim, but must be available upon request.

Within the infusion industry, providers occasionally utilize data collection forms to ensure they are gathering appropriate documentation to support the Medicare claim. These "provider created" data collection forms are not sufficient by themselves to document medical necessity, even when affixed with the physician's signature. Any information they contain must be corroborated by documentation in patient's medical record. The type of records that need to be obtained will depend on underlying medical condition which requires treatment with HPN (Table 12.1).

TABLE 12.1
Medicare Documentation Criteria

Situation A—Massive Small Bowel Resection

The medical records should document:

- Details and date of surgery

Suggested additional documentation:

- Admission health and physical
- Progress notes
- Discharge summary
- Operative report

Situation B—Short Bowel Syndrome

The medical records should document:

- Cause of short bowel syndrome
- Patient's oral intake
- Patient's enteral output
- Patient's urine output

Suggested additional documentation:

- Admission health and physical
- Progress notes
- Discharge summary
- Operative report
- Intake and output records
- Diagnostic test results:
    - Serum electrolytes
    - Other pertinent tests

Situation C—Bowel Rest

The medical records should document:

- Condition that requires bowel rest
- How long the physician anticipates the beneficiary will need bowel rest

Suggested additional documentation:

- Admission health and physical
- Progress notes
- Discharge summary
- Diagnostic test results

Situation D—Complete Mechanical Small Bowel Obstruction

The medical records should document:

- Presence of obstruction
- Surgical options

Suggested additional documentation:

- Admission health and physical
- Progress notes
- Discharge summary
- Diagnostic test results
- Operative report

(*Continued*)

TABLE 12.1 (*Continued*)
Medicare Documentation Criteria

Situation E—Severe Malabsorption

The medical records should document:

- Cause of malabsorption

Suggested additional documentation:

- Admission health and physical
- Progress notes
- Discharge summary
- Diagnostic test results:
  - Serum albumin
  - 72 fecal fat
- Other pertinent tests
- Nutritional assessment
- Weight history

Situation F—Severe Motility Disturbance

The medical records should document:

- Cause of motility disturbance
- Three-month weight history
- Serum albumin level
- Prokinetic medication history
- Nuclear isotope of x-ray motility study

Suggested additional documentation:

- Admission health and physical
- Progress notes
- Discharge summary
- Diagnostic test results:
  - Serum albumin
  - Small bowel motility study
- Nutritional assessment
- Medication records
- Weight history

Situation G and H—Other Qualifying Condition and Failed Tube Trial

The medical records should document:

- Three-month weight history
- Serum albumin level
- Enteral nutrition attempts

Suggested additional documentation:

- Admission health and physical
- Progress notes
- Discharge summary
- Operative reports
- Diagnostic test results
- Details of enteral nutrition trial
- Nutritional assessment
- Medical records
- Weight history

Source: Adapted from National Government Services, Jurisdiction B, Durable Medical Equipment Education and Training, Policy Education. September 2013. www.ngsmedicare.com (accessed April 2, 2015).

MEDICARE COVERAGE LIMITATIONS: COVERAGE PROVISIONS

The patient must meet two initial conditions in order for Medicare Part B to cover HPN (called TPN in Medicare literature):

1. Have a *permanent* severe pathology of the gastrointestinal tract which does not allow absorption of sufficient nutrients to maintain weight and strength commensurate with overall health status, and
2. A condition of the *small intestine* and/or its exocrine glands which significantly impairs absorption or
3. A motility disorder of the stomach and/or intestine that impairs the ability of nutrients to be transported through the GI system

The medical record must include *objective evidence* supporting the clinical diagnosis. The medical record must also reflect that, in the judgement of the attending physician, the impairment is of a long and indefinite duration, defined as ≥90 days. Coverage does allow for improvement in the patient's condition sometime in the future. Permanence does not require a medical judgement that the impairment necessitating the therapy will persist throughout the patient's remaining years.

Maintenance of weight and strength commensurate with overall health status *must* require infusion of parenteral nutrition. Adequate nutrition must not be possible by modifying the nutrient composition of an oral/enteral diet or by utilizing medications that treat the etiology of the malabsorption (e.g., pancreatic enzymes, bile salts, broad-spectrum antibiotics for bacterial overgrowth, prokinetic medications for reduced motility, etc.).

MEDICARE COVERAGE LIMITATIONS: COVERED SITUATIONS

HPN is covered in any of the following situations. For criteria A–F, Medicare recognizes the conditions are severe enough that the patient would not be able to maintain weight and strength on *only* oral intake or via enteral feeding tube. HPN is noncovered for patients who do not meet these criteria.

Situation A. Massive small bowel resection within the past three months leaving ≤5 feet of small bowel beyond the Ligament of Treitz.

Situation B. Short Bowel Syndrome defined as severe fluid and electrolyte losses where GI output is greater than 50% of oral/enteral intake when taking 2.5–3 L per day, and urine output is less than 1000 mL per day.

Situation C. Need for bowel rest for at least 3 months and receiving PN providing 20–35 calories/kg/day for the treatment of the following:

1. Symptomatic pancreatitis with/without pancreatic pseudocyst
2. Severe exacerbation of regional enteritis
3. Proximal enterocutaneous fistula where tube feeding distal to the fistula is not possible

Situation D. Complete mechanical small bowel obstruction where surgery is not an option.

Situation E. Significant malnutrition (defined as 10% weight loss over 3 months or less and serum albumin ≤3.4 g/dL) with very severe fat malabsorption. Documentation must show the patient received an oral/enteral diet of at least 50 g of fat/day, and during the diet test period, fecal fat output exceeded 50% of intake as measured by a standard 72 h fecal fat test.

Situation F. Significant malnutrition (as defined in Situation E, above) in the presence of a severe motility disturbance of the small intestine and/or stomach which is unresponsive to prokinetic medication (defined as the presence of daily symptoms of nausea and vomiting while taking maximum doses). The motility disorder must be demonstrated either scintigraphically (solid meal gastric emptying study where the isotope fails to reach the right colon by 6 h after ingestion) or radiographically (where the pellet fails to reach the right colon by 6 h following administration). These studies must be performed when the patient is not acutely ill and is not on any medications which reduce bowel motility.

Patients who fail to meet Situations A–F above, must have malnutrition in the presence of a less severe condition that does not respond to modification of oral/enteral nutrition and to pharmacologic intervention as follows:

Situation G. The patient has malnutrition as defined as a 10% weight loss over 3 months or less and a serum albumin ≤3.4 g/dL, and

Situation H. A disease and clinical condition has been documented as being present and has not responded to altering the manner of delivery of appropriate nutrients (e.g., slow infusion through a gastric or jejunal feeding tube).

A failed trial of enteral tube feeding must be documented before coverage for parenteral nutrition will be considered under Situations G and H. Examples of these less severe conditions include but are not limited to

- Moderate fat malabsorption where fecal fat exceeds 25% of intake of at least 50 g of fat per day as measured by a standard 72-h fecal fat test
- Diagnosis of malabsorption with objective confirmation by methods other than a 72 h fecal fat test
- Gastroparesis where the isotope or pellet fails to reach the jejunum in 3–6 h, or where the results of manometric motility studies demonstrate abnormal gastric emptying, and which is unresponsive to prokinetic medication
- Small bowel dysmotility demonstrated by a gastric to right colon transit time between 3 and 6 h, which is unresponsive to prokinetic medications
- Small bowel resection leaving greater than 5 feet of small bowel beyond the Ligament of Treitz
- Short bowel syndrome that is not as severe as described in Situation B
- Mild-to-moderate exacerbation of regional enteritis, or an enterocutaneous fistula
- Partial mechanical small bowel obstruction where surgery is not an option

For a tube feeding trial to be considered a failure, a concerted effort must be made to place the tube, with the tip appropriately placed (postpyloric in cases of gastroparesis) and verified by radiology or documented placement by endoscopy or an open surgical procedure. The trial of enteral nutrition must also include attention to appropriate formula selection, infusion rate, dilution and documented trial of alternative formulas to address the side effect of diarrhea.

In addition to the permanence and medical necessity criteria, Medicare lists guidelines for the actual HPN formula. The ordering physician must document the need for an HPN formula outside the range of 0.8–1.5 g of amino acids per kilogram per day, final dextrose concentration less than 10% or lipid use greater than 1500 g each month. Daily caloric intake (parenteral, enteral, and oral) of 20–35 calories per kilogram per day is considered adequate to maintain appropriate body weight. The ordering physician must also document the need for caloric intake outside this range.

Medicare Part B determines that HPN consists of amino acids, dextrose, electrolytes, vitamins, and trace minerals. Lipids are billed separately. Documentation of continued medical necessity must be available upon request. Intra-dialytic parenteral nutrition (IDPN) is rarely covered under Part B, as the patient must concurrently meet criteria as determined in Situations A–H.

A careful review and understanding of the current Medicare policy is of utmost importance in managing documentation and claim submission to assure accuracy. The home infusion provider (supplier) must also obtain a detailed written order (DWO) before submitting the claim, and it must be available upon request. If the claim for payment is submitted prior to receiving the DWO, the claim will be denied as not reasonable or necessary. Someone other than the ordering physician may produce the DWO, however, the prescribing physician must review, sign, and date the document. The order must include the patient's name, physician's name, date of the order, start date (if different from the order date), detailed description of the items and physician signature and date (signature and date stamps are not allowed). "Date of order" is defined as the date the supplier was contacted by the physician (for verbal orders) or, in the case of written orders, the date entered by the physician. The written order must also include dosage or concentration (if applicable), route of administration, frequency of use, and duration of infusion. The detailed description in the written order may be either a narrative description or a brand name.

It is expected that the ordering physician will see the patient within 30 days of start of HPN, and periodically after start of care. For patients with long-term (>90 days) or lifetime requirements, continued medical necessity must be documented by the physician at least annually, and the home infusion provider must maintain copies of follow-up evaluations as proof of continued need for HPN.

Medicare can become primary insurance after two years of documented disability through the Social Security Administration. As consumers move from commercial insurance or Medicaid to Medicare Part B criteria, it is essential that physicians and health care providers keep scrupulous records that support Situations A–H as previously described. Part B beneficiaries that have a 60-day lapse in provision of HPN must be evaluated as a new start and supporting documentation must be again obtained by the HPN supplier.

MEDICARE PART D

In 2003, Congress enacted the Medicare Modernization Act, which established a prescription drug benefit. This optional coverage, for which beneficiaries pay an additional premium, is called Medicare Part D. Limited coverage of HPN ingredients is possible under the Part D provision for those who do not meet the Part B guidelines. Under Medicare Part D, the coverage of each drug/solution in the HPN formula can be separately billable but coverage is dependent on the Part D formulary and policy requirements. There can also be coverage under Part D for other IV medications and IV solutions that patients may require. Payment of a dispensing fee is also possible, but the consumer bears responsibility for all supplies and equipment. Of note, Intraperitoneal Nutrition (IPN) solutions where amino acids are compounded with the dialysate cannot be billed separately under Part D. Only facilities licensed under the *Part B ESRD* benefit can bill for the IPN dialysate; additional charges for amino acid supplementation will be denied. These limitations emphasize the importance of full secondary policies or Medicare Advantage Part D plans for additional coverage.

MEDICAID

Medicaid was signed into law in 1965 by President Lyndon B. Johnson as Title 19, which made comprehensive health care available to millions of Americans who may not have otherwise afforded it. Medicaid is considered to be an entitlement program for defined types of individuals and groups who may be of low income. In 1997, the Medicaid program expanded by enabling the states to extend health coverage to more uninsured children through the creation of the State Children's Health Insurance Program (SCHIP), and expanded again in 2003 by providing Part D prescription drug benefits for Medicaid enrollees through the implementation of the Medicare Modernization Act. During this same time, CMS allowed states to arrange a capitated payment to private managed care organizations for the development of *Managed Medicaid*. Since the passage of the Affordable Care Act (2010), which allowed states to expand their Medicaid programs, an increase of 22% of the national Medicaid patient population has been reported.[5]

HPN is generally covered under both Medicaid and Managed Medicaid programs if the HPN is determined to be medically necessary by the physician. Medicaid plans, whether traditional or managed, may require prior authorization in order to secure coverage. Prior authorization is usually obtained by submitting clinical documentation to justify the need along with the current prescription. Authorization is awarded for a specific period of time after which updated documentation must be submitted for reauthorization. The HPN may be reimbursed on the major medical side of contracting or through pharmacy contracted line-item billing, which requires itemization of all individual HPN components. Ongoing assessment and updating of the clinical documentation is necessary to ensure continued authorization. This requires clinical input from the physician and the home nutrition support team.

In conclusion, HPN is a covered benefit through Medicare Parts B, C, and D, through commercial insurers and through Medicaid programs. Each has individual nuances, but all require physician determination of medical necessity. As stated previously, all nutrition support clinicians should have a basic understanding of how HPN is covered by commercial and government payers and recognize they have the responsibility for accurate, timely documentation as required.

Regardless of the payer, reimbursement verification should be completed before providing service with an explanation of coverage as well as out-of-pocket expenses. Supporting records, verification of benefits, and authorization should be obtained by the home care provider prior to start of care, and the patient's ability to afford the copayment must also be considered. Financial issues must be discussed with patients prior to hospital discharge so they understand out-of-pocket expenses and accept financial responsibilities for their HPN. The home care team must work in tandem with the consumer, family, medical team, and insurers to ensure ongoing, optimal care and continued medical necessity as indicated by the consumer's condition. The home and hospital teams should also work together to find solutions for the minimally or unfunded patients whose life may be dependent upon receiving PN.

RESOURCES

IDPN/IPN Coverage under Medicare Part D, Memo to Part D Sponsors. https://www.cms.gov/Medicare/Prescription-Drug-Coverage/PrescriptionDrugCovContra/Downloads/IDPN-IPNCoverageunderMedicarePart-D.pdf (accessed March 31, 2015).

Medicare National Coverage Determinations Manual, Chapter 1, Part 3 (Sections 170–190.34) Coverage Determinations. https://www.cms.gov/Regulations-and-guidance/Guidance/Manuals/downloads/ncd103c1_Part3.pdf (accessed February 3, 2015).

National Coverage Determination (NCD) for Enteral and Parenteral Nutritional Therapy (180.2). http://www.cms.gov/medicare-coverage-database/details/ncd-details.aspx?NCDId=242&bc=AgAAQAAAAAAA&ncdver=1 (accessed October 1, 2014).

National Government Services, Jurisdiction B, Durable Medical Equipment Education and Training, Policy Education. September 2013. www.ngsmedicare.com (accessed April 2, 2015).

Total Parenteral Nutrition Net Course. Cigna Healthcare Medicare DMERC, Region D. www.cignamedicare.com/webtraining (accessed December 15, 2014).

REFERENCES

1. Patient Protection and Affordable Care Act. www.healthcare.gov (accessed March 15, 2015).
2. Durfee, S. M., Adams, S. C., Arthur, E. et al. A.S.P.E.N. Standards for nutrition support: Home and alternate site care. *Nutrition in Clinical Practice* 2014;29:542–555.
3. Kelly, D. 2015. Home parenteral nutrition in the USA. In *Home Parenteral Nutrition*, 2nd Edition, eds. F. Bosetti, M. Staun, and A. van Gossum, 25–29. Boston: CAB International.
4. Greaves, J. Medicare update: Navigating through reimbursement of home enteral nutrition therapy. *Support Line* 2011;33(1):24–27.
5. Noyes, B. Medicaid—An increasing slice of the payer pie. *Infusion* 2015;21(5):14–16.

13 Nutrition Services in the Outpatient Setting

The RDN Private Practice

David Orozco, MS, RDN, LD

CONTENTS

INTRODUCTION

Many people can benefit from nutrition care/diet intervention in the outpatient setting.

To enhance the patient's care on a day-to-day outpatient setting, it is important to team up with a registered dietitian nutritionist (RDN) within a practice or within the community. Diabetes, GI (gastrointestinal) diseases such as IBS (irritable bowel syndrome) and IBD (inflammatory bowel disease), heart disease, and weight loss are just a few of the many conditions that can be treated with nutrition care provided by an RDN. The RDN can work with patients in groups or individually to help reduce chronic medical complications, improve and enhance the patient's level of care and outcomes, and provide a source of outpatient connection that would otherwise be difficult to receive in an inpatient setting. Often, the RDN in the hospital has limited time to spend with the patient in providing individualized diet instructions for home, which makes referral to the outpatient RDN invaluable. For the RDN working outside the hospital, referral sources can be from hospitals, home care, individuals, or physician or clinic practices. Patients may self-refer as well.

This chapter will provide information for the RDN and for other healthcare professionals on working with an RDN. For the RDN, this may provide you with concepts you may use in creating or building a private practice. For other healthcare professionals, this information may help you find an RDN and design the practice option that fits your practice/clinic best.

RDN Practice Settings

There can be several approaches health professionals can take to work with RDNs. Two key steps to consider would be the type of practice the RDN has, and the type of work relationship that would fit best for both parties. An RDN may have a private office to see patients individually and/or as a group. The RDN may be a contracted provider for Medicare, Medicaid, or other commercial insurance plans or patients may self-pay to see the RDN in their own office. RDNs may alternatively use the physician's office and work as an independent contractor and/or work as an employee for the practice. Other RDNs offer a combination of options as both an independent contractor or as a part-time employee with clinic hours at a practice sight location. Whichever the type of relationship, the nutrition and diet counseling and therapy are beneficial for patient outcomes.

For an RDN contemplating private practice, consider what practice area to focus in (e.g., general, diabetes, weight management, renal, enteral nutrition, eating disorders, sports nutrition, oncology, allergies, etc.). For the healthcare provider working with the RDN, consider whether his/her practice fits with the services the practice provides. Also, it is important to determine if a practice wants to work with the RDN as an independent contractor seeing patients in the practice, or separately at the RDNs office.

Similarly, the RDN may have a specialty such as diabetes or GI disease and want to focus only on this area. In this case, the RDN will want to seek out those practices that would provide the best fit for their expertise. Depending on the practice, the RDN may want to work in the office or be available in the RDN practice office separate from the referral source. There is no one way to provide nutrition care in the outpatient setting and it is best to decide what works best for the practice, the RDN and the patient.

Financial Agreements

The next step is to determine what financial agreement would be necessary. Some facilities bill for the RDNs services, some RDNs bill insurance or the patient for their services directly, and some practices have a combination. It is also important to make sure the RDN is licensed, maintains professional liability, maintains their continuing education hours, and is in good ethical standing. This helps reduce liabilities for both parties and provides some assurance that patients receive reliable science-based and up-to-date counseling services that maximize patient outcomes. More information on billing will be provided later in this chapter.

Location

One of the simplest methods to start working with an RDN is bringing them onboard as an independent contractor seeing patients at the practice location. In this type of work relationship, the RDN conducts nutrition consults in an office within the practice. The RDN maintains their own hours and schedule, and can coordinate with office staff for room and scheduling if necessary. The practice can decide how involved they want their staff to be in this process. In most cases, physicians provide the space and allow the RDN to maintain their own schedule to reduce the workload on their staff. In turn, the RDN provides a nutrition evaluation note for each visit, which is important to add to the patient's chart and medical information. Having the RDN in the practice office helps the physicians and staff communicate more readily about client or patient cases, thus increasing the possibility for better patient outcomes and greater level of care.

RDN in Office as Staff or Independent Contractor

Having an RDN in-house can enhance patient care in several ways. The physician can refer patients directly to the RDN during consults, or for follow-up visits so nutrition recommendations, goals, and patient care can occur faster and increase patient adherence and enhance (or improve) health outcomes. Another important benefit of having the RDN in-house is that patient information such as laboratory data, past medical and family history, and medication lists can easily be obtained by the RDN in-house to help customize and enhance medical nutrition advise and therapy approaches. This also allows improved communication between the patient and physician since in several instances patient's medications can affect nutrition recommendations. An important benefit of having an RDN in-house is that the private patient information stays in-house, and it's easier to meet HIPAA (Health Insurance Portability and Accountability Act) compliance. The main differences with the RDN as staff or as an independent contractor RDN include type of office hours and level of control by practice, payment or reimbursement of services, and type of outcomes and expectations for the practice patients. However, this can be managed by developing a contract and patient outcome guidelines by the practice that helps explain expectations, and by building a relationship and level of trust over time.

There are several additional added benefits of having an RDN either on staff or within the practice as an independent contractor. The RDN can also provide nutrition and fitness clinics and classes on various topics such as diabetes, cardiovascular diseases, weight management, eating disorders, digestive disorders, and many other nutrition and preventive related topics throughout the year to both patients and staff. Additionally, RDNs can help provide nutrition information, updates, and tips that can be included in patient medical health records, practice website, email blasts, newsletters, and patient brochures and flyers. The benefits of employing or contracting with an RDN in-house can truly enhance a practice and patient outcomes, especially now that so much of insurance and the Affordable Care Act is driven by prevention and patient outcomes.

RDN Private Practice

A medical practice can also choose to simply refer patients out to an RDN with their own private practice. This alternative decreases the burden on the practice to have another employee on the payroll, less staffing and scheduling issues, and reduces the liability of the practice. The RDN will usually have his/her own office space he/she rents off-sight or even near or within the same building as the medical practice. In this case the RDN is completely working independently and receives referrals from various sources such as medical practices and doctors, other health professionals, the Internet, or from word-of-mouth from other clients. The independent RDN private practice model is typically one of the easiest routes medical doctors and facilities choose to team up with. The RDN sees their own patients, practices independently, and has their own liability, office space, and bills for their services independently from the physician's office. To obtain more information regarding business models for RDNs working in physicians' offices, the publication "RDNs in the New Primary Care: A Toolkit for Successful Integration," published in 2016 by the Academy of Nutrition and Dietetics, may be helpful.

Professional Obligations

All RDNs must maintain their registration and/or licensure and continuing education as well as keeping current with the latest science-based information, which can enhance patient care and public safety. When deciding to work with an RDN it is important to determine if they have licensure, registration, and liability insurance, and what their specialization or area of expertise. Understanding the RDN's expertise can also help a practice group or physician match their patients with someone that understands their medical conditions or complications, such as diabetes, renal disease, cardiovascular issues, or cancer. This is why it's important to find an RDN and not just a nutritionist. Someone who does not have the RDN credentials could be anyone claiming to be a nutrition expert, and more importantly would not be legally allowed to be a provider for insurance or submit claims to insurance. The next section looks at these differences.

NUTRITIONIST VS. REGISTERED DIETITIAN NUTRITIONIST

The route to becoming an RDN is by attending an ACEND (Accreditation Council for Education in Nutrition and Dietetics) accredited university and program. An RDN receives a verification statement after completing a minimum of an undergraduate and supervised practice didactic program in dietetics, and can only be credentialed as an RDN after completing the national examination administered by the Council on Dietetics Registration CDR. In order for an RDN to practice nutrition or dietetics, or to bill Medicare/Medicaid for nutrition services, such as medical nutrition therapy and nutrition counseling, the RDN has to be registered and in most cases licensed by the state in which they practice. Therefore, a doctor or healthcare practice looking to team up with a nutritionist, should confirm that they are an RDN and have to knowledge, skills sets, and training to work with clients and patients. The only verification of this is proof of registration through the CDR "Online Credential Verification Search" section of their website at http://www.cdrnet.org/about/who-is-a-registered-dietitian-rd, or through their state license certificate website.

PROFESSIONAL LIABILITY INSURANCE

Professional liability insurance is important for an RDN to have as well as any health professional working with the public. In many cases it's not legally required for an RDN to have professional liability, yet most do and it is common throughout the dietetics and nutrition profession.

EXPERTISE AND SCOPE OF PRACTICE

There are two different credentials and five certifications in specialty areas within the nutrition and dietetics profession (http://www.cdrnet.org/about accessed on January 2015) and several other specialty area certifications offered by other organizations (list of certifications below). It is therefore important that a physician or medical practice understand what the scope of practice and the standards of professional practice are within the RDN profession, as well as to discern what specialties or level of certifications an RDN may have. In addition, many RDNs like to focus on certain areas of expertise and have advanced level training and experience that may be better suited for a practice. The physician or medical practice should take the time to interview the RDN and determine whether the RDN would be a good fit for their practice type and clients. For example, endocrinologists would benefit with an RDN that may have a CDE (Certified Diabetes Educator®) credential, or has several years of experience working as a diabetes educator and with diabetes patients. This can be helpful when understanding the interactions of medications to food, appetite, weight, and blood sugar responses. An RDN with at least two years experience working with a specific clientele or patient population can provide greater insight to the medical team, such as more specific dietary recommendations, counseling ideas, behavioral tips, and information. More importantly, knowing an RDN's level of expertise or scope of practice helps the medical practice attain more improved health outcomes and better understanding of patient behavior and lifestyle barriers to change.

Specialties or Certifications

- CDR—http://www.cdrnet.org/about
- Diabetes—http://www.diabeteseducator.org/About/credit.html
- Sports and Fitness—http://www.acsm.org/certification
- Nutrition Support—http://www.nutritioncare.org/nbnsc/
- Cancer Nutrition Specialty—http://www.oncologynutrition.org
- Integrative and Functional Nutrition—http://integrativerd.org
- Culinary and Food Industry—http://www.foodculinaryprofs.org
- Nutrition and Aging—http://www.hadpg.org
- Pediatric Nutrition—http://www.pnpg.org

Managing a Private Practice

Patient Forms: HIPAA Compliance, Privacy Forms, Sharing Data, and Storage

It is beneficial for a physician or medical group planning to work with the RDN to integrate nutrition information and assessments into their various medical forms. The RDN captures patient medical and nutritional status that includes diet history, physical activity level, BMI (body mass index), biochemical information, past medical and possibly psychological or emotional history and other client personal or professional information. In addition, many RDN's also ask for information about the client's diet and typical meal patterns, food choices, as well as lifestyle questions that can help the RDN determine goals, therapy types, and counseling methods in order to maximize the client or patient's outcomes.

Patient privacy and protection of information should continue seamlessly through the referral process and on to the RDN. The medical practice or physician would probably already be incorporating HIPAA compliant and privacy information and language in all forms, and in managing the collection of those forms and client records. If the medical practice or physician has legal and liability concerns with incorporating the independent RDN contractor, then that RDN would need to maintain their own HIPAA compliance forms and manage all patient records within HIPAA standards and regulations. The independent RDN should provide their own HIPAA compliance and privacy information forms to the patient on their first visit. It is also critical and customary to use secure online and digital methods when sending patient data and information, and it is vital to patient privacy that sensitive medical information be shared in a method that is secure and safe. The physician or medical practice working with an independent RDN contractor should verify that their practice maintains patient data securely online, and does not share information in a nonsecure method. If the physician or medical practice hires the RDN, they should have the same level of access as any other staff personnel in order to help provide the client or patient with the best level of nutrition and dietary therapy possible.

Forms: Referral, Assessment, and Tracking

As part of the initial nutrition consultation, the RDN may receive a written or faxed physician referral. The RDN may choose to create a referral form or modify a form from one such as listed in Figure 13.1.

Assessment forms help the RDN get a better understanding of the client's or patient's nutritional and dietary history, as well as their general health and treatment plan. Just as medical forms help the medical team improve patient outcomes, so do the nutrition assessment forms. RDNs are able to get an understanding of meal patterns, why patients choose certain foods, obstacles to change, and

Referral for Medical Nutrition Therapy (MNT)

Date:	Patient name:
Day time phone number:	Insurance: (Attach copy of front & back of card)
DOB:	Home address: Zip:

Above is referred for medical nutrition therapy as a necessary part of medical treatment and prevention of complications for diagnoses listed.

Referral Needs: ☐ New Diagnosis ☐ New treatment plan ☐ New complication

Special Needs: ☐ Language ☐ Hearing/Speech/Vision ☐ Learning/Processing

☐ Other:

✓ Check all diagnoses that apply to this referral

✓	ICD-9	ICD-9 Description	✓	ICD-9	ICD-9 Description
☐			☐		
☐			☐		
☐			☐		
☐			☐		
☐			☐		
☐			☐		
☐			☐		
☐			☐		
☐			☐		
☐			☐		
☐			☐		
☐			☐		
☐			☐		
☐			☐		
☐			☐		

✓ Lab work (Please attach or complete) BP ___/___

Hct/ Hgb	FBS &/or pc	Hgb A1c	Total Chol	HDL LDL	Non HDL	Trig	Ua Micro Albumin/Cr	BUN/ Cr	EGFR	Na/K	Phos/ PTH	Vit D

✓ Exercise/Activity Plan

☐ Release: may walk 20-30 min 5-7 x/week or ____________________________

☐ Not Released: ____________________________

✓ Medications – Please attach list

Physician signature X______________________MD/DO Phone ________________

NPI: ______________ ______________________ Fax ________________

Print MD/DO Name

The information requested above is Protected Health Information (PHI), and is the minimum necessary to execute delivery of patient services. Please understand as a link in the "Chain of Trust", all PHI will remain confidential as mandated by the Treatment, Payments, and Healthcare Operation Laws mandated by HIPAA.

FIGURE 13.1 Referral for MNT. (Downloadable is the MNT Referral form—free to members of the Academy of Nutrition and Dietetics, www.eatrightpro.org.)

even emotional or lifestyle issues that affect the way a client eats or chooses foods. In the nutrition assessment form there are some key elements necessary to capture from the client or patient such as

- Demographic information—name, address, gender, date of birth, phone, and email
- Biometrics—measurements, height, current weight, laboratory values
- Medical history—medical conditions or diagnoses, medications, supplement use
- Insurance information
- Diet history—appetite, diet history, digestive concerns, eating patterns, food choices, drinks, typical foods, food aversions, allergies, or intolerances, alcohol consumption
- Physical activity—types and levels of activity
- Work/life balance
- Reason for visit or nutrition and health goals

Also included in the initial assessment form is nutrition focused physical assessment to identify and stratify incidence of malnutrition. An experienced RDN will be able to narrow the information and be able to capture additional information from the client or patient at the time of the initial nutrition assessment visit. An example of a nutrition assessment form that can be adopted to fit with an RDN and practice is found in Figure 13.2.

It is important to note that capturing patient nutrition information is extremely helpful so long as there are procedures in place that help the RDN enhance nutrition advice. For instance, it is a good idea to have assessment forms integrated within the practice so the patient fills out one set of documents from the beginning. This allows the RDN be a team member and extract pertinent nutrition and medical data that enhances their ability to provide sound nutrition advise and counseling. Having procedures such as incorporating the assessment form with initial patient documents also helps reduce the amount of forms the client or patient has to complete. It keeps information in one place, reduces privacy concerns, it is more secure, and information is shared by all team members, which only enhances patient care and outcomes.

(a) **Nutrition Evaluation Form**

Name:______________________ DOB: ____/____/____ Age: ________

❑ Male ❑ Female Marital Status: ❑ S ❑ M ❑ D ❑ W ❑ Separated

Address:______________________

Home Phone (____)______________ Work Phone (____)______________

Email:______________________

Height: ______ ft. ______ in Current Weight: ________ lb Lowest Adult Weight: ________ lb

Please answer the following questions:

How would you describe you appetite? ( ) Excellent ( ) Good ( ) Fair ( ) Poor

Have your eating habits changed within the past several days/weeks/months: ( ) Yes ( ) No

If yes, list changes ______________________

Are you following any diets/food plans?

Weight Loss	( ) Yes ( ) No	Low fat/Low Cholesterol	( ) Yes ( ) No
Diabetes	( ) Yes ( ) No	Low Sodium/No Salt	( ) Yes ( ) No
Other	( ) Yes ( ) No		

If other, please describe: ______________________

Have you experienced any of these symptoms during the past few days/weeks/months?

Nausea	( ) Yes ( ) No	Heartburn	( ) Yes ( ) No
Vomiting	( ) Yes ( ) No	Abdominal Pains	( ) Yes ( ) No
Diarrhea	( ) Yes ( ) No	Bloating/Cramps	( ) Yes ( ) No
Constipation	( ) Yes ( ) No	Other Illness	( ) Yes ( ) No

Are you experiencing any symptoms now? ( ) Yes ( ) No

If yes, please explain ______________________

Are you a vegetarian? ( ) Yes ( ) No If yes, do you eat any of the following?

Eggs	( ) Yes ( ) No	Cheese	( ) Yes ( ) No
Yogurt	( ) Yes ( ) No	Milk	( ) Yes ( ) No
Poultry	( ) Yes ( ) No	Fish	( ) Yes ( ) No

Please list any food allergies or food intolerance:______________________

Are there foods you dislike? ______________________

If so, why? ______________________

What are your favorite foods or snacks? ______________________

Who does the cooking at home? ______________ Who does the food shopping? ______________

How often during the week do you eat out? ______________________

How often do you bring your own meals or leftovers to work? ______________________

Do you avoid eating any foods because of cultural or religious practices? ( ) Yes ( ) No

If yes, please specify: ______________________

FIGURE 13.2 (a and b) Assessment form. (Adapted from Orozco, D., td wellness, LLC. With permission.)

(Continued)

(b) Please circle any illness or complications you have had:

Hypertension	Osteoporosis	Cancer
High Cholesterol	Arthritis	Migraines
Over Weight/Obese	Back or Joint Pains	IBS/IBD/Chron's
High Triglycerides	Sleep Apnea	Other: ____________
Hypothyroidism	Asthma	Other: ____________

Please list any medications you are taking: ____________ ____________

____

____

____________ ____________

Are you taking any of the following?

Vitamin/mineral supplements ( ) Yes ( ) No Name: ____________

Herbal supplements/medications ( ) Yes ( ) No Name: ____________

Have you ever or do you smoke? ( ) Yes ( ) No

If yes: Less than 10/day ( ) 10-20/day ( ) More than 20/day ( )

If quit, how long ago? ____________

How often do/did you drink any of the following: beer, wine, wine coolers, hard liquor, mixed drinks, malt liquor (Leave blank if you don't)? Daily ( ) Weekly( ) Monthly( ) Never ( )

Are you able to do physical activity? ( ) Yes ( ) No

If you can, how often are you active? ____________

Please list types of exercises/activities you enjoy? ____________

____

What prevents you from doing regular physical activity? ____________

____

Type of work/school: ____________

____

Number of hours/week: ____________

What was your lowest adult body weight? ________ lb

What is your goal weight? ________ lb

What is your confidence level in changing your eating patterns (scale 1-10)? ____________

What is your confidence level in changing your physical activity level (scale 1-10)? ____________

What is your confidence level in maintaining weight loss (scale 1-10)? ____________

Rate your eating patterns:

A = Contributes Most to Wt-gain, B = Contributes Somewhat to Wt-Gain, C = Contributes Least to Wt-Gain

________ Eating and/or snacking constantly throughout the day

________ Choosing unhealthy foods (ie: Fast Food, Candy, Fried Food)

________ Eating or snacking late

________ Long gaps between meals – 5 or more hours between meals

________ Skipping meals

________ Eating in response to stress or emotions (positive or negative)

________ Eating at social or business functions (ie: family, friends, celebrations, gatherings, holidays, etc.)

________ Eating large portions

________ Eating too fast

FIGURE 13.2 (Continued) (a and b) Assessment form. (Adapted from Orozco, D., td wellness, LLC. With permission.)

PATIENT PAYMENT AND AGREEMENT FORMS

Often clients cancel, reschedule appointments, their insurance denies claims, or co-pays are not collected. For the independent RDN contractor, it is good practice to maintain some type of patient payment and cancellation policy. For instance, if people cancel less than 24 h prior to an appointment or arrive more than a reasonable time late (more than 10–15 min late), it may be helpful to have a policy that states the client will have to reschedule their appointment and charged a certain reasonable cancellation or rescheduling fee. Often, clients forget appointments or have last minute changes in their schedule; therefore it is important to also have some type of an appointment reminder system. Whether it is a sophisticated scheduling software programs available to private practices, or a computer calendar program such as MS Outlook or Mac iCal and independent RDN contractor can incorporate in their own practice, it is important to create a system in place where appointments are made, reminders are sent, and patient follow-up can be established. This not only helps with improved patient outcomes, it makes strong and sound business sense. Clients and patients appreciate the reminders and can better make appointments, which is a simple planning step in any practice that improves the customer satisfaction and the motivation to make change.

PATIENT OR CLIENT HANDOUTS

Regardless of whether the RDN is employed by the practice or is an independent contractor, the best tools to have on hand are simple and easy to read education materials and handouts. The RDN is a valuable resource to have in help developing tips sheets, guidelines, and nutrition information on a range of topics specific to the practice. These handouts can be distributed to patients and clients during consults with the physician, while they wait in the lobby or waiting room, or while visiting the practice's website. These educational materials can aid in RDN referrals, or they can be part of an online blog or newsletter that clients can receive as an added benefit or perk from being a member of the practice. These handouts can serve as great marketing tools as well. Short tips can be included into social media and help increase traffic to a practice. Handouts and educational materials also help the patient better understand their goals and supplement visit information. For example, the RDN can provide monthly or quarterly education sessions on nutrition for diabetes, blood fats, and weight management and offer education material that summarize or outlines the major nutrition topics or goals the patients need to remember. The patient can then work with the RDN one-on-one with these education materials to individualize the patient's care to meet their specific goals.

COMPENSATION

There are several approaches to RDN compensation, but working with an RDN as an independent contractor is simply easier for the practice to allow the RDN to manage their own patient billing and payment arrangement. The independent RDN should evaluate their time spent in providing the services as well as the expertise required to set pricing. If contracted with an insurance provider, rates are already established and the RDN will be paid at the contracted rate. Therefore, the RDN must decide if he/she will include accepting insurance coverage in the practice or will require self-pay only. Additionally, consults may be priced differently for initial and follow up and for group classes. Services provided such as body composition assessment or indirect calorimetry are often provided outside of the consult. This is a business decision and must be carefully evaluated for cost/benefit.

MAINTAINING PRACTICE

Continuing Education

It should be the responsibility of the RDN to stay current in practice and maintain continuing education as required. Most states require licensure for RDNs, and each state may require yearly continuing education credits to ensure the RDN is meeting their current competencies. Some states do not have licensure, however, the RDN must maintain a minimum of 75 continuing education hours in 5 years to maintain the registration with CDR (Commission on Dietetic Registration).

Specializations

The RDN may have additional certifications in specialty areas such as sports, gerontology, oncology, pediatrics, and renal.

- Board-certified specialist in renal nutrition
- Board-certified specialist in sports dietetics

- Board-certified specialist in pediatric nutrition
- Board-certified specialist in gerontological nutrition
- Board-certified specialist in oncology nutrition

These are certifications that require rigorous training and several years of experience, accented with a board examination. Other specialty certifications can include

- Certificate of Training in Adult Weight Management Program
- Certificate of Training in Childhood and Adolescent Weight Management Program
- Certification Diabetes Educator (CDE)
- Certified Nutrition Support Clinician (CNSC)
- Fitness Certifications
    - American College of Sports Medicine
    - National Academy of Sports Medicine
    - American Council on Exercise
- Eating Disorders
    - International Association of Eating Disorder Professionals Foundation (iaedp)

And many other RDNs seek various other types of specialties and health-related certifications or degrees. Certifications are a great mutual benefit for both the RDN and the physician or practice working with them. They add various levels of specialization and care for patients, such as

- Increased marketability for both the practice and RDN
- Focus on care for specific disease state, condition, or diagnosis
- Improved multidisciplinary team approach to patient care
- Preventive approaches to care
- Reduce patient costs and enhanced patient outcomes
- Availability to specific education, information, and resources

Advanced Training

The difference between an advanced and specialized RDN is that an advanced RDN has a broader knowledge level, skill set, and abilities of the professional. The advanced RDN would probably have a minimum of about eight years of experience, and may or may not have a specialization or additional certifications, but they can work independently and autonomously, making quicker decisions on a broader level than a specialist. In most cases, advanced level RDNs take on more management or leadership type roles. Advanced level RDNs create or develop programs and are involved at the strategic level compared to a specialist that may be involved in the implementation of the program. It may be beneficial for the physician or practice to hire an advanced practice RDN, especially if the practice is thinking of creating weight management, diabetes, or cardiovascular type programs requiring the management of employees, certification or accreditation of programs, finding grant funding, working with billing, and scheduling and managing patient attendance and outcomes among many other components of these types of programs. Advanced level RDNs would be better equipped and trained to help establish a nutrition program or manage a team of health professionals than a beyond entry level practitioner. It may be worth the investment to enhance practice outcomes and increase revenue.

Insurance Coverage

The Basics

Many RDNs around the country are providers for most major insurance plans such as Medicare, Medicaid, Anthem/Blue Cross Blue Shield, Aetna, United Healthcare, Cigna, Humana, and others.

However, insurance plans vary greatly from state to state on the type of nutrition services covered. In many instances, they follow the Medicare/Medicaid model to cover for medical nutrition therapy for diabetes and renal disease. Still, several plans are now starting to see the benefits of preventive medicine and starting to cover more nutrition services for various conditions or for prevention. More importantly, it's beneficial for the RDN to be included in covered benefits when working with physicians or a practice group, as this could help enhance patient outcomes and prevent expensive and timely procedures.

Therefore, whether the RDN is an independent contractor or employee of a practice, they should understand the basic requirements for becoming a provider for insurance plans.

Obtaining the National Provider Identification number or (NPI) is the first step in seeking reimbursement from an insurance company as a Medical Nutrition Therapy (MNT) provider. An NPI may be obtained for an individual RDN or a group NPI may be obtained, which will allow the independent contractor RDN hire other RDNs to work with him/her to see clients or patients. This can be accomplished by accessing the National Plan and Provider Enumeration System (NPPES—https://nppes.cms.hhs.gov/NPPES/Welcome.do.

An RDN who is an independent contractor, may obtain an Employer Identification Number (EIN) or tax ID number (https://sa1.www4.irs.gov/modiein/individual/index.jsp). This helps the RDN use the EIN instead of their personal social security number for payment with the insurance companies and CMS.

For those RDNs who desire to enroll as a Medicare provider, the information is available at: http://www.cms.gov/Medicare/Provider-Enrollment-and-Certification/MedicareProviderSupEnroll/ (accessed on 3/27/2015). Applying to be an MNT provider with one of the major insurance companies usually requires that he/she registers with CAQH, but to be able to register, the RDN must first ask the insurance company to invite them to enroll in the CAQH system otherwise the application process cannot begin. The CAQH is a clearinghouse database and organization that stores the RDN information, which is accessed by insurance companies to review the RDN qualifications, licensure, liabilities, location, and specialties. Additionally, if the RDN will be working with children, uninsured, or very low-income populations, then it would be wise to have them enroll with Medicaid. The RDN should visit their state Medicaid website to begin the provider enrollment process.

These are the basics steps for the RDN to become a provider for most major insurance companies and Medicare and Medicaid. A more detailed explanation of the process can be found through the "Registered Dietitian Billing Guide 2010" (9) (*Academy of Nutrition and Dietetics, Registered Dietitian Billing Guide* 2010: http://www.eatrightpro.org/~/media/eatrightpro%20files/practice/coding%20coverage%20compliance/billing_guide_2010_full_version.ashx, accessed on 3/27/2015 at). Each insurance company as well as Medicare will have varying contractual obligations, such as location of patient office visits, registration of multiple locations, billing rates, and more. It is recommended that the RDN and physician or medical practice visit the Academy of Nutrition and Dietetics to help with more information on becoming an insurance provider and credentialing. (http://www.eatrightpro.org/resources/practice/getting-paid/getting-started-with-payment, accessed on 3/27/2015).

Marketing

Embracing Social Media Early On

One cannot underestimate the power and immense benefits of getting connected on Social Media soon enough! Social media provides an enormous sounding board and advocacy for the nutrition professional. So much misinformation is out there that it's vital for the RDN to embrace social media early on and provide credible and sound science or evidence-based information to drown out those unreliable and non-credible voices. Social media is therefore a practical advocacy channel as well as a major and practically free, or at least very inexpensive form of marketing and advertising.

For the RDN and medical practice team, it is wise to build a respected and reputable group on social media. The recommendation is to start with one social media outlet first, such as Facebook, LinkedIn, or Twitter. This way the RDN or practice can understand how social media works, how to build connections and groups, and build greater recognition both for the RDN and for the practice (11) (*Food and Nutrition Magazine*, Are you a #SocialPro? http://www.foodandnutrition.org/Social-Pro/, Accessed on 3/27/2015).

Website or Blog?

Websites and Blogs can be extremely helpful in marketing services, but they are not extremely necessary for the small independent contractor RDN starting out. For the small RDN independent contractor or employees it is more important to be on social media and create a Facebook, Twitter, LinkedIn accounts before embarking on building a website or blog. However, as the practice or the physician or medical group where the RDN is employed grows, it may be wise to start small with a blog and build from there. There are numerous advantages to developing a blog versus a website.

- Blogs are quick, simple, and free. (12) (C/Net.com, "Top 5 Blog Sites by C/Net and PC World Magazine": http://www.cnet.com/news/top-five-blog-platforms/, accessed on 3/27/15 at)
  - Blogger.com
  - Wordpress.com
  - Typepad.com
  - Squarespace.com

Building a website takes a great deal of work, understanding of code, and graphic design. One may have to invest a little more time and money learning what programs are best, where to host, and how much to pay. Setting up a blog can be fairly easy and quick. One can set up the blog to link to social media, and this is where the real benefit is. Linking blogs to social media helps increase traffic to the blog and to social media sites. Be sure to use evidence-based or science-based information, stick to facts and information, and avoid controversial or negative posts and blogs. More importantly, a blog is a great way to help enhance information delivery to the patients of a medical practice. Therefore, it is a great idea to have the RDN employee or independent contractor help develop, update, or maintain a blog or social media. A blog can also be linked to a practice website if one already exists, other health professionals in the practice can also contribute their expertise and information, and therefore enhance patient care.

NETWORKING AND VOLUNTEERING

Networking with other RDNs and health professionals is vital to keeping on the pulse with current knowledge and honing counseling techniques for the RDN. Networking with registered dietitian nutritionists and with other health professional groups can also enhance practice knowledge, marketing skills stay up-to-date on new trends and ideas within nutrition and dietetics profession. The RDN is able to gain greater insight into what's going on related to billing, coding, blogging, patient care, and finding the latest resources for patient information and research. It is therefore beneficial to both the practice and the RDN to schedule time to attend monthly or quarterly local or state association meetings, specialty group workshops or webinars, community focused events such as runs, walks, or cooking demonstrations, or attend annual national conferences.

It is equally important to allow the RDN time to volunteer to hone leadership and interdisciplinary skills. The RDN is able to make connections with other colleagues, which can lead to possible grant or research opportunities, as well as gaining a strong connection with their community. Volunteering allows the RDN an avenue to network, build relationships, and possibly seek awards and honors over time. These types of relationships, honors, or awards can be shared by the practice and enhance the credibility within health professions as well. It is also a mainstay of the Academy of Nutrition and Dietetics (Academy of Nutrition and Dietetics, Leadership: http://www.eatrightpro.org/resources/leadership/volunteering, accessed on 3/27/15).

RESOURCES

Brown-Riggs, C. The patient centered medical home—The dietitian's role in the healthcare model that improves diabetes outcomes. *Today's Dietitian Magazine*, accessed on 3/27/15: http://www.todaysdietitian.com/newarchives/080112p26.shtml

Meeting the Need for Obesity Treatment: A Toolkit for the RD/PCP Partnership. https://www.eatright.org/shop/product.aspx?id=6442473941

Section III

Summary

14 Nutrition, Diet, and Health
For Further Consideration

Carol Ireton-Jones, PhD, RDN, LD, CNSC, FAND, FASPEN

CONTENTS

Nutrition care in the outpatient setting may be the key to disease prevention. It is hard to name a disease process that does not have a nutrition component. Diabetes, GI diseases, osteoporosis and cancer can all be treated and prevented with good nutrition. Malnutrition continues to be a problem while the incidence of overweight and obesity rises. New techniques may allow for genetic manipulations that prevent disease or nutrition therapies that positively affect genes. This has already begun. The gut microbiome has an ever-increasing importance in unlocking better health. What one eats makes a difference in health, performance, and quality of life.

HEALTHY EATING

Healthy eating is actually pretty complex. In fact, what is healthy eating? Healthy eating or a healthy diet might be defined consumption of a variety of foods that meet an individual's nutrient needs. Is there one healthy diet? The U.S. Dietary Guidelines and My Plate give suggestions for including nutritious foods and understanding portion sizes [1,2]. According to U.S. News and World reports, the DASH diet comes up as "Best Overall Diet" several years in a row based on nutritional value, ease of use, and effectiveness to help manage chronic disease. Based on well-controlled human research studies dating back to the mid-1990s, there is strong evidence to support that lowering sodium and increasing potassium, calcium, and magnesium can be effective for lowering blood pressure [3]. These nutrients are the backbone of the DASH Eating Plan which incorporates fresh, wholesome food such as fruits and vegetables, low-fat dairy, nuts and low-fat protein sources. Cindy Kleckner, RDN (Cooper Aerobics Center, Dallas, Texas) coauthor *DASH Diet for Dummies and Hypertension Cookbook for Dummies* suggests if one wants to take charge of their health, to try the DASH difference, a powerful medicine that doesn't come in a pill.

MALNUTRITION

In the United States, a large majority of individuals do not meet their nutrient needs. Malnutrition is present in children, adults, and the elderly in many socioeconomic levels. In U.S. hospitals the prevalence of malnutrition in the hospital is 13%–88% (pediatric and adult patients), long-term care—21%–51% and outpatient or homecare—13%–30% [4]. Improving food accessibility as well as nutrition interventions for disease treatment and prevention are needed to improve nutrition status. This is a focus for organizations such as the American Society for Parenteral and Enteral Nutrition (www.nutritioncare.org), the Academy of Nutrition and Dietetics (www.eatright.org), and the Alliance to Advance Patient Nutrition (www.malnutrition.com).

OVERWEIGHT AND OBESITY

The majority of the adult U.S. population is overweight or obese [5]. This trend is occurring in children as well as with approximately one-third of children considered overweight or obese [5]. Weight management is not covered specifically in this book; however, the chapter on diabetes management is certainly applicable. There are many diet plans and programs as well as surgical procedures for weight loss. Weight loss is a journey and requires expert guidance. Working with a registered dietitian/nutritionist (RDN) can demystify the process and provide the support and expertise needed for weight loss and maintenance. See Chapter 13 to find an RDN.

NUTRIGENOMICS

Is the secret to nutrition in our genes? Nutrigenomics is a common term used to refer to nutritional genomics—the study of nutrient and gene interactions which encompasses both nutrigenetics and nutrigenomics. Nutrigenetics relates to how DNA variations affect the response to and metabolism of nutrients (gene/nutrient), while nutrigenomics is the effect of nutrients on genes (nutrient/gene) [6–8]. Phenylketonuria (PKU), an inborn error of metabolism, is an example of nutrigenetics. By knowing that the amino acid phenylalanine cannot be metabolized, it can be avoided and the deleterious effects of PKU obviated. Understanding how certain nutrients affect gene expression will allow for optimal food choices by modifying food or nutrient intake to produce positive health outcomes [7,8]. Genetic tests that provide actionable information are available for weight management, nutrient metabolism, and others [7]. Research in the field of nutrigenomics continues to enhance the knowledge and applicability of this complex science to the development of an individualized, optimal diet [7,8].

THE GUT MICROBIOME

"You are what you eat" is a quote from Anthelme Brillat-Savarin who wrote, in *Physiologie du Gout, ou Meditations de Gastronomie Transcendante, 1826*: "Dis-moi ce que tu manges, je te dirai ce que tu es." [Tell me what you eat and I will tell you what you are] [9]. This old quote has new life especially as it relates to the human gut microbiota. This microbiota comprises trillions of microorganisms that have many functions including immune function and metabolism [9–12]. The type and amount of food consumed effects the microbiota and may have a crucial role in obesity, diabetes, and diseases such as inflammatory bowel disease (see Chapter 4) [11,12]. The microflora is also affected by medications. Antibiotics have been shown to decrease the gut bacteria although a recent study showed that while this may affect immune competence, glucose tolerance was not affected [13]. Probiotics and prebiotics are being used to influence the gut microbiome; however, much more research is needed [11,12]. The future of nutrition, prevention, and disease management may be based on managing and modifying the gut microbiota [11,12].

SUMMARY

Nutrition is ever changing and evolving, with some of the "discoveries" turning out to be fine tuning of previously known therapies through better research techniques. Today, the best advice may be to eat fresh foods as often as possible, be active and avoid stress—easier said than done. Most importantly, it is up to each individual to make the choice of good health. And, to see an expert in the evidence-based practice of nutrition. It pays now and in the long-run!

RESOURCES

DASH Diet for Dummies and Hypertension Cookbook for Dummies.
The American Society for Parenteral and Enteral Nutrition (www.nutritioncare.org).
The Academy of Nutrition and Dietetics (www.eatright.org).
The Alliance to Advance Patient Nutrition (www.malnutrition.com).

REFERENCES

1. http://www.cnpp.usda.gov/DietaryGuidelines, accessed 12.17.15.
2. http://www.choosemyplate.gov/MyPlate, accessed 12.17.15.
3. http://www.dummies.com/how-to/content/dash-diet-for-dummies-cheat-sheet.html, accessed 12.17.15.
4. Academy of Nutrition and Dietetics, Executive Summary: Malnutrition, 2015.
5. http://www.niddk.nih.gov/health-information/health-statistics/Pages/overweight-obesity-statistics.aspx, accessed 12.17.15.
6. West AA, Caudill MA. Applied choline-omics: Lessons from human metabolic studies for the integration of genomics research into nutrition practice. *J Acad Nutr Diet* 2014;114(8):1242–50.
7. DeBusk R. The role of nutritional genomics in developing an optimal diet for humans. *Nutr Clin Prac* 2010;25(6):627–33.
8. Camp KM, Trujillo E. Position of the Academy of Nutrition and Dietetics: Nutritional genomics. *J Acad Nutr Diet* 2014;114(2):299–312.
9. http://www.phrases.org.uk/meanings/you-are-what-you-eat.html, accessed 12.17.15.
10. Wu H, Tremaroli V, Backhed F. Linking microbiota to human disease: A systems biology perspective. *Trends Endocrinol Metab* 2015;26(12):758–70.
11. Mullin GE. *The Gut-Balance Revolution*. New York: Rodale, 2015.
12. Cresci GA, Bawden E. Gut microbiome: What we do and don't know. *Nutr Clin Prac* 2015;30(6):734–46.
13. Mikkelsen KH, Frost M, Bahl MI et al. Effects of antibiotics on gut microbiota, gut hormones, and glucose metabolism. *PLoS One* 2015;10(11):e0142352.

Index

H

I

J

K

L

Q

R

S

T

U

V